METHODS IN MOLECULAR BIOLOGY

Series Editor
John M. Walker
School of Life and Medical Sciences
University of Hertfordshire
Hatfield, UK

For further volumes:
http://www.springer.com/series/7651

For over 35 years, biological scientists have come to rely on the research protocols and methodologies in the critically acclaimed *Methods in Molecular Biology* series. The series was the first to introduce the step-by-step protocols approach that has become the standard in all biomedical protocol publishing. Each protocol is provided in readily-reproducible step-by-step fashion, opening with an introductory overview, a list of the materials and reagents needed to complete the experiment, and followed by a detailed procedure that is supported with a helpful notes section offering tips and tricks of the trade as well as troubleshooting advice. These hallmark features were introduced by series editor Dr. John Walker and constitute the key ingredient in each and every volume of the *Methods in Molecular Biology* series. Tested and trusted, comprehensive and reliable, all protocols from the series are indexed in PubMed.

Geminiviruses

Methods and Protocols

Edited by

Francisco Murilo Zerbini

Dep. de Fitopatologia, Universidade Federal de Viçosa, Viçosa, Brazil

Elvira Fiallo-Olivé and Jesús Navas-Castillo

Instituto de Hortofruticultura Subtropical y Mediterránea 'La Mayora' (IHSM-UMA-CSIC), Algarrobo-Costa, Málaga, Spain

Humana Press

Editors
Francisco Murilo Zerbini
Dep. de Fitopatologia
Universidade Federal de Viçosa
Viçosa, Brazil

Elvira Fiallo-Olivé
Instituto de Hortofruticultura Subtropical y Mediterránea 'La Mayora' (IHSM-UMA-CSIC)
Algarrobo-Costa, Málaga, Spain

Jesús Navas-Castillo
Instituto de Hortofruticultura Subtropical y Mediterránea 'La Mayora' (IHSM-UMA-CSIC)
Algarrobo-Costa, Málaga, Spain

ISSN 1064-3745 ISSN 1940-6029 (electronic)
Methods in Molecular Biology
ISBN 978-1-0716-4456-0 ISBN 978-1-0716-4454-6 (eBook)
https://doi.org/10.1007/978-1-0716-4454-6

This Humana imprint is published by the registered company Springer Science+Business Media, LLC, part of Springer Nature.
The registered company address is: 1 New York Plaza, New York, NY 10004, U.S.A.

Preface

Geminiviruses represent a unique and economically impactful group of plant viruses, characterized by their geminate particle structure and small, circular, single-stranded DNA genomes. Infecting key crops such as maize, cotton, cassava, beans, and tomatoes, they pose a major challenge across tropical and subtropical regions. This group stands out as one of the most diverse within the virosphere, and, along with nanoviruses, they represent the only "true" DNA plant viruses. Their replication strategy, which involves abundant double-stranded DNA intermediates, facilitates the amplification and cloning of full-length genomes. Consequently, geminiviruses are a focal point of both basic and applied virology research, with an active "geminivirology" community worldwide.

This book compiles a comprehensive collection of protocols essential for geminivirus research, ranging from foundational methods—such as DNA extraction and inoculation assays—to advanced techniques in cloning, sequencing, phylogenetic and recombination analysis, diagnostics, and virus-host interaction studies. Our goal is for this resource to support the geminivirus research community as a practical laboratory guide and serve as a valuable "one-stop-shop" for researchers new to geminiviruses, facilitating the establishment of a robust geminivirus research program.

Viçosa, Brazil
Algarrobo-Costa, Málaga, Spain

Francisco Murilo Zerbini
Elvira Fiallo-Olivé
Jesús Navas-Castillo

Contents

Contributors

NEIL BOONHAM • *School of Natural and Environmental Sciences, Agriculture Building, Newcastle University, Newcastle upon Tyne, UK*

ALVIN CRESPO-BELLIDO • *Department of Ecology, Evolution and Natural Resources, School of Environmental and Biological Sciences, Rutgers, The State University of New Jersey, New Brunswick, NJ, USA*

HUI DU • *Ministry of Agriculture Key Laboratory of Molecular Biology of Crop Pathogens and Insects, Zhejiang Key Laboratory of Biology and Ecological Regulation of Crop Pathogens and Insects, Institute of Insect Sciences, Zhejiang University, Hangzhou, China*

MIN DU • *State Key Laboratory for Biology of Plant Diseases and Insect Pests, Institute of Plant Protection, Chinese Academy of Agricultural Sciences, Beijing, China*

CHRISTIANE ELIZA MOTTA DUARTE • *National Institute of Science and Technology in Plant-Pest Interactions/BIOAGRO, Universidade Federal de Viçosa, Viçosa, MG, Brazil; Glycobiology and Cell Signaling Laboratory, Universidade do Estado de Minas Gerais, Passos, MG, Brazil*

SIOBAIN DUFFY • *Department of Ecology, Evolution and Natural Resources, School of Environmental and Biological Sciences, Rutgers, The State University of New Jersey, New Brunswick, NJ, USA*

ELVIRA FIALLO-OLIVÉ • *Instituto de Hortofruticultura Subtropical y Mediterránea 'La Mayora' (IHSM-UMA-CSIC), Consejo Superior de Investigaciones Científicas, Algarrobo-Costa, Málaga, Spain*

MADISON T. FLASCO • *Section of Plant Pathology and Plant-Microbe Biology, School of Integrative Plant Science, Cornell AgriTech at the New York State Agricultural Experiment Station, Cornell University, Geneva, NY, USA; Plant Pathology and Crop Physiology, Louisiana State University, Baton Rouge, LA, USA*

ELIZABETH PACHECO BATISTA FONTES • *National Institute of Science and Technology in Plant-Pest Interactions/BIOAGRO, Universidade Federal de Viçosa, Viçosa, MG, Brazil; Dep. de Bioquímica e Biologia Molecular/BIOAGRO, Universidade Federal de Viçosa, Viçosa, MG, Brazil*

MARC FUCHS • *Section of Plant Pathology and Plant-Microbe Biology, School of Integrative Plant Science, Cornell AgriTech at the New York State Agricultural Experiment Station, Cornell University, Geneva, NY, USA*

ELISA GARZO • *Instituto de Ciencias Agrarias (ICA), Consejo Superior de Investigaciones Científicas (CSIC), Madrid, Spain*

VICTOR GOLYAEV • *Tropical Crop Improvement Laboratory, Crop Biotechnics, Department of Biosystems, KU Leuven, Leuven, Belgium; Leuven Plant Institute (LPI), KU Leuven, Leuven, Belgium*

BIANCA GOUVEIA-MAGESTE • *National Institute of Science and Technology in Plant-Pest Interactions/BIOAGRO, Universidade Federal de Viçosa, Viçosa, MG, Brazil; Dep. de Tecnologia de Alimentos, Universidade Federal de Viçosa, Viçosa, MG, Brazil*

VICTORIA J. HOYLE • *Section of Plant Pathology and Plant-Microbe Biology, School of Integrative Plant Science, Cornell AgriTech at the New York State Agricultural Experiment Station, Cornell University, Geneva, NY, USA*

DIRK JANSSEN • *IFAPA, Centro La Mojonera, La Mojonera, Spain*

Anders Kvarnheden • *Department of Plant Biology, Linnean Centre for Plant Biology, Swedish University of Agricultural Sciences, Uppsala, Sweden; Chair of Plant Health, Institute of Agricultural and Environmental Sciences, Estonian University of Life Sciences, Tartu, Estonia*

Cristiano Lacorte • *Embrapa Recursos Genéticos e Biotecnologia, Brasília, DF, Brazil*

João Paulo Batista Machado • *National Institute of Science and Technology in Plant-Pest Interactions/BIOAGRO, Universidade Federal de Viçosa, Viçosa, MG, Brazil; Instituto de Ciências Agrárias, Universidade Federal de Viçosa, Florestal, MG, Brazil*

Darren Patrick Martin • *Division of Computational Biology, Department of Integrative Biomedical Sciences, Institute of Infectious Diseases and Molecular Medicine, University of Cape Town, Cape Town, South Africa*

Devang Mehta • *Leuven Plant Institute (LPI), KU Leuven, Leuven, Belgium; Experimental Systems Biology Laboratory, Division of Crop Biotechnics, Department of Biosystems, KU Leuven, Leuven, Belgium*

Heyam S. Mohammed • *Instituto de Hortofruticultura Subtropical y Mediterránea 'La Mayora' (IHSM-UMA-CSIC), Consejo Superior de Investigaciones Científicas, Algarrobo-Costa, Málaga, Spain; Botany Department, Faculty of Science, University of Khartoum, Khartoum, Sudan*

Aránzazu Moreno • *Instituto de Ciencias Agrarias (ICA), Consejo Superior de Investigaciones Científicas (CSIC), Madrid, Spain*

Brejnev Muhizi Muhire • *Division of Computational Biology, Department of Integrative Biomedical Sciences, Institute of Infectious Diseases and Molecular Medicine, University of Cape Town, Cape Town, South Africa*

Jesús Navas-Castillo • *Instituto de Hortofruticultura Subtropical y Mediterránea 'La Mayora' (IHSM-UMA-CSIC), Consejo Superior de Investigaciones Científicas, Algarrobo-Costa, Málaga, Spain*

Jim Nygren • *Department of Plant Biology, Linnean Centre for Plant Biology, Swedish University of Agricultural Sciences, Uppsala, Sweden*

Anelise F. Orílio • *Dep. de Fitopatologia/BIOAGRO, Universidade Federal de Viçosa, Viçosa, MG, Brazil*

Ayane F. F. Quadros • *Dep. de Fitopatologia/BIOAGRO, Universidade Federal de Viçosa, Viçosa, MG, Brazil*

Roberto Ramos-Sobrinho • *Laboratory of Entomology and Phytopathology, Molecular Plant Virology, State University of the North Fluminense Darcy Ribeiro, Rio de Janeiro, Brazil*

Simone G. Ribeiro • *Embrapa Recursos Genéticos e Biotecnologia, Brasília, DF, Brazil*

Philippe Roumagnac • *UMR PHIM, CIRAD, Montpellier, France; PHIM Plant Health Institute, Univ Montpellier, CIRAD, INRAE, Institut Agro, IRD, Montpellier, France*

Leticia Ruiz García • *IFAPA, Centro La Mojonera, La Mojonera, Spain*

Fredy Davi Albuquerque Silva • *National Institute of Science and Technology in Plant-Pest Interactions/BIOAGRO, Universidade Federal de Viçosa, Viçosa, MG, Brazil*

Gonçalo Silva • *Natural Resources Institute, University of Greenwich, Chatham Maritime, UK*

Tripti Singhal • *Amity Institute of Virology & Immunology, Amity University Uttar Pradesh, Noida, India*

Ashish Srivastava • *Amity Institute of Virology & Immunology, Amity University Uttar Pradesh, Noida, India; Department of Plant Pathology, University of Minnesota Twin Cities, Saint Paul, MN, USA*

HERVÉ VANDERSCHUREN • *Plant Genetics Lab, TERRA Research and Teaching Centre, Gembloux Agro BioTech, University of Liège, Gembloux, Belgium; Tropical Crop Improvement Laboratory, Crop Biotechnics, Department of Biosystems, KU Leuven, Leuven, Belgium; Leuven Plant Institute (LPI), KU Leuven, Leuven, Belgium*
ARVIND VARSANI • *The Biodesign Center for Fundamental and Applied Microbiomics, Center for Evolution and Medicine, School of Life Sciences, Tempe, AZ, USA; Structural Biology Research Unit, Department of Integrative Biomedical Sciences, University of Cape Town, Observatory, Cape Town, South Africa*
ANDREZA H. VIDAL • *Embrapa Recursos Genéticos e Biotecnologia, Brasília, DF, Brazil*
XIAO-WEI WANG • *Ministry of Agriculture Key Laboratory of Molecular Biology of Crop Pathogens and Insects, Zhejiang Key Laboratory of Biology and Ecological Regulation of Crop Pathogens and Insects, Institute of Insect Sciences, Zhejiang University, Hangzhou, China*
YU-MENG WANG • *Ministry of Agriculture Key Laboratory of Molecular Biology of Crop Pathogens and Insects, Zhejiang Key Laboratory of Biology and Ecological Regulation of Crop Pathogens and Insects, Institute of Insect Sciences, Zhejiang University, Hangzhou, China*
XIULING YANG • *State Key Laboratory for Biology of Plant Diseases and Insect Pests, Institute of Plant Protection, Chinese Academy of Agricultural Sciences, Beijing, China*
ELHAM YAZDKHASTI • *Department of Plant Biology, Linnean Centre for Plant Biology, Swedish University of Agricultural Sciences, Uppsala, Sweden*
SYED SHAN-E-ALI ZAIDI • *Plant Genetics Lab, TERRA Research and Teaching Centre, Gembloux Agro BioTech, University of Liège, Gembloux, Belgium; INRAE & UMR 1332 Biologie du fruit et Pathologie, University of Bordeaux, Villenave d'Ornon Cedex, France*
FRANCISCO MURILO ZERBINI • *Dep. de Fitopatologia/BIOAGRO, Universidade Federal de Viçosa, Viçosa, MG, Brazil*
XUEPING ZHOU • *State Key Laboratory for Biology of Plant Diseases and Insect Pests, Institute of Plant Protection, Chinese Academy of Agricultural Sciences, Beijing, China; State Key Laboratory of Rice Biology, Institute of Biotechnology, Zhejiang University, Hangzhou, China*

[illegible]

Chapter 1

Extraction of Geminivirus and Associated Satellite DNA from Leaf Samples

Elvira Fiallo-Olivé, Heyam S. Mohammed, Francisco Murilo Zerbini, and Jesús Navas-Castillo

Abstract

The isolation of DNA from geminiviruses and their associated DNA satellites in plant leaf samples is a key step, as high-quality DNA preparations are essential for studies related to the characterization of geminivirus genomes and their interactions with host plants. The protocol outlined in this chapter describes a methodology based on the use of cetyltrimethylammonium bromide (CTAB) that facilitates the efficient extraction of total nucleic acids from plant tissues. The DNA obtained through this protocol finds direct application in various molecular techniques such as polymerase chain reaction, Southern blot, dot blot, and rolling-circle amplification. Additionally, the obtained DNA remains stable for years when stored at −20 °C, even after periods at room temperature. In essence, this extraction protocol is simple and useful for both experienced researchers and those introducing themselves to the study of geminiviruses and DNA satellites.

Key words Nucleic acid extraction, CTAB protocol, Geminiviruses, DNA satellites

1 Introduction

Geminiviruses (family *Geminiviridae*) are plant viruses with circular, single-stranded DNA genomes and a distinct twinned particle structure [1]. These viruses pose a serious threat to global agriculture, affecting crops like maize, cassava, and beans, and are primarily transmitted by insect vectors such as whiteflies, leafhoppers, and aphids. The diseases they cause lead to significant yield losses, reduced produce quality, and economic challenges for farmers [2–4]. Understanding the molecular and biological aspects of geminiviruses is crucial for developing effective management strategies, including the breeding of resistant crops and integrated pest management approaches that minimize environmental risks.

A critical step in studying geminiviruses and their associated DNA satellites is extracting high-quality DNA from plant tissues.

Francisco Murilo Zerbini et al. (eds.), *Geminiviruses: Methods and Protocols*, Methods in Molecular Biology, vol. 2912,
https://doi.org/10.1007/978-1-0716-4454-6_1,

This chapter outlines a cetyltrimethylammonium bromide (CTAB)-based protocol specifically designed for geminiviral studies, which efficiently isolates nucleic acids from plant samples. The protocol uses H-buffer, a solution containing the cationic surfactant CTAB, Tris–HCl, EDTA, sodium chloride, and glucose, to disrupt plant cells and release nucleic acids, followed by purification using chloroform-isoamyl alcohol, isopropanol precipitation, and ethanol washing. The resulting DNA is suitable for various molecular techniques, including polymerase chain reaction (PCR), Southern blot, dot blot, and rolling-circle amplification (RCA), and remains stable for long-term storage at −20 °C.

In summary, this extraction method provides researchers with a reliable tool for studying geminiviruses, associated DNA satellites, and their interactions with host plants.

2 Materials

Prepare all solutions using ultrapure water and analytical grade reagents. Prepare and store all reagents at room temperature unless indicated otherwise.

2.1 Reactive and Solutions

1. Liquid nitrogen.
2. H-Buffer: 100 mM Tris–HCl, pH 8.0, 20 mM ethylenediaminetetraacetic acid (EDTA), 1.4 M sodium chloride (NaCl), 2% cetyltrimethylammonium bromide (CTAB), 0.5 M glucose. Prepare a stock solution of 50 mL (2.5 mL of 2 M Tris–HCl, pH 8.0, 2.0 mL of 500 mM EDTA, 17.5 mL of 4 M NaCl, 10 mL of 10% CTAB, 12.5 mL of 2 M glucose, and 5.5 mL of water). *See* **Note 1**.
3. Extraction buffer: 500 μL extraction buffer consists of 450 μL of H-Buffer, 50 μL of 100 mM dithiothreitol (DTT), 0.2 μL 2-mercaptoethanol. This solution should be prepared at the moment of beginning the process and the solution that is not used must be discarded.
4. 2 M Tris–HCl, pH 8.0: Add 24.228 g Tris base to 60 mL of water and shake until solute is dissolved. Adjust the pH to 8.0 with concentrated HCl, bring final volume to 100 mL with water, and autoclave.
5. 500 mM EDTA: Add 14.612 g EDTA to 80 mL of water. Dissolve and adjust the volume to 100 mL with water, and autoclave.
6. 4 M NaCl: Add 23.376 g NaCl to 70 mL of distilled water. Dissolve and adjust the volume to 100 mL with water, and autoclave.

7. 10% CTAB: 10 g CTAB in 100 mL of water and dissolve using a magnetic stirrer.
8. 2 M glucose: 36.032 g glucose in 80 mL of water, dissolve using magnetic stirrer until glucose has completely dissolved, adjust the volume to 100 mL with water. Then, filter the solution.
9. 100 mM DTT: 7.71 g in 50 mL water, aliquot in 2.0 mL tubes and store at −20 °C.
10. Chloroform:isoamyl alcohol (24:1, v/v): Mix 24 mL of chloroform and 1.0 mL of isoamyl alcohol.
11. Isopropanol.
12. 70% ethanol.

2.2 Required Material and Equipment

1. Pestle and mortar.
2. Bench microcentrifuge.
3. Shaker for microcentrifuge tubes.
4. Vortex.

3 Methods

1. Place the leaf sample (10–50 mg) in a mortar and grind in the presence of liquid nitrogen until the tissue is powdered, or grind directly in a 1.5 mL Eppendorf tube using a micropestle. If using a mortar, transfer the powdered tissue to a 1.5 mL Eppendorf tube. *See* **Note 2**.
2. Add 500 μL of freshly prepared Extraction Buffer.
3. Incubate samples at 60 °C for 1 h with shaking.
4. Allow the samples to cool, then add 500 μL of chloroform-isoamyl alcohol (24:1) and mix using a vortex.
5. Spin at the highest speed (14,000 rpm) in a bench centrifuge for 5 min at 4 °C.
6. Carefully, transfer the upper phase (approximately 350 μL, avoiding debris) to a new 1.5 mL tube and add 0.8 volumes of isopropanol (approximately 280 μL).
7. Mix briefly using a vortex or by inverting the tubes up and down twice. A precipitate should be visible.
8. Spin at highest speed (14,000 rpm) in a bench centrifuge for 10 min at 4 °C to pellet the nucleic acids.
9. Discard the supernatant and wash pellets with 70% ethanol.
10. Spin at the highest speed (14,000 rpm) in a bench centrifuge for 5 min at room temperature.

11. Air dry the pellets at room temperature for at least 5 min, then dissolve the pellets in 100 μL of water. *See* **Note 3**.
12. Store samples at −20 °C. *See* **Note 4**.

4 Notes

1. An improvement of traditional CTAB-based methods is the addition of glucose in the extraction buffer, which prevents browning from polyphenolic compounds and enhances the quality of DNA for molecular analysis [5].
2. As an alternative to using a mortar or Eppendorf tube, the homogenization of the leaf samples can be carried out with an electronic homogenizer (e.g., FastPrep). For this, place leaf samples in 2-mL Eppendorf tubes containing H-buffer, and follow the device instructions. This option is particularly useful when working with a high number of samples or hard tissues from woody plants.
3. This protocol extracts both DNA and RNA; however, RNA does not interfere with most subsequent applications such as PCR, RCA, and dot blot hybridization. An RNase treatment step can be included to completely eliminate RNA if desired.
4. Although this protocol typically yields DNA suitable for direct use in other procedures, working with some wild plants may require diluting the obtained DNA (1/10 or even 1/50) to improve amplification by PCR or RCA.

Acknowledgments

This work was supported by grants from the Ministerio de Ciencia e Innovación (MICINN, Spain) (PID2021-128445OA-I00/AEI/10.13039/501100011033), cofinanced by the European Regional Development Fund, and the i-COOP program from Consejo Superior de Investigaciones Científicas (CSIC, Spain) (COOPB22030) to E.F.O.

References

1. Fiallo-Olivé E, Lett JM, Martin DP et al (2021) ICTV virus taxonomy profile: *Geminiviridae*. J Gen Virol 102:001696
2. Varma A, Malathi VG (2003) Emerging geminivirus problems: a serious threat to crop production. Ann Appl Biol 142:145–164
3. Fiallo-Olivé E, Navas-Castillo J (2023) Begomoviruses: what is the secret(s) of their success? Trends Plant Sci 28:715–727
4. Rao GP, Reddy MG (2020) Overview of yield losses due to plant viruses. In: Awasthi LP (ed) Applied plant virology. Academic Press, Cambridge, MA
5. Permingeat HR, Romagnoli MV, Sesma JI et al (1998) A simple method for isolating DNA of high yield and quality from cotton (*Gossypium hirsutum* L.) leaves. Plant Mol Biol Report 16:89

Chapter 2

Mechanical Sap Transmission of Geminiviruses

Francisco Murilo Zerbini

Abstract

Mechanical sap transmission is the simplest, quickest, and most cost-effective method to transmit geminiviruses (and indeed any plant virus) from one plant to another. However, a significant number of geminiviruses, which are phloem-restricted in their hosts, are not transmitted in this form. For those geminiviruses which do invade the mesophyll, mechanical transmission is possible. The procedure consists of grinding virus-infected plant material (usually leaves) in a buffer solution and rubbing the plant sap onto the surface of the leaves of a healthy plant, which have been sprinkled with an abrasive powder. Injury to the epidermal cells (maximized by the presence of the abrasive powder) allows viral particles to enter the cell and initiate infection.

Key words Phosphate buffer, Carborundum, Celite, Reducing agents, Chelating agents

1 Introduction

Grafting is the guaranteed means of transmitting a virus from one plant to another [1]. However, results take time and it is impossible to graft botanically unrelated species. The use of insect vectors is an often used alternative. Transmission via buffered plant extract (mechanical sap transmission) is much simpler and faster than grafting or the use of insect vectors. Several geminiviruses are mechanically transmissible, including African cassava mosaic virus (ACMV), bean dwarf mosaic virus (BDMV), bean golden yellow mosaic virus (BGYMV), and Sida micrantha mosaic virus (SimMV) [2–5]. However, other geminiviruses of great economic importance are not transmitted in this way, including bean golden mosaic virus (BGMV), tomato yellow leaf curl virus (TYLCV), tomato severe rugose mosaic virus (ToSRV), beet curly top virus (BCTV), and maize streak virus (MSV) [6–10]. The impossibility of transmitting a virus mechanically is associated with viral infection restricted to the vascular tissues [11, 12]. Since mechanical inoculation reaches only cells of the epidermis and palisade parenchyma,

Francisco Murilo Zerbini et al. (eds.), *Geminiviruses: Methods and Protocols*, Methods in Molecular Biology, vol. 2912,
https://doi.org/10.1007/978-1-0716-4454-6_2,

viruses restricted to the vasculature will not be able to establish a systemic infection following mechanical inoculation.

Some basic precautions must be taken for a virus to be successfully transmitted via plant extract. First, it is essential that the pH of the extract is maintained close to optimum for the stability of the viral particle. This optimum pH is close to neutral for most geminiviruses. It is also necessary to minimize the activity of oxidative enzymes and phenolic compounds, which can destabilize the viral particle due to modifications in the capsid protein. The use of a buffer solution containing reducing or chelating agents is the most common way to satisfy these requirements. Phosphate buffers are the most used for mechanical transmission, as they are relatively inert and do not cause harmful effects to viral particles. Among the most commonly used reducing and chelating agents are sodium sulfite, betamercaptoethanol, EDTA, polyvinylpyrrolidone (PVP) or sodium diethyldithiocarbamate (Na-DIECA). Once the plant extract has been prepared, it must be quickly used for inoculation, as even with the precautions mentioned above, the viability of the virus in the extract is limited. Finally, it must be ensured that plant cells will allow viral particles to enter. In other words, cells must be injured but not killed, as dead cells will not allow viral replication. This objective is achieved by the use of an abrasive powder such as silicon carbide, commercially named Carborundum 600 (600 mesh) or diatomaceous earth (Celite). The abrasive should be sprayed onto the leaves prior to inoculation, or it can be mixed with buffered plant extract (which is more practical when the number of plants to be inoculated is very large).

All the precautions mentioned above must be taken extra when the plant from which the extract is prepared contains high concentrations of phenolic and/or oxidative compounds (e.g., tomato, pepper, most woody plants). Mechanical transmission may be of low efficiency in these cases.

2 Materials

1. Ice-cold (2–5 °C) inoculation buffer: 0.1 M potassium phosphate buffer pH 7.2, containing 0.01 M sodium sulfite (Na_2SO_3) (*see* **Note 1**).
2. Porcelain mortar and pestle recently removed from the freezer (*see* **Note 2**).
3. Gauze (*see* **Note 3**).
4. Carborundum, 600 mesh (*see* **Note 4**).
5. Source plants (infected by a geminivirus).
6. Healthy plants to be inoculated.

3 Methods

1. Mark the pot or batch of pots BEFORE inoculation with labels, indicating the plant species being inoculated, the inoculator and the date.
2. Sprinkle Carborundum 600 on the leaves of the plants to be inoculated (*see* **Notes 5** and **6**).
3. Collect a young, symptomatic leaf from the source plant (*see* **Note** 7) and grind it in the mortar, in the presence of buffer, in an approximate ratio of 1:5 (leaf weight: volume of buffer solution) (*see* **Note 8**).
4. Wet the gauze in the inoculum and apply it with low pressure on the leaf, minimizing damage to tissues and cells (*see* **Note 9**).
5. Inoculated plants should be kept in a greenhouse; the appearance of symptoms should be observed periodically as the symptom may change over time.

4 Notes

1. This is a general buffer solution that will work for most geminiviruses (indeed, for most plant viruses). The relevant parameters of a buffer solution are the nature of the salt (monovalent or divalent, weakly or strongly dissociated), the ionic strength and the pH. In addition, for viral mechanical transmission, reducing or chelating agents are almost always used. Phosphate salts with monovalent cations (sodium or potassium) are ideal as they are inert and are not affected by chelating agents (such as EDTA). A 0.1 M buffer is usually capable of maintaining the pH for most plant extracts, but a 0.05 or even a 0.02 M buffer can also be used. The pH of the buffer is usually close to neutral, but could be above neutral (up to 8) is the plant extract is acidic (e.g., *Capsicum* peppers). Sodium sulfite is an efficient reducing agent which does not affect the viral particles and is not toxic, unlike stronger agents such as betamercaptoethanol.
2. If porcelain mortar and pestles are not available, a simple alternative is to grind the leaves inside plastic bags.
3. Instead of gauze or cheesecloth, cotton balls can also be used. It is also possible to rub the leaves directly with the porcelain pestle, or even with one's fingers (in this case, use latex gloves!).
4. A common and equally effective alternative is Celite, the commercial name for finely ground diatomaceous earth. Celite is

>90% silica, approx. 4% aluminium oxide and 2% iron oxide. Carborundum is >98% silicon carbide.

5. When using Carborundum, the amount of powder to be sprinkled on the leaves is very small. As a rule of thumb, if the powder is visible on the surface of the leaves, then too much was applied. Applying too much powder will increase the magnitude of injury and may kill the cells.
6. Sprinkling the leaves directly is most efficient when inoculating a small number of plants. If hundreds of plants are being inoculated, a better strategy is to add the abrasive directly to the buffered plant sap.
7. For the best results, the youngest fully developed leaves should be used as inoculum sources, as they have a high viral load and low concentrations of phenolic compounds and free radicals. However, other parts of the plant can also be used, such as roots, fruit or seeds.
8. It is advisable, but not essential, to use a standard buffer:leaf proportion for mechanical sap inoculation. A 5:1 ration is most efficient in keeping the pH stable and the viral concentration in the inoculum sufficiently high to assure transmission.
9. Apply enough pressure so that it can be felt as you place two fingers under the leaves being inoculated. If no pressure is felt, no injury will be caused and the efficiency of the inoculation will be low. Too much pressure will kill most cells.

References

1. Matthews REF (1991) Plant virology, 3rd edn. Academic, San Diego
2. Jovel J, Reski G, Rothenstein D, Ringel M, Frischmuth T, Jeske H (2004) *Sida micrantha* mosaic is associated with a complex infection of begomoviruses different from *Abutilon mosaic virus*. Arch Virol 149:829–841
3. Stanley J, Townsend R, Curson SJ (1985) Pseudorecombinants between cloned DNAs of two isolates of cassava latent virus. J Gen Virol 66:1055–1061
4. Gilbertson RL, Hidayat SH, Martinez RT, Leong SA, Faria JC, Morales FJ, Maxwell DP (1991) Diferentiation of bean-infecting geminiviruses by nucleic acid hybridization probes and aspects of bean golden mosaic in Brazil. Plant Dis 75:336–342
5. Bock KR, Woods RD (1983) Etiology of African cassava mosaic disease. Plant Dis 67:994–995
6. Bennett CW, Esau K (1936) Further studies on the relation of the curly top virus to plant tissues. J Agric Res 53:595–620
7. Czosnek H, Ber R, Antignus Y, Cohen S, Navot N, Zamir D (1988) Isolation of tomato yellow leaf curl virus, a geminivirus. Phytopathology 78:508–512
8. Storey HH (1928) Transmission studies of maize streak disease. Ann Appl Biol 15:1–25
9. Figueira AR, Costa AS (1986) Attempts at mechanical transmission of bean golden mosaic virus from Brazil (in Portuguese). Fitopatol Bras 11:433–442
10. Fernandes JJ, Carvalho MG, Andrade EC, Brommonschenkel SH, Fontes EPB, Zerbini FM (2006) Biological and molecular properties of *Tomato rugose mosaic virus* (ToRMV), a new tomato-infecting begomovirus from Brazil. Plant Pathol 55:513–522

11. Morra MR, Petty ITD (2000) Tissue specificity of geminivirus infection is genetically determined. Plant Cell 12:2259–2270
12. Wang HL, Gilbertson RL, Lucas WJ (1996) Spatial and temporal distribution of bean dwarf mosaic geminivirus in *Phaseolus vulgaris* and *Nicotiana benthamiana*. Phytopathology 86:1204–1214

Chapter 3

Cloning of Complete Geminivirus Genomes by Rolling Circle Amplification (RCA)

Francisco Murilo Zerbini

Abstract

Rolling circle amplification (RCA) revolutionized geminivirology before high-throughput sequencing. Using the DNA polymerase of phage phi29 and random primers, it is a simple isothermal reaction which will amplify circular DNA without any prior knowledge of its sequence. It is thus ideal to clone complete geminivirus genomes. The procedure outlined here has been used in the author's laboratory for more than 15 years and has allowed the cloning of thousands of full-length genomes. It consists of three parts: first, the RCA reaction itself; second, the analysis of RCA products with restriction enzymes, to identify an enzyme that will cleave the genome at a single site; and third, the ligation of the linearized genome to a plasmid vector, followed by *E. coli* transformation. The whole procedure will normally take 3 days.

Key words Begomoviruses, RCA, Plasmid, *E. coli*, Full-length clone

1 Introduction

The genome of begomoviruses is composed of one or two circular, single-stranded DNA (ssDNA) molecules, each with approximately 2600 nucleotides. However, in infected plants, the "replicative form" (RF) of the viral genome (double-stranded circular DNA) is present in a higher concentration than ssDNA. Replication of the viral genome occurs in the nucleus of infected cells, through a mechanism called "rolling circle".

In the early days of "geminivirology", DNA extraction from purified virions [1, 2] or RF extraction [3] were the methods of choice to obtain the complete viral genome. The procedures were time-consuming and inefficient, but allowed for the cloning of the complete genome without prior sequence information. In the 1990s, amplification of the viral genome via polymerase chain reaction (PCR) using overlapping oligonucleotides [4] became the standard strategy for cloning the geminivirus genome. Amplification via PCR allows cloning of the complete genome much more

Francisco Murilo Zerbini et al. (eds.), *Geminiviruses: Methods and Protocols*, Methods in Molecular Biology, vol. 2912, https://doi.org/10.1007/978-1-0716-4454-6_3,

quickly and efficiently. However, there must be prior information about the sequence of the viral genome for the synthesis of oligonucleotides [4].

In the early 2000s, several companies began commercializing a high-fidelity DNA polymerase from the bacteriophage phi29 [5, 6]. This bacteriophage replicates using the same rolling circle mechanism used by geminiviruses. The phi29 DNA polymerase is capable of carrying out all stages of the replication process, using a double-stranded circular DNA template molecule and oligonucleotides with a random sequence. It was soon realized that such a strategy could be used for the amplification of begomovirus RF (circular dsDNA) [7]. In fact, the use of phi29 phage DNA polymerase allows the amplification of the complete viral genome, without prior sequence information, from a total DNA extract from an infected plant. This technique, which was named "rolling circle amplification" (RCA), made it possible to clone complete viral genomes from dozens or even hundreds of samples in a matter of days [8]. Amplification generates a multimeric molecule containing several units of the viral genome. Cloning is carried out after cleavage of this molecule with an enzyme that cuts the viral genome in just one site, releasing the monomeric genomes from the multimeric molecule [7, 8].

RCA is currently the standard for cloning circular DNA viral genomes, and has allowed the discovery of new species and genera of geminiviruses as well as new families of plant, fungal, and animal viruses with circular, ssDNA genomes.

2 Materials

1. Total DNA extracted from a geminivirus-infected plant (*see* Chap. 1).
2. Micropipettes (P20, P200, and P1000) and tips (200 and 1000 μL).
3. Disposable latex gloves.
4. phi29 DNA polymerase and accompanying enzyme buffer (*see* **Note 1**).
5. Thioprotected random hexamers (*see* **Note 2**).
6. Triphosphate deoxynucleotide mix (dATP, dCTP, dGTP, and dTTP).
7. Bovine serum albumin (BSA), 10%.
8. Water bath or thermocycler.
9. Agarose gel electrophoresis apparatus.
10. Ethidium bromide, 10 mg/mL in water.
11. Restriction enzymes.

12. Incubator (37 °C).
13. Plasmid vector.
14. T4 DNA ligase.
15. Electroporator and "electrocompetent" cells.
16. Sterile Petri dishes.
17. Solid and liquid LB or 2xYT culture media.
18. Ampicilim (100 mg/mL).
19. X-Gal (5-bromo-4-chloro-3-indolyl-β-d-galactopyranoside) (20 mg/mL).
20. IPTG (100 mM).

3 Methods

1. To a 0.5 mL microfuge tube, add:
   (a) 1.0 μL of DNA extracted from a geminivirus-infected plant.
   (b) 1.0 μL of enzyme buffer.
   (c) 1.0 μL of thioprotected random hexamers.
   (d) 1.0 μL of BSA.
   (e) 1.0 μL of dNTP mix.
   (f) 0.3 μL of the phi29 DNA polymerase enzyme.
   (g) 4.7 μL of autoclaved Milli-Q water.
2. Incubate at 30 °C for 18–20 h in a water bath or thermocycler (*see* **Note 3**), followed by 65 °C for 10 min (to inactivate the enzyme). Store the reaction at -20 °C until electrophoresis is performed.
3. Amplification is verified through electrophoretic analysis in an agarose gel (0.7%) prepared in 0.5× TBE, using a 1 μL aliquot of the reaction. Electrophoresis is performed at 100 V, until the front reaches 0.5 cm from the end of the gel. Transfer the gel to a vat containing diluted ethidium bromide solution (50 μL of 10 mg/mL ethidium bromide in 100 mL of water) (*see* **Note 4**), and incubate at room temperature for 10 min. Observe and photograph the gel under ultraviolet light.
4. For enzymatic cleavage of the RCA product (*see* **Note 5**), prepare the following rection in a 0.5 mL microfuge tube:
   (a) 3.0 μL of DNA amplified by RCA.
   (b) 1.5 μL of restriction enzyme buffer (10×).
   (c) 0.5 μL of restriction enzyme (1u/μg of DNA).

(d) 10.0 μL of autoclaved Milli-Q water for a total reaction volume of 15 μL.

5. Incubate at 37 °C for 2 h (some enzymes are incubated at different temperatures; check the manufacturer's instructions). The cleavage pattern is verified using electrophoretic analysis in an agarose gel (0.7%) as described in Subheading 3, **step 3**. If an approx. 2700 nt band is present, proceed to the next step.
6. For ligation of the RCA product to the vector plasmid, prepare the following reaction in a 0.5 mL microfuge tube:
   (a) 5 μL of RCA product cleaved with the appropriate restriction enzyme.
   (b) 1 μL of pBluescript KS+ plasmid vector (pKS+) cleaved with the same enzyme and dephosphorylated (*see* **Note 6**).
   (c) 0.3 μL of T4 DNA ligase.
   (d) 1 μL of enzyme buffer (10x).
   (e) 2.7 μL of autoclaved Milli-Q water.
7. Incubate at 4 °C for 16 h.
8. Purification of the ligation product (*see* **Note 7**):
   (a) Bring the ligation reaction volume to 50 μL with autoclaved Milli-Q water.
   (b) Add 500 μL of n-butanol and vortex for 1 min.
   (c) Spin at 13,000 *g* for 10 min at 4 °C, discarding the supernatant.
   (d) Dry the pellet in a SpeedVac for 10 min.
   (e) Resuspend in 4 μL of autoclaved Milli-Q water.
9. Bacterial transformation (*see* **Note 8**):
   (a) Label the tubes (0.5 μL microfuge tubes) and keep them at −80 °C for 5 min.
   (b) Place the plates with solid LB medium in the incubator at 37 °C.
   (c) Warm up the liquid LB medium without antibiotics to 37 °C.
   (d) Thaw the competent cells (100 μL) on ice.
   (e) Add 1.0 μL of the purified ligation product (*see* Subheading 3, **step 8**). Mix gently. Do not pipette up and down. Competent cells are extremely fragile and can be damaged during this step.
   (f) Transfer the entire volume to the electroporation cuvette. Keep the cuvette on ice.

(g) Dry the cuvette completely before electroporation; electroporate at 2.5 kV/25 μF/200 Ω.

(h) Transfer the entire volume of the cuvette to a microcentrifuge tube (1.5 mL) and add 500 μL of LB medium without antibiotics, preheated to 37 °C; incubate at 37 °C for 1 h without shaking.

(i) Prepare 10 μL of IPTG, 40 μL of X-Gal, and 100 μL of LB with ampicillin per plate, and spread on the plates (*see* **Note 9**).

(j) Spin the bacterial cells at 13,000 *g* for 1 min, discard the supernatant and resuspend the cells in 100 μL of LB medium without antibiotics.

(k) Plate the entire volume in LB medium with X-Gal and ampicillin.

(l) Incubate the plates at 37 °C for 12–16 h.

10. Transfer white colonies to liquid LB medium with ampicillin, grow at 37 °C for 12–16 h and extract plasmids using a commercial kit to confirm the transformation.

4 Notes

1. The enzyme is available commercially either as a stand-alone product or as part of kits. Either option will work. Kits will include other items such as the random hexamers and dNTPs, depending on the manufacturer. Using a kit will reduce liquid handling time, thus minimizing the likelihood of errors, but will increase costs.

2. Use of "thioprotected" primers is essential for the success of the reaction. This is because of the proofreading, 3′–5′ exonuclease activity of phi29 DNA polymerase, which degrades non-protected primers and drastically reduces the reaction yield [6]. Thioprotected primers have thiophosphate linkages at the two 3′ terminal nucleotides (5′-NpNpNpNpsNpsN-3′).

3. The RCA reaction is isothermal, that is, it occurs at a constant temperature. Thus, the use of a thermal cycler is not necessary. However, if the laboratory has a thermocycler, its use is recommended due to greater precision in temperature adjustment.

4. Ethidium bromide is a known carcinogen, and should be handled with extreme care. A number of alternative "safer" dyes are available, but they cost more and are not really safer (every intercalating dye is inherently hazardous).

5. If RCA is being used to clone a known, previously sequenced geminivirus, the restriction enzyme to be used can be determined by analyzing the sequence and looking for an enzyme

with a single cleavage site. If, however, the reaction is being performed to amplify the genome of a newly detected virus which has not yet been fully sequenced, then a number of enzymes will have to be tested by cleavage of the RCA product. Typically, 5–10 enzymes are tested in separate reactions. After the cleavage reaction, the result is analyzed by agarose gel electrophoresis. Cleavage of the geminivirus genome at just one site produces a fragment with approximately 2700 nucleotides (nt). Enzymes that cleave the viral DNA at more than one site produce smaller fragments, the sum of which must be approximately 2700 nt. There are also cases in which only one of the genomic components of bipartite begomoviruses (DNA-A or DNA-B) is cleaved. In this case, a 2700 nt fragment is observed together with the band corresponding to the amplified and uncut DNA, which migrates much more slowly in the gel. Finally, there are cases in which one component is cleaved in a single site and the other component at multiple sites, or both components are cleaved at multiple sites, generating complex band patterns which should add up to approximately 5400 nt. Even more complex patterns may arise if RCA is performed directly from field samples, which may be infected by more than one begomovirus. *See* Fig. 1.

6. Many different vectors can be used, and the one listed here is simply a suggestion. But regardless of the vector, it must have been cleaved with the same enzyme used to cleave the RCA product, and dephosphorylated to prevent self-ligation. For cleavage and dephosphorylation, prepare the following reactions:
   (a) 300 ng of plasmid DNA, 4 μL of enzyme buffer (10×), 1 μL of restriction enzyme, and autoclaved Milli-Q water up to 40 μL. Incubate at 37 °C for 2 h.
   (b) To 40 μL of the cleavage reaction, add 5 μL of enzyme buffer (10x), 1 μL of calf intestinal alkaline phosphatase, and 4 μL of autoclaved Milli-Q water. Incubate at 37 °C for 30 min. Add another 1 μL of enzyme and incubate at 37 °C for another 30 min. Incubate at 65 °C for 10 min to inactivate the enzyme. Purify the cleaved plasmid DNA using a commercial kit, according to the manufacturer's instructions.
7. This step is necessary when the transformation is carried out by electroporation, to remove the salt present in the enzyme buffer. If the salt is not removed, the electric shock will be amplified, killing the bacterial cells.
8. For electroporation, bacterial cells are subjected to an electrical pulse of approximately 2400 volts/cm, which induces the formation of small pores in the cell membrane through which the

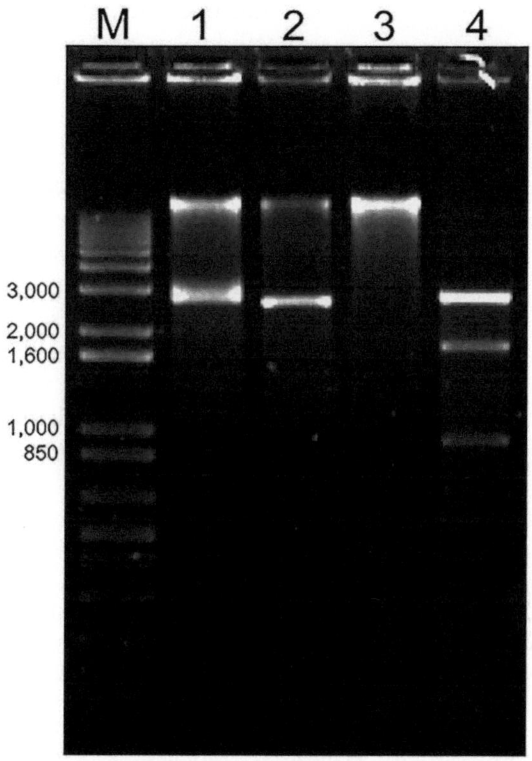

Fig. 1 Cleavage of rolling circle amplification (RCA) products obtained from geminivirus-infected plants. (1) RCA products from a plant infected with begomovirus X, digested with ApaI. One of the components was cleaved at just one site, producing a fragment with approximately 2700 nucleotides (nt). The other component was not cleaved, which is indicated by the presence of a high molecular weight band, corresponding to uncleaved RCA product. (2) RCA products of begomovirus X digested with BamHI. One of the components was cleaved at just one site, producing a fragment with slightly less than 2700 nucleotides (nt). The other component was not cleaved. The smaller size of the digested component suggests that it is a DNA-B. (3) RCA products from a plant infected with begomovirus Y, digested with SpeI. None of the two components was cleaved. (4) RCA products of begomovirus Y digested with BamHI. One of the components was cleaved at just one site, producing a fragment with approximately 2700 nt. The other component was cleaved at two sites, producing fragments with approximately 1700 and 900 nt. M, Size marker (in nt)

DNA penetrates the cell. The transformation efficiency using electroporation is greater than that obtained through heat shock, ranging from 10^9–10^{10} transformed colonies per μg of plasmid DNA. This is the recommended method when attempting to clone full-length geminivirus genomes, due to the large size of the recombinant plasmids (>6000 nt). Bacterial transformation methods are based on the fact that bacterial cells treated with $CaCl_2$ undergo structural changes in the cell wall and become capable of absorbing DNA in solution when subjected to an electrical or thermal shock. Cells treated in this way are called "competent", but they become extremely sensitive to any mechanical damage and should be handled gently.

9. The antibiotic to be used depends on the chosen plasmid vector. The vector suggested here (pBLUESCRIPT KS+) has an ampicillin resistance gene. The use of IPTG and X-Gal is to allow for blue/white selection of bacterial colonies, but only when the plasmid vector contains the *lacZ* gene which encodes β-galactosidase. In these cases, empty vectors will express *lacZ* and the encoded protein will process X-Gal, forming a blue precipitate (thus, blue colonies in the agar plates). Recombinant vectors have a disrupted *lacZ*. With no β-galatosidase, X-Gal is not processed and the colonies grow white.

References

1. Sequeira JC, Harrison BD (1982) Serological studies on cassava latent virus. Ann Appl Biol 101:33–42
2. Stanley J, Gay MR (1983) Nucleotide sequence of cassava latent virus DNA. Nature 301:260–262
3. Gilbertson RL, Faria JC, Hanson SF, Morales FJ, Ahlquist PG, Maxwell DP, Russell DR (1991) Cloning of the complete DNA genomes of four bean-infecting geminiviruses and determining their infectivity by electric discharge particle acceleration. Phytopathology 81:980–985
4. Patel VP, Rojas MR, Paplomatas EJ, Gilbertson RL (1993) Cloning biologically active geminivirus DNA using PCR and overlapping primers. Nucleic Acids Res 21:1325–1326
5. Garmendia C, Bernad A, Esteban JA, Blanco L, Salas M (1992) The bacteriophage phi 29 DNA polymerase, a proofreading enzyme. J Biol Chem 267:2594–2599
6. Dean FB, Nelson JR, Giesler TL, Lasken RS (2001) Rapid amplification of plasmid and phage DNA using phi29 DNA polymerase and multiply-primed rolling circle amplification. Genome Res 11:1095–1099
7. Inoue-Nagata AK, Albuquerque LC, Rocha WB, Nagata T (2004) A simple method for cloning the complete begomovirus genome using the bacteriophage phi29 DNA polymerase. J Virol Met 116:209–211
8. Haible D, Kober S, Jeske H (2006) Rolling circle amplification revolutionizes diagnosis and genomics of geminiviruses. J Virol Met 135:9–16

Chapter 4

Biolistic Inoculation of Plants with Geminivirus Infectious Clones

Cristiano Lacorte, Andreza H. Vidal, and Simone G. Ribeiro

Abstract

The propagation of viruses in laboratory-controlled conditions is an essential step in studying viruses' molecular and biological properties. For geminiviruses, the main methods of inoculation are agroinoculation and biolistics. Here, we describe the protocol for inoculating self-ligated cloned geminivirus inserts into plants using particle bombardment. This method is convenient for the characterization of the cloned virus, as the exact clones used for sequence analysis can be used for the inoculation of the plants.

Key words Biolistics, Cloned virus, Particle bombardment, Gene gun

1 Introduction

The study of molecular and biological properties of viruses relies on their propagation to healthy plants in laboratory-controlled conditions. Although propagation by mechanical inoculation, grafting, and through vectors are commonly used in plant virology studies, in the case of geminiviruses, the inoculation of cloned virus components is the prevailing method of viral propagation for virus-host interaction studies. It is widely used for virus isolation and identification, host range and pseudorecombination evaluation, functional studies of viral genes and mutants, access to the host response to the virus infection, and resistance screening in germplasm accessions.

There are two main inoculation methods to inoculate cloned complete geminivirus genomes into plants: agroinoculation and biolistics.

For agroinoculation, a geminivirus full-length genome dimer or a partial dimer (containing two copies of the geminivirus origin of replication) is cloned between the T-DNA borders of a binary vector and introduced into *Agrobacterium tumefaciens* cells, which will transfer this T-DNA into plant cells [1].

Francisco Murilo Zerbini et al. (eds.), *Geminiviruses: Methods and Protocols*, Methods in Molecular Biology, vol. 2912, https://doi.org/10.1007/978-1-0716-4454-6_4,

In the biolistics approach, the cloned geminivirus genetic material is precipitated on gold metal microparticles and directly delivered to plant cells by particle bombardment using a gene gun [2]. Several forms of viral genomic DNA can be used to coat the particles for inoculation:

1. Undigested recombinant dimeric or a partial dimer genome cloned into a plasmid cloning vector or binary vector.
2. DNA digests of recombinant plasmid where full-length monomer or dimeric genome virus inserts are excised or linearized by a restriction enzyme.
3. DNA digests of recombinant plasmid where full-length monomer virus genome inserts were excised by restriction enzyme and then self-ligated.

In our laboratory, we have successfully been using self-ligated DNA digests of monomer virus genome inserts to inoculate geminiviruses belonging to three genera, including *Begomovirus* (tomato chlorotic mottle virus, bean golden mosaic virus, tomato severe rugose virus, corchorus mottle virus, sida micrantha mosaic virus, and macroptilium yellow mosaic virus), *Citlodavirus* (passionfruit chlorotic mottle virus), and *Topilevirus* (tomato geminivirus 1). Plants from different botanical families, comprising Solanaceae (*Nicotiana benthamiana N. tabacum*, *Capsicum annum*, *Solanum lycopersicon*, and *Nicandra physaloides*), Fabaceae (*Glycine max* and *Phaseolus vulgaris*), Malvaceae (*Sida glasiovii* and *S. rhombifolia*), Passifloraceae (*Passiflora edulis*), and Brassicaceae (*Arabidopsis thaliana*) were successfully infected using bombardment with self-ligated geminivirus inserts [3–6]. This type of DNA preparation has the advantage that the exact clone used for sequencing can be used for biolistics inoculation without further cloning steps. However, the full-length viral DNA genome must be cloned in a unique restriction enzyme site within the virus genome.

2 Materials

2.1 Viral DNA Preparation for Bombardment

1. A plasmid containing a full-length monomer of a geminivirus genome (*see* **Note 1**).
2. 1.5 mL microfuge tubes.
3. Ultrapure water (e.g., Milli-Q purified water).
4. Restriction enzyme (RE) (the same restriction nuclease used for cloning).
5. 10X restriction enzyme buffer (use a compatible buffer for the RE according to manufacturers' instructions).
6. Temperature-controlled water or dry bath incubator.

7. 10X Bovine Serum Albumin (BSA 1 mg/mL).
8. T4 DNA ligase.
9. 10X T4 DNA ligase buffer (use a compatible buffer for the T4 ligase according to manufacturer's instructions).
10. Absolute ethanol.
11. Microcentrifuge.
12. 70% ethanol.
13. 3 M sodium acetate, pH 5.2.
14. Reagents and apparatuses for agarose gel electrophoresis: Agarose, 1X TAE buffer (Tris-acetate-EDTA—40 mM Tris, 20 mM Acetate, and 1 mM EDTA) (*see* **Note 2**), 10X loading buffer (10 mM Tris–HCl (pH 7.6), 60 mM EDTA, 0.03% bromophenol blue, 60% glycerol), SYBR Safe or other DNA gel stain, commercial DNA molecular weight marker, horizontal agarose gel electrophoresis tray and comb, electrophoresis power supply, and gel documentation system.

2.2 Preparation of Plant Material

1. Plant seeds.
2. Small pots, about 6 cm in height and 10 cm in diameter.
3. Mixture of commercial substrate and potting soil 1:1.

2.3 Biolistic Inoculation of Geminiviruses

1. Gold particles (M10).
2. 2.5 M $CaCl_2$ (filter sterilized).
3. 0.1 M spermidine (filter sterilized).
4. 50% glycerol, sterile (autoclaved).
5. Absolute ethanol.
6. Sterile water.
7. Isopropanol.
8. Geminivirus DNA preparation.
9. 1.5 mL microfuge tubes.
10. Vortex mixer.
11. Ultrasonic bath (*see* **Note 3**).
12. Desiccating chamber (e.g., a petri dish with silica desiccant).
13. Particle bombardment device (*see* **Note 4**).
14. Carrier membranes (Kapton® film) and membrane supports.
15. Rupture disks (Kapton® film).
16. Healthy plants to be inoculated, properly labeled (*see* **Note 5**).
17. Moist chamber (e.g., a plastic box with a layer of water and covered with a transparent plastic film).

3 Methods

This method uses the particle bombardment technique to inoculate plants with self-ligated digests of cloned geminivirus genomes. The presented protocol yields enough DNA for four precipitations for DNA-A and DNA-B components of bipartite begomoviruses and two for monopartite geminiviruses. The DNA preparation is enough to inoculate 24 plants in the first case and 12 plants in the second. The procedures described in the protocol are outlined in Figs. 1 and 2.

3.1 Viral DNA Preparation for Bombardment

1. Set up the digestion reaction: 10.5 μg plasmid containing a full-length monomer of geminivirus DNA (*see* **Note 6**), 10 μL of the appropriate 10X reaction buffer, 10 μL 10X BSA (*see* **Note 7**), 4 units of the proper RE per μg of DNA, ultrapure water to a final volume of 100 μL.
2. Incubate the reaction mixture at 37 °C overnight (*see* **Note 8**).
3. Load and run 2 μL of the digested DNA on a 0.8% agarose gel in 1X TAE to check if the digestion was complete; if the digestion is incomplete, add more RE (1–1.5 RE units per μg of DNA to the reaction); incubate at 37 °C for 2 h.
4. Set up the ligation reaction: 98 μL digested DNA, 20 μL 10X T4 DNA ligase buffer, 7.5 units of T4 DNA ligase, and water to a final volume of 200 μL. Incubate at 16 °C overnight (*see* **Note 9**).
5. Load and run 4 μL of the ligated DNA on a 0.8% agarose gel in 1X TAE to check if the ligation was successful.

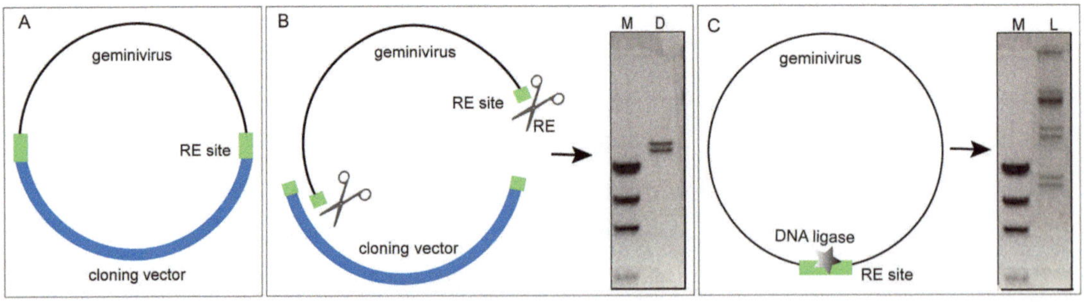

Fig. 1 Schematic representation of the geminivirus DNA preparation for inoculation by particle bombardment. (**a**) Recombinant plasmid with full-length geminiviral genome cloned in a unique restriction endonuclease (RE) site. (**b**) The viral insert is excised from the plasmid by digestion with the single-cutter RE and analyzed by agarose gel electrophoresis. (**c**) Ligation of the fragments corresponding to the viral genome (empty vector DNA is also present as a byproduct). The ligation mix is checked by agarose gel electrophoresis analysis. M: DNA molecular weight marker; D: RE digested fragments, L: ligated fragments

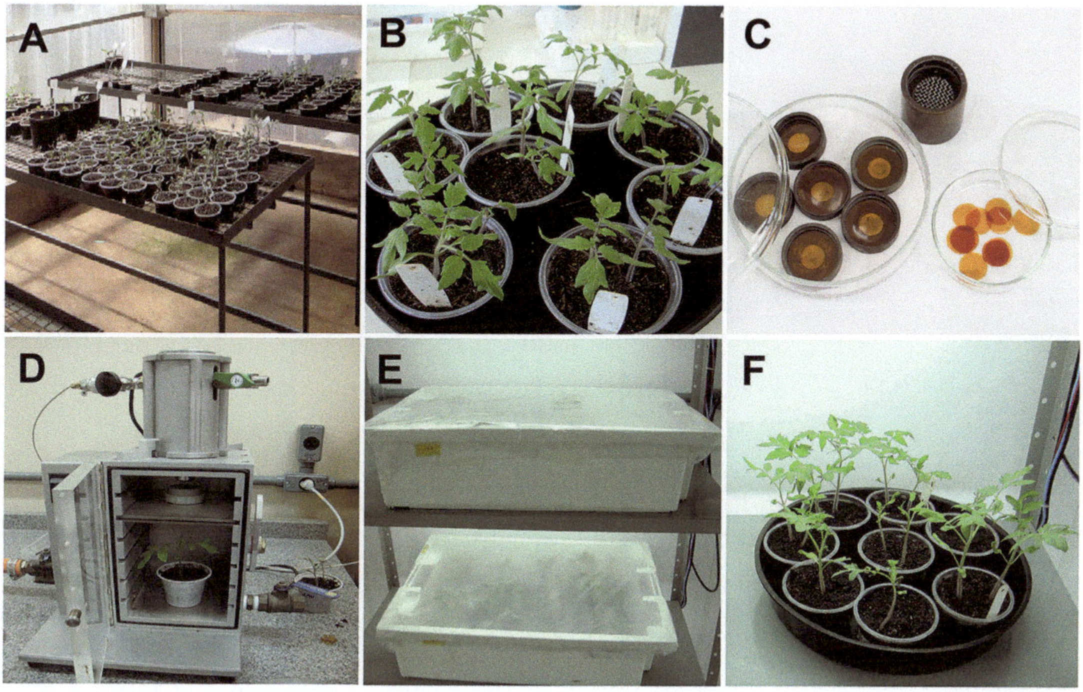

Fig. 2 Inoculation of tomato plants with geminivirus using particle bombardment. (**a**) Tomato seedlings cultivated in the greenhouse. (**b**) Plants are labeled and kept in the laboratory for 24 h before inoculation. (**c**) DNA/particles are precipitated and distributed on the macrocarriers. (**d**) Plants are placed inside the particle bombardment device's chamber for inoculation. (**e, f**) After bombardment, plants are kept in a moist chamber and then cultivated in a growth chamber

6. Precipitate the DNA by adding 20 μL of 3 M sodium acetate, pH 5.2, and 400 μL (2 volumes) of absolute ethanol; mix well and leave at −20 °C for 1 h.
7. Centrifuge at 13,000–16,000 *g* for 15 min; discard the supernatant and wash the pellet with 400 μL of 70% ethanol.
8. Centrifuge at 13,000–16,000 *g* for 15 min; discard the supernatant and dry the pellet.
9. Resuspend the DNA with 10 μL of water (1 μg DNA per μL).
10. Use 2.5 μL of DNA-A and 2.5 μL of DNA-B for bipartite begomoviruses (total of 5 μg) or 5 μL (5 μg) for monopartite geminiviruses for each precipitation (*see* **Note 10**).

3.2 Preparation of Plant Material

1. Sow one or two seeds of the plants you want to inoculate in small pots filled with 1:1 substrate and soil; for plants with tiny seeds, sow seeds in a seed tray and later transplant the seedlings to the pot.
2. Keep the plants in an insect-proof greenhouse or growth chamber (Fig. 2a). For most plants use plantlets with 1–2 true leaves for the inoculation; for *Nicotiana benthamiana* and

Arabidopsis thaliana, use one plantlet with 4–5 true leaves and 8–10 rosette leaves, respectively, and one plant per pot; most plants (e.g., tomato and *N. benthamiana*) can be grown at 24–25 °C. *Arabidopsis* should be cultivated at 22 °C.

3. Transfer the plants to the laboratory 24 h before inoculation (Fig. 2b) (*see* **Note 5**).

3.3 Biolistic Inoculation of Geminiviruses

3.3.1 Preparation of the Gold Particles

1. Weigh 60 mg of gold particles in a 1.5 mL microfuge tube.
2. Add 1 mL of 70% ethanol; mix for 10–15 min.
3. Centrifuge at 3000 *g* for 5 min and remove the supernatant.
4. Add 1 mL of sterile water and centrifuge at 3000 *g* for 5 min.
5. Add 500 μL of absolute ethanol, mix thoroughly and centrifuge for 1 min.
6. Remove the supernatant and repeat this ethanol washing step.
7. Add 1 mL of sterile 50% glycerol and store at −20 °C for up to a year.

3.3.2 Precipitation of the DNA on the Gold Microparticles

1. Mix the particle suspension vigorously in the vortex mixer.
2. Remove 50 μL of the particle suspension and transfer to a 1.5 mL tube.
3. Add 5 μL of viral DNA preparation (1 μg/μL); in the case of bipartite begomoviruses, mix 2.5 μL of DNA-A and 2.5 μL of DNA-B and add the mixture to the particle suspension.
4. Mix thoroughly, open the tube and add, while mixing, 50 μL of $CaCl_2$ and 20 μL of spermidine.
5. Close the tube and continue mixing for 10 min (notice the flocculation of the precipitated DNA).
6. Centrifuge at 3000 *g* for 10 s.
7. With a pipette, carefully remove and discard the supernatant.
8. Add 150 μL of 100% ethanol and mix briefly by flicking the tube with the finger.
9. Repeat this ethanol washing step.
10. Add 24 μL of absolute ethanol and mix vigorously.
11. Place the tube for 3–4 s in an ultrasonic bath (*see* **Note 3**).
12. Distribute aliquots of 3 μL onto the center of the six macrocarriers (Fig. 2c); using the pipette tip, keep mixing the particle/DNA suspension while taking the aliquots.
13. Place the membrane and support in a desiccating chamber for 5–10 min.

3.3.3 Plant Inoculation by Particle Bombardment

1. Turn on the vacuum source and the particle bombardment device.
2. Open the helium valve and set the pressure to 850 psi (5860 kPa) (*see* **Note 11**).
3. Separate the rupture membranes and keep them in a Petri dish with isopropanol.
4. Place the rupture disk and the macrocarrier on the gene gun device.
5. Place the pot with the plant to be inoculated in the chamber of the particle bombardment device at 2–5 cm from the macrocarrier (Fig. 2d); make sure the first plants to be inoculated are the controls (i.e., macrocarriers with particles only, no DNA) (*see* **Note 12**).
6. Close the chamber's door, open the vacuum valve, and evacuate the chamber until the vacuum gauge reaches 20–25 inHg (508–635 mmHg).
7. Open the helium valve and trigger the rupture membrane buster.
8. Open the air valve to release the vacuum pressure.
9. Remove the pot with the plant and immediately transfer it to a moist chamber (Fig. 2e).
10. Remove and discard the used macrocarrier and disrupted membranes.
11. Restart the procedure to inoculate the next plant.
12. When finished with the inoculations, turn off the vacuum pump and the device, close the helium valve, and release any pressure left in the tubing; clean the device's chamber with 70% ethanol.
13. Keep the inoculated plants in a growth chamber with a 12-h photoperiod at 25 °C; after 24 h, remove the plants from the moist chamber.
14. Cultivate the plants and observe any symptoms, which should appear after 7–15 days; compare the virus-inoculated plants with the mock-inoculated controls (plants inoculated with particles only) for the appearance of symptoms.
15. To confirm the presence of the inoculated virus, analyze the plants through PCR or hybridization.

4 Notes

1. The full-length viral genome must be cloned in a unique restriction endonuclease site (*see* Chap. 2). Other types of cloned virus such as undigested DNA or DNA digests of

recombinant dimeric or a partial dimer genome cloned into a plasmid vector or binary vector can also be used. Besides cloned virus, preparations of total DNA from infected plants or RCA products can be used. In the latter cases, the inoculation can result in mixed infections since other DNA viruses might be present in the preparations.

2. To obtain a 1X working solution of TAE buffer, dilute stock 50X TAE buffer (2 M Tris base, 0.05 M EDTA, 1 M acetic acid pH 8.2–8.4).
3. The ultrasonic bath helps disrupt larger aggregates of particles/DNA. These courser clumps can damage the target leaf tissue and reduce the inoculation efficiency. If an ultrasonic bath is unavailable, particle aggregates can be disrupted by vigorously mixing and pressing the sedimented clumps with a pipette tip.
4. There are different devices for particle bombardment, although the principles are the same for most inoculation devices. The PDS-1000/He Biolistic Particle Delivery System and the Helios Gene Gun System are some commercially available models (https://www.bio-rad.com/en-us/category/biolistic-particle-delivery-systems). The model we use is a custom-made device similar to the PDS-1000/He [7]. Other systems, such as the Particle Inflow Gun, can also be used for virus inoculation [8]. Follow manufacturers' recommendations for the specific device.
5. The plants should be healthy and well irrigated. Keep the plants in the laboratory for 24 h before inoculation. Ensure not to wet the leaves, as a film of water on the leaves will drastically reduce the particle penetration into the cells.
6. Set up one reaction for each component in the case of bipartite begomoviruses.
7. Check the composition of the RE reaction buffer. If it already contains BSA, omit the BSA addition.
8. Most RE work at an optimal temperature of 37 °C. However, check the temperature recommended by the manufacturer.
9. A high volume in the ligation mixture will favor the self-ligation of virus-excised fragments to form closed, circular, double-stranded DNA molecules that resemble geminivirus replicative forms. The ligation reaction can also generate virus genome concatemers. Self-ligated or concatemer vector molecules may also be produced.
10. The DNA preparation for bombardment can be scaled up, and the resuspended DNA can be stored at −20 °C for later use.
11. The optimal pressure may vary according to the plant species and the size of the plant being inoculated. A pressure of

approximately 850 psi works well for the species tested in our laboratory.

12. A set of plants should be inoculated as negative controls (typically 4–5 plants). For these plants, the procedure is done with macrocarriers containing only particles, without DNA. These control plants should be the first to be treated and placed in a separate moist chamber, reducing the risk of cross-contamination. All the pots should be labeled, indicating the plant species, the target construct, and the date of inoculation.

Acknowledgments

We thank all present and former lab members who performed biolistic inoculation with geminiviruses and helped to improve this protocol. Financial support was provided by grants from Embrapa (Empresa Brasileira de Pesquisa Agropecuária), CNPq (Conselho Nacional de Desenvolvimento Científico e Tecnológico), and FAP-DF (Fundação de Apoio à Pesquisa do Distrito Federal).

References

1. Grimsley N, Hohn T, Davies J, Hohn B (1987) *Agrobacterium*-mediated delivery of infectious maize streak virus into maize plants. Nature 325:177–179
2. Gilbertson RL, Faria JC, Hanson SF, Morales FJ, Ahlquist PG, Russell MD (1991) Cloning of the complete DNA genomes of four bean-infecting geminiviruses and determining their infectivity by electric discharge particle acceleration. Phytopathology 81:980–985
3. Ribeiro SG, Martin DP, Lacorte C, Simões IC, Orlandini DRS, Inoue-Nagata AK (2007) Molecular and biological characterization of tomato chlorotic mottle virus suggests that recombination underlies the evolution and diversity of Brazilian tomato begomoviruses. Phytopathology 97:702–711
4. Blawid R, Fontenele RS, Lacorte C, Ribeiro SG (2013) Molecular and biological characterization of corchorus mottle virus, a new begomovirus from Brazil. Arch Virol 158:2603–9260
5. Fontenele RS, Lamas NS, Lacorte C, Lacerda ALM, Varsani A, Ribeiro SG (2017) A novel geminivirus identified in tomato and cleome plants sampled in Brazil. Virus Res 240:175–179
6. Fontenele RS, Abreu RA, Lamas NS, Alves-Freitas DMT, Vidal AH, Poppiel RR, Melo FL, Lacorte C, Martin DP, Campos MA, Varsani A, Ribeiro SG (2018) Passion fruit chlorotic mottle virus: molecular characterization of a new divergent geminivirus in Brazil. Viruses 10:169
7. Rech EL, Vianna GR, Aragão FJ (2008) High-efficiency transformation by biolistics of soybean, common bean and cotton transgenic plants. Nat Protoc 3:410–418
8. Finer JJ, Vain P, Jones MW, McMullen MD (1992) Development of the particle inflow gun for DNA delivery to plant cells. Plant Cell Rep 7: 323–328

Chapter 5

Agroinoculation of Plants with Geminiviruses

Anelise F. Orílio

Abstract

Agroinoculation refers to the introduction of genetic information from plant viruses into leaves or other organs of the host plant through *Agrobacterium tumefaciens*. Agroinoculation of geminiviruses requires the insertion of tandem copies of the genome between the T-DNA borders of an *Agrobacterium* binary vector. The technique is applicable to most plant species and is limited only by the host range of the virus and of the *A. tumefaciens* strain. Herbaceous plants can be easily agroinoculated using a needleless syringe. The successful agroinoculation of plants with begomoviruses involves the preparation of *A. tumefaciens* competent cells, the transformation of *A. tumefaciens* with the cloned tandem copy of the viral genome, and the agroinoculation procedure itself. This chapter describes a straightforward protocol for the agroinoculation of a cloned infectious begomovirus into plants.

Key words *Agrobacterium*, Infectious clone, Binary vector, Electroporation

1 Introduction

Agrobacterium tumefaciens is a plant pathogenic, soil-borne bacterium, able to induce the development of plant tumors or galls. It is well-known due to its exceptional capability to accomplish inter-kingdom genetic transfer [1]. *A. tumefaciens* has been adapted for either transient or stable transformation of plasmid DNAs in plants utilizing modified binary vectors [2].

Agroinoculation is the term used to refer to the technique of introducing genetic information from plant viruses into leaves or other organs of the host plant through *A. tumefaciens* [3]. The rescue of virus infection from this inoculation is referred to as agroinfection [4]. The technique relies on the natural T-DNA transfer mechanism of disarmed (non-oncogenic) *A. tumefaciens* strains, and any T-DNA binary vector may be used. Agroinoculation has been used successfully for a wide variety of plant viruses, including geminiviruses [5–8].

Agroinoculation of viruses with circular DNA genomes requires the insertion of tandem multimeric copies of the genome

Francisco Murilo Zerbini et al. (eds.), *Geminiviruses: Methods and Protocols*, Methods in Molecular Biology, vol. 2912, https://doi.org/10.1007/978-1-0716-4454-6_5,

between the T-DNA borders of an *Agrobacterium* binary vector [9]. The construction of infectious clones of geminiviruses should comprise two origins of replication to enhance their ability to infect the host cells. Once inside the plant cells, the begomovirus construct undergoes transcription and replication. The genetic material of interest is expressed, and the virus starts replicating, following its natural infection cycle.

Three frequently employed methods for introducing plasmids of interest into *A. tumefaciens* are electroporation, the freeze/thaw method, and triparental mating [10]. Electroporation stands out as the most effective method. It employs electrical pulses to generate aqueous pores in the lipid membrane of bacteria. These pores are large enough to facilitate the passage of DNA molecules into the cells. The efficiency of this method is influenced by the control of electric field strength, pulse duration, and the size of the plasmid [11].

The agroinoculation technique has proven especially useful when the virus or its genome cannot be manually inoculated to the plants, thereby allowing the in vivo assay of cloned material. The technique is applicable to most plant species and is limited only by the host range of the virus or the *A. tumefaciens* strain. Herbaceous plants like *Nicotiana benthamiana*, tobacco, and tomato can be readily infiltrated with *A. tumefaciens* inoculum using a needleless syringe.

Three steps are necessary to achieve agroinfection of plants with begomovirus clones: (i) Preparation of *A. tumefaciens* competent cells; (ii) Transformation of *A. tumefaciens* with the cloned tandem multimeric copy of the viral genome; and (iii) Agroinoculation of plants. The following is a straightforward procedure for the agroinoculation of a cloned infectious begomovirus into plants.

2 Materials

1. *Agrobacterium tumefaciens* strain GV3101.
2. Four-week-old *Nicotiana benthamiana* plants.
3. Luria-Bertani (LB) broth/agar medium for growing the agrobacterium cultures supplemented with the appropriate antibiotics.
4. Autoclaved/sterile milli-Q water.
5. Autoclaved/sterile 10% (v/v) glycerol in milli-Q water.
6. Autoclaved/sterile 2 L Erlenmeyer flasks.
7. Autoclaved/sterile centrifuge tubes.
8. Autoclaved/sterile 5 mL, 1 mL, 200 μL pipet tips.
9. Autoclaved/sterile 1.5 mL microfuge tubes.

10. Shaker/incubators set to 28 °C.
11. High-speed tabletop cooled centrifuge.
12. Spectrophotometer for measuring culture optical density at 600 nm.
13. Cuvettes, 2 mm.
14. Electroporator.
15. Agrobacterium induction buffer: 10 mM 4-morpholineethanesulfonic acid (MES) pH 5.5, 10 mM $MgCl_2$, 150 μM acetosyringone.
16. One mL syringes without needle.

3 Methods

3.1 Preparation of Agrobacterium tumefaciens *Competent Cells*

Important: All the procedures listed below should be carried out aseptically.

1. From a frozen bacteria glycerol stock (−80 °C) streak it on an LB-agar plate with antibiotics (for strain GV3101, rifampicin and gentamicin), let it grow for 2 days at 28 °C (*see* **Notes 1** and **2**).
2. The following morning, pick an isolated colony to inoculate 5 mL of liquid LB (*see* **Note 3**); incubate for 8–12 h with shaking at 28 °C.
3. On the same day, in the afternoon, inoculate 20 mL of LB with the 5 mL of the culture (final 25 mL); incubate for 24 h with shaking at 28 °C.
4. Use 10 mL of the grown culture to inoculate the next 500 mL LB; transfer to two flasks, with 250 mL each (so that it aerates more and grows better) and incubate overnight with shaking at 28 °C.
5. Starting in the morning, monitor the OD_{600} every hour until it reaches the range 0.5–0.8 (*see* **Note 4**).
6. Once cells reach OD_{600} of 0.5–0.8, immediately chill on ice for 10–15 min (the rest of the protocol should be carried out on ice).
7. Centrifuge for 10 min at 5000 *g* at 4 °C; remove as much of the supernatant as possible.
8. Add 5 mL of ice-cold water and resuspend the pellet carefully, so as not to make bubbles; complete with 245 mL ice-cold water.
9. Centrifuge for 10 min at 5000 *g* at 4 °C and gently pour off the water.

10. Add 5 mL of ice-cold water, resuspend the pellet carefully and complete with 120 mL of ice-cold water.
11. Centrifuge for 10 min at 5000 *g* at 4 °C and remove all supernatant.
12. Add 5 mL of ice-cold water, resuspend the pellet in two tubes (10 mL), add up to 40 mL of ice-cold water and transfer all to a smaller tube.
13. Centrifuge for 10 min at 5000 *g* at 4 °C and remove all supernatant.
14. Add 5 mL of ice-cold 10% glycerol, resuspend the pellet, add 20 mL more of ice-cold 10% glycerol.
15. Centrifuge for 10 min at 5000 *g* at 4 °C.
16. Resuspend the pellet in 2.5 mL of ice-cold 10% glycerol; prepare 50 μL aliquots in 1.5 mL microtubes and throw them in liquid N_2.
17. Store at −80 °C; cells are good for at least 6 months.
18. Check the transformation efficiency (*see* **Note 5**).

3.2 Transformation of the Begomovirus Clones into Agrobacterium tumefaciens by Electroporation

1. Prepare purified binary vector containing the tandem dimeric copy of the begomovirus genome at a concentration of approximately 20 ng/μL in sterile water (*see* **Note 6**).
2. Thaw the electro-competent *Agrobacterium tumefaciens* cells on ice.
3. Mix 1 μL of binary vector with 50 μL GV3101 *A. tumefaciens* competent cells in a 1.5 mL microfuge tube on ice.
4. Transfer the mixture into a chilled 2 mm electroporation cuvette; shake cells to bottom, tapping down to eliminate air bubbles.
5. Set the electroporator to 2500 V, 200 Ω, 25 μF.
6. Snap cuvette into proper orientation, push the pulse button, wait for the beep; the time constant should read about 5.
7. Add 950 μL LB to cuvette, mix, immediately transfer 1 mL to sterile 1.5 mL microfuge tube.
8. Incubate at 28 °C, with shaking, for 2–3 h.
9. Plate 200 μL of the cells on LB + antibiotics (selective media) plates.
10. Incubate the plate, inverted, at 28 °C for 2–3 days.
11. Select isolated colonies, confirm the transformation by polymerase chain reaction (PCR) testing, and inoculate them into 5 mL of LB medium containing the appropriate antibiotics; the medium should be supplemented with 10 mM MES at pH 5.5

and 20 μM acetosyringone; incubate the cultures at 28 °C for 2 days with continuous shaking at 200 rpm.

12. Store the clones in 15% sterile glycerol at −80 °C.

3.3 Agrobacterium-Mediated Inoculation of Plants

1. Grow agrobacterium clones from a 1:100 dilution of an aliquot stored at −80 °C in LB medium supplemented with the necessary antibiotics (*e.g.*: 50 μg/mL kanamycin, 25 μg/mL rifampicin, 20 μg/mL gentamicin), 10 mM MES pH 5.5 and 20 μM acetosyringone, at 28 °C, with shaking, for 2 days.
2. Harvest bacterial cells by centrifugation at 3000 *g* for 15 min at room temperature.
3. Resuspend cells until reaching an OD_{600} of 0.5 in 10 mM MES buffer pH 5.5, 10 mM $MgCl_2$ and 150 μM acetosyringone.
4. Incubate the cultures for at least 2 h at room temperature; in the case of a bipartite begomovirus, mix equal volumes of the two corresponding cultures for the DNA-A and DNA-B clones.
5. Infiltrate with gentle pressure into the abaxial surface of *N. benthamiana* leaves of plants at the 3–5 leaf stage with a 1 mL needleless syringe (*see* **Note** 7).
6. After agroinoculation, keep the plants in a growth chamber (25 °C day and 20 °C night, 70% relative humidity, with a 16 h photoperiod) or an insect-proof glasshouse (*see* **Note 8**).
7. Symptoms in susceptible plants will show up after approximately 15–21 days post inoculation.

4 Notes

1. Bacterial stocks are maintained frozen at −80 °C in 15% glycerol for long-term storage. Never thaw frozen bacterial stocks. Use a sterile loop, sterile wooden stick or sterile disposable pipette to scrape the surface of the frozen mixture in the stock tube.
2. The *Agrobacterium tumefaciens* strains we use is GV3101, which has resistance to both rifampicin (25 μg/mL, in the chromosome) and gentamicin (20 μg/mL, in a helper plasmid). This protocol can be used for any other strains, such as C58, LBA4404, and GV2260.
3. To grow the agrobacteria for cell preparation in LB-broth, the use of antibiotics, such as rifampin and gentamicin, is optional. However, it is important to avoid contamination.
4. Be attention with OD measure, after it reaches 0.3, it is normal to quickly increases (in a matter of minutes).

5. When preparing a new batch of competent cells, remember to include a negative control (i.e., plate cells without adding a plasmid) to check for contamination. Additionally, perform a positive control by testing a plasmid known to transform well in other competent cells to verify the transformability of your cells. Compare the colony yield from your freshly prepared competent cells with commercially available cells or previous homemade batches to ensure optimal efficiency.
6. Approximately 20 ng/μL of plasmid is an ideal concentration, if too high the cells will be killed by the electrical impulse.
7. *N. benthamiana* is chosen due to its susceptibility to agroinoculation and the ability to support begomovirus replication. Any other host of the virus can be used.
8. Agroinfected material, bacterial stocks and cultures should be sterilized by autoclaving for 20 min at 15 psi on liquid cycle before disposal.

References

1. Chilton MD, Drummond MH, Merio DJ, Sciaky D, Montoya AL, Gordon MP, Nester EW (1977) Stable incorporation of plasmid DNA into higher plant cells: the molecular basis of crown gall tumorigenesis. Cell 11: 263–271
2. Horsch RB, Fraley RT, Rogers SG, Sanders PR, Lloyd A, Hoffmann N (1984) Inheritance of functional foreign genes in plants. Science 223: 496–498
3. Abrahamian P, Hammond RW, Hammond J (2020) Plant virus-derived vectors: applications in agricultural and medical biotechnology. Annu Rev Virol 7:513–535
4. Grimsley N, Hohn B, Hohn T, Walden R (1986) "Agroinfection", an alternative route for viral infection of plants by using the T-DNA plasmid. Proc Natl Acad Sci USA 83: 3282–3286
5. Grimsley N, Hohn T, Davies JW, Hohn B (1987) Agrobacterium-mediated delivery of infectious maize streak virus into maize plants. Nature 325:177–179
6. Klinkenberg FA, Stanley J (1990) Encapsidation and spread of *African cassava mosaic virus* DNA-A in the absence of DNA-B when agroinoculated to *Nicotiana benthamiana*. J Gen Virol 71:1409–1412
7. Czosnek H, Kheyr-Pour A, Gronenborn B, Remetz E, Zeidan M, Altman A, Rabinowitch HD, Vidavsky S, Kedar N, Gafni Y, Zamir D (1993) Replication of tomato yellow leaf curl virus (TYLCV) DNA in agroinoculated leaf-disks from selected tomato genotypes. Plant Mol Biol 22:995–1005
8. Trenado HP, Orílio AF, Marquez-Martin B, Moriones E, Navas-Castillo J (2011) Sweepoviruses cause disease in sweet potato and related *Ipomoea* spp.: fulfilling Koch's postulates for a divergent group in the genus *Begomovirus*. PLoS One 6:e27329
9. Ferreira PT, Lemos TO, Nagata T, Inoue-Nagata AK (2008) One-step cloning approach for construction of agroinfectious begomovirus clones. J Virol Methods 147:351–354
10. Wise AA, Liu Z, Binns AN (2006) Three methods for the introduction of foreign DNA into *Agrobacterium*. Methods Mol Biol 343:43–53
11. Mersereau M, Pazour GJ, Das A (1990) Efficient transformation of *agrobacterium tumefaciens* by electroporation. Gene 90:149–151

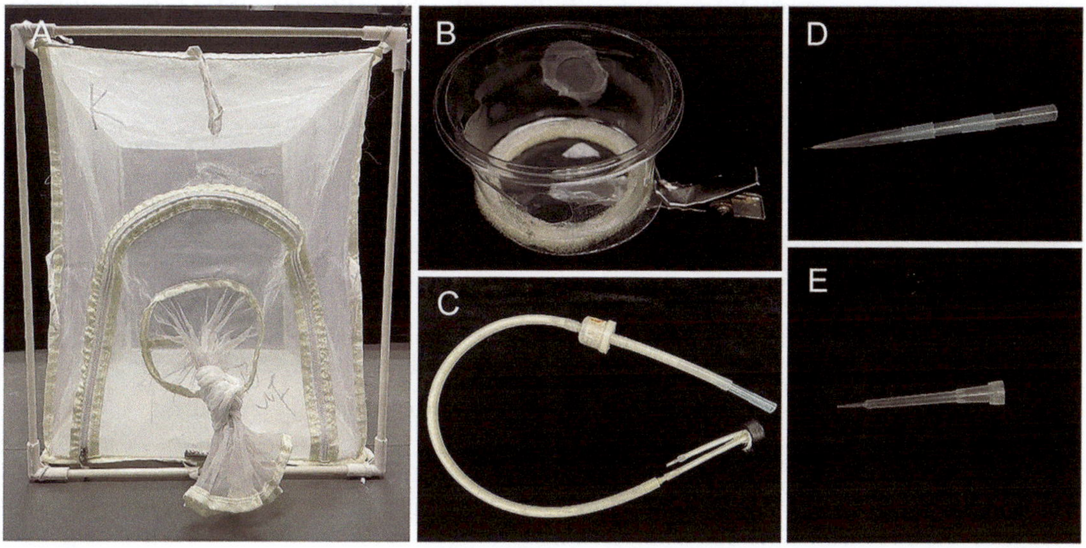

Fig. 1 Materials used in this protocol. (**a**) Nylon mesh cage. (**b**) Clip-cage. (**c**) Aspirator. (**d**) Dissection needle. (**e**) Capillary pipette tips

7. Glass bottle.
8. Dissection needle: it was made with an acupuncture needle and a 1 mL pipette tip (Fig. 1d).
9. Dissecting microscope.
10. Glass tube.
11. Parafilm.

2.3 Molecular Biological Materials

2.3.1 Reagents

1. Lysis buffer: 10 mM Tris–HCl (pH 8.4), 0.45% NP40, 50 mM KCl, 0.45% Tween-20, 0.2% Gelatin, 60 mg/L Proteinase K.
2. Ice.
3. 10 × PCR Buffer (Mg^{2+} Plus).
4. dNTPs (2.5 mM).
5. r*Taq* enzyme.
6. Sterile ddH_2O.
7. 10 × *Taq* I Buffer.
8. *Taq* I enzyme.
9. 3% Bovine serum albumin (BSA).
10. 50 × TAE buffer.
11. Agar.
12. LB liquid medium: 1 g tryptone, 0.5 g yeast extract, 1 g NaCl (for LB agar plate: add extra 1.5 g agar), add ddH_2O to 100 mL. Autoclaved for 15 min.

13. Resuspension buffer: 10 mM MES, 10 mM $MgCl_2$, 200 μM acetosyringone (pH 5.7).
14. Imidacloprid.
15. 1× phosphate-buffered saline (PBS) buffer (pH 7.4).
16. 4% paraformaldehyde.
17. 0.4% Triton X-100.
18. Anti-TYLCV CP antibody (provided by Professor Xue-Ping Zhou from the Institute of Biotechnology, Zhejiang University).
19. Alexa Fluor 488-conjugated secondary antibody (Earthox).
20. 4′,6-diamidino-2-phenylindole (DAPI) (Abcam).
21. Chloroform.
22. Ethanol.
23. Glacial acetic acid.
24. 0.01% Sodium dodecyl sulfate (SDS).
25. 30% Formamide.
26. Fluoroshield mounting medium.
27. Phenol.
28. Isopropanol.
29. Nuclease-free water.
30. Agarose.
31. Sucrose.
32. Rabbit/mouse pre-immune serum.
33. Hybridization buffer: 20 mM Tris–HCl (pH 8.0), 0.9 M NaCl, 0.01% SDS, and 30% formamide.

2.3.2 Consumables

1. Ceramic beads.
2. PCR tubes.
3. Syringe.
4. Pipette tips.
5. 12 mL tubes.
6. 50 mL centrifuge tubes.
7. Capillary pipette tips (the pipette tips were drawn to a fine point of 0.5 μm in diameter before use) (Fig. 1e).
8. Glass slide.
9. Cover glass.

2.3.3 Kits

1. Plant genomic DNA extraction kit.
2. SYBR Premix Ex Taq II (Takara).
3. T7 high-yield transcription kit.

2.3.4 Instruments

1. Tissue Lyser.
2. High speed centrifuge.
3. Temperature-controlled water bath.
4. Refrigerator.
5. PCR Amplifier.
6. DNA gel electrophoresis apparatus.
7. Vertical pressure steam sterilizer.
8. Constant temperature incubator.
9. Constant temperature shaker.
10. Pipette.
11. Nanodrop (Thermo Fisher).
12. CFX96™ Real-Time PCR Detection System (Bio-Rad).
13. LSM 780 confocal microscope (Zeiss).
14. FemtoJet (Eppendorf).

2.3.5 Primers

Primers	Sequences (5′-3′)
mt*COI* F	TGRTTYTTTGGTCATCCVGAAGT
mt*COI* R	TTACTGCACTTTCTGCCACATTAG
TYLCV-PCR F	GTCGAAGCGACCAGGCGATA
TYLCV-PCR R	GGTTCTCATACTTGGCTGCCTCC
actin-qRT-PCR F	GGAAAAGCTTGCCTATGTGG
actin-qRT-PCR R	CCTGCAGCTTCCATACCAAT
β-actin-qRT-PCR F	TCTTCCAGCCATCCTTCTTG
β-actin-qRT-PCR R	CGGTGATTTCCTTCTGCATT
TYLCV-qRT-PCR F	GAAGCGACCAGGCGATATAA
TYLCV-qRT-PCR R	GGAACATCAGGGCTTCGATA

3 Methods

3.1 Maintenance of Whitefly

1. Maintain the populations of whitefly on cotton plants in climate chambers at 26 ± 1 °C, 14 h/10 h dark photoperiod and 70 ± 10% relative humidity.

2. Approximately 3 weeks later, transfer cotton leaves carrying whitefly pseudopupa to fresh cotton plants. After 7 days, whitefly adults within 7 days post-emergence were obtained and used for virus transmission experiments (*see* **Note 2**).

3.2 Whitefly Species Identification

1. Monitor the purity of whitefly culture every three generations by PCR-restriction fragment length polymorphism (PCR-RFLP) and mtCO1 sequencing analysis as follows (**steps 2–12**) [18] (*see* **Note 3**).
2. Whitefly DNA extraction was performed according to **steps 3–7**.
3. Add appropriate amounts of ceramic beads and lysis buffer (*see* **Note 4**) into PCR tube.
4. Place the collected whiteflies on ice to numb them. Pick the whiteflies into the PCR tube with the needle of a syringe.
5. Put the samples into the Tissue Lyser, set the parameter to 60 Hz, 120 s and grind twice.
6. Centrifuge the samples for 1 min and place them in 65 °C water bath for 2 h.
7. Centrifuge the samples for 10 s and place them in 100 °C water bath for 10 min. Whitefly DNA solution can be used for PCR immediately or stored at −20 °C.
8. Use the DNA samples obtained above as templates to perform PCR reaction (primers are listed in Subheading 2.3.5).
9. Set up a PCR reaction (total volume 25 μL) as follows: 2.5 μL of 10×PCR Buffer (Mg^{2+} Plus), 2 μL of dNTPs (2.5 mM), 0.5 μL of each primer (10 μM each), 0.5 μL of r*Taq* enzyme, 2 μL of DNA template, and 17 μL of ddH_2O.
10. Use the following PCR cycling parameters: 1 cycle at 94 °C for 3 min (pre-denaturation), 35 cycle, each consisting of 30 s at 96 °C (denaturation), 30 s at 50 °C (annealing) and 60 s at 72 °C (extension, 1 min/kb), and 1 cycle at 72 °C for 10 min (extension).
11. Set up a digestion (total volume 10 μL) as follows: 1 μL of 10 × *Taq* I Buffer, 1 μL of 0.1% BSA, 0.2 μL of *Taq* I enzyme, 5 μL of PCR product, and 2.8 μL of ddH_2O. Incubate the samples at 65 °C for 1 h.
12. Perform DNA gel electrophoresis and observe the bands.

3.3 Preparation of Tomato Plants Infected with Virus

Use agrobacterium-mediated inoculation to obtain TYLCV-infected tomato plants as follows:

1. Streak a LB agar plate (50 μg/mL kanamycin, 50 μg/mL rifampicin) with agrobacteria containing TYLCV from a frozen stock. Incubate the plate upside down at 28 °C until colonies appear.

2. Inoculate one colony into 3 mL LB liquid medium (50 μg/mL kanamycin, 50 μg/mL rifampicin). Incubate at 28 °C with shaking at 200 rpm for 24 h.
3. Transfer 200 μL of the culture to 20 mL of LB liquid medium (50 μg/mL kanamycin, 50 μg/mL rifampicin). Incubate at 28 °C with shaking at 200 rpm for 12 h.
4. Centrifuge the cells at 1700 g for 10 min at room temperature. Discard the supernatant and resuspend the pellet in resuspension buffer and the final OD_{600} was set to 1.0. Keep the suspension liquid at room temperature for 3 h.
5. Infiltrate the suspension liquid into leaves of tomato at the 3–4 true leaf stage with 1 mL needleless syringe. When the virus-inoculated tomato plants were cultivated to the 7–8 true leaf stage, examine the plants by inspection of the typical symptoms and PCR (primers are listed in Subheading 2.3.5). Genomic DNA extraction was performed using Plant Genomic DNA Kit. Select 2–3 samples with correct band size for sequencing. Plants confirmed to be infected with TYLCV were taken for use in experiments (*see* **Note 5**).

3.4 Acquisition of Virus by Whiteflies

1. Collect whitefly adults within 7 days post-emergence in dactylethrae and identify sex under dissecting microscope. Transfer the whiteflies into a clip-cage attached to the central leaf of the TYLCV-infected tomato plant, each cage contains ten adults of the same sex.
2. After 48 h acquisition access periods (AAP) (*see* **Note 6**), collect adults in glass bottles and examine for virus by PCR. Whitefly DNA extraction was performed according to **steps 3–7** of Subheading 3.2 (*see* **Note 7**).

3.5 Transmission of Virus by Whiteflies

1. After 48 h TYLCV acquisition, transfer 4 (sex ratio 1:1) whitefly adults into a clip-cage attached to an uninfected tomato seedling at the 2–3 true-leaf stage to feed for 48 h.
2. Remove whitefly adults from tomato plants and spray the plants with imidacloprid (50 mg/L) to kill the eggs.
3. After 30 days, evaluate the status of plant infection based on symptoms and PCR as described above (*see* Subheading 3.2, **step 5**).

3.6 Dissection of Whitefly Organs

3.6.1 Midgut

1. Place the whiteflies collected in glass bottle on ice to numb them.
2. Transfer a female whitefly on a clean glass slide and drop 10 μL of 1 × PBS buffer.

3. Hold the chest of whitefly down with a dissection needle and slowly cut the abdomen with another dissection needle, pulling out the midgut.
4. Suck out the midgut with the drawn capillary pipette tip and transfer it to clean 1 × PBS buffer for washing 2–3 times (*see* **Note 8**).

3.6.2 Hemolymph

1. Repeat **steps 1–2** of Subheading 3.6.1.
2. After dissecting the midgut according to **step 3** of Subheading 3.6.1, gently squeeze the abdomen of the whitefly remnant to make the hemolymph flow out as much as possible.
3. Suck out 8 μL liquid and transfer it to a PCR tube containing 20 μL lysis buffer.

3.6.3 Primary Salivary Glands

1. Repeat **steps 1–2** of Subheading 3.6.1.
2. Hold the chest of whitefly down with a dissection needle and slowly pull off the head with another dissection needle, picking out the primary salivary glands at the junction of the head and chest.
3. Suck out the primary salivary glands with the drawn capillary pipette tip and transfer it to clean 1 × PBS buffer for washing 2–3 times (*see* **Note 8**).

3.7 Analysis of Virus Quantity in Whiteflies

1. Follow the steps in Subheading 3.6 and **steps 3–7** in Subheading 3.2 to dissect the tissues of whitefly and extract DNA (*see* **Note 9**). Then use the samples to quantity the virus by qRT-PCR (primers are listed in Subheading 2.3.5). The *β-actin* gene of *B. tabaci* was used as the reference gene (*see* **Note 10**).
2. Set up a qRT-PCR reaction (total volume 20 μL) as follows: 10 μL of 2 × SYBR Green Premix, 0.8 μL of each primer (10 μM each), 2 μL of DNA template, and 6.4 μL of ddH_2O.
3. Use the following PCR cycling parameters: 1 cycle at 95 °C for 30 s (pre-denaturation), 40 cycle, each consisting of 5 s at 95 °C (denaturation) and 34 s at 60 °C (extension). Add the following reaction to detect the dissolution curve of the primer when using for the first time: 1 cycle at 95 °C for 15 s, 1 cycle at 60 °C for 15 s, and heating up to 95 °C at 0.5 °C/s. Each treatment should be repeated three times.
4. Calculate qRT-PCR data using $2^{-\Delta CT}$ as normalized to whitefly *β-actin*.

3.8 Immuno-fluorescence Detection of Virus in Whitefly Tissues

1. Follow the steps in Subheading 3.6 to dissect the tissues of whitefly and fixed with 4% paraformaldehyde for 2 h.
2. Discard the 4% paraformaldehyde and wash with 1 × PBS for three times.

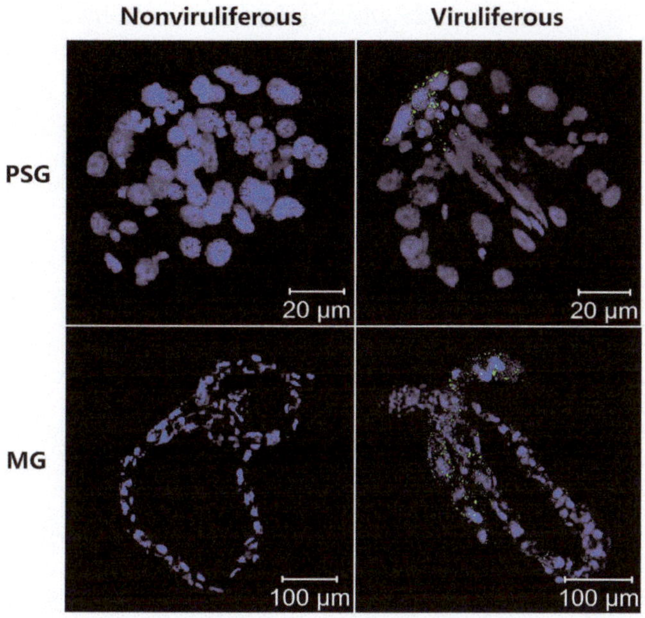

Fig. 2 Virus signals (green) in *Bemisia tabaci* MEAM1 primary salivary gland (PSG) and midgut (MG) detected by immunofluorescence assay. Signals of *Tomato yellow leaf curl virus* (TYLCV) CP were shown in green. TYLCV virions were detected by use of a mouse anti-CP monoclonal antibody and goat anti-mouse IgG labeled with Dylight 488 (green) secondary antibody. The nuclei were stained with 4′,6 diamidino-2-phenylindole (blue)

3. Permeabilize the samples with 0.4% Triton X-100 for 1 h.
4. Discard the fluid and wash with 1 × PBS for three times.
5. Block the samples with 3% BSA to for 2 h.
6. Discard the fluid and wash with 1 × PBS for three times.
7. Incubate the samples overnight with anti-TYLCV CP monoclonal antibody at a 1:400 dilution in 3% BSA at 4 °C.
8. Discard the fluid and wash with 1 × PBS for three times.
9. Incubate the samples with Alexa Fluor 488-conjugated secondary antibody at a 1:400 dilution in 3% BSA for 2 h at room temperature.
10. Discard the fluid and wash with 1 × PBS for three times.
11. Transfer tissues onto glass slide. Drop 4 μL of DAPI and cover the cover glass (*see* **Note 11**).
12. Examine with an LSM 780 confocal microscope (Fig. 2).

3.9 FISH

1. Follow the steps in Subheading 3.6 to dissect the tissues of whitefly and fixed in Carnoy's fixative (chloroform-ethanol-acetic acid, V: V: V = 6:3:1) for 5 min.

2. Discard the fixative and hybridize the tissues overnight at 37 °C in hybridization buffer containing 10 pmol of fluorescent probe per mL.
3. Wash the tissues in 1 × PBS buffer three times, mount them in fluoroshield mounting medium with DAPI.
4. Image the samples on a LSM780 confocal microscope. Use non-viruliferous whiteflies as controls.

3.10 Membrane Feeding of dsRNA or Antibody

1. Amplify DNA templates by PCR using primers with the T7 promoter at both ends (*see* **Note 12**).
2. Use the T7 high-yield transcription kit to synthesize dsRNA as manual described.
3. Purify dsRNA with phenol: chloroform extraction, isopropanol precipitation.
4. Resuspend dsRNA in nuclease-free water.
5. Determine the quality and concentration of the dsRNA with 2% agarose gel electrophoresis and Nanodrop.
6. Collect whitefly adults within 7 days post-emergence from cotton plants. A group of 250 adults were collected into a glass bottle.
7. For dsRNA feeding, release whiteflies into membrane feeding chamber (a glass tube of which one end was covered with a double layer of parafilm filled with artificial diet and the other end with a layer of gauze) with 15% sucrose solution containing 200 ng/μL dsRNA for 48 h. Use ds*GFP* as a control.
8. For antibody feeding, release whiteflies into membrane feeding chamber with antibody and 15% sucrose solution (mixed with a dilution rate of 1:50) for 24 h. Use rabbit/mouse pre-immune serum as control.
9. Measure the silencing efficiency of dsRNA and the results of antibody feeding in whiteflies by qRT-PCR (*see* **Note 13**) and Western blot respectively.

3.11 Microinjection

1. Follow the **steps 1–6** in Subheading 3.10 to obtain purified dsRNA and whitefly adults.
2. For dsRNA microinjection, inject approximately 6 nL of purified dsRNA (8 μg/μL) into the thorax of each female whitefly adult using capillary and FemtoJet. Use ds*GFP* as a control.
3. After injection, keep whiteflies on cotton plants for 3 days for recovery.
4. Verify the efficiency of dsRNA-mediated gene silencing by qRT-PCR.

4 Notes

1. Other begomoviruses and cryptic species of whiteflies can be used. As plant host, any plant cultivar that can be infected with begomovirus can be used. In this chapter, we use these objects as examples.
2. The newly emerged (7 days post-emergence) whitefly adults are very active, and have a high feeding frequency, so they have high transmission efficiency of virus. The older whitefly adults also can transmit the virus, but their efficiency is lower.
3. The purity of the whitefly cultures was identified every 2--3 months. Whitefly cultures must be kept free of pathogens, parasites, and other insects such as aphids which can reduce the amount of whitefly populations or the transmission efficiency of the virus.
4. Add about 4–8 ceramic beads according to the number of whiteflies. A single whitefly is usually added with 20 μL of lysis buffer and several whiteflies are added with 100 μL of lysis buffer.
5. In this section, infected plants can be inoculated using either agrobacterium-mediated inoculation or viruliferous whiteflies (Subheading 3.5).
6. Acquisition access periods of begomoviruses by whiteflies should be determined by actual combination. For example, for MEAM1 whiteflies, it was able to detect viral nucleic acid in some whiteflies 10 min after feeding on TYLCV-infected tomato plants, but for other viruses such as TYLCCNV and TbCSV, the process took a longer time [19, 20]. The amount of virus acquired is not necessarily proportional to the length of the acquisition access period.
7. The DNA extraction methods of whitefly tissues are the same as that of adults. According to our experience, 30 μL of lysis buffer is usually added to the midguts, 10 μL of lysis buffer is usually added to the hemolymph and 20 μL of lysis buffer is usually added to the primary salivary glands.
8. Washing is to avoid contamination by impurities such as hemolymph. Since whitefly tissue is extremely tiny, the amount of fluid inhaled during each transfer is minimized to obtain a larger concentration of samples.
9. For virus quantification in the whole body, we usually collect 15 female whiteflies as one sample for DNA extraction. For virus quantification in the tissues, we usually collect 20 midguts or 30 primary salivary glands from dissected whiteflies as one sample, and collect hemolymph from four female whiteflies as one sample.

10. When quantify the virus abundance in infected plants by qRT-PCR, the plant *actin* gene was used as the reference gene.
11. Cover the cover glass gently to avoid bubbles interfering with the observation.
12. When select the DNA template sequences for the synthesis of dsRNA, pay attention to avoiding the homologous sequences in the transcriptomes of whiteflies.
13. Primer amplification segments should be selected to avoid overlapping with dsRNA sequences.

Acknowledgments

Financial support for this paper was provided by the National Natural Science Foundation of China (32161143008, 31925033 & 32102188).

References

1. Navas-Castillo J, Fiallo-Olivé E, Sánchez-Campos S (2011) Emerging virus diseases transmitted by whiteflies. Annu Rev Phytopathol 49:219–248
2. Harrison BD, Barker H, Bock KR et al (1977) Plant viruses with circular single stranded DNA. Nature 270:760–762
3. Lazarowitz SG (1992) Geminiviruses: genome structure and gene function. Crit Rev Plant Sci 11:327–349
4. Brown JK, Zerbini FM, Navas-Castillo J et al (2015) Revision of begomovirus taxonomy based on pairwise sequence comparisons. Arch Virol 160:1593–1619
5. Zerbini FM, Briddon RW, Idris A et al (2017) ICTV virus taxonomy profile: *Geminiviridae*. J Gen Virol 98:131–133
6. De Barro PJ, Liu SS, Boykin LM et al (2011) *Bemisia tabaci*: a statement of species status. Annu Rev Entomol 56:1–19
7. Liu SS, Colvin J, De Barro PJ (2012) Species concepts as applied to the whitefly *Bemisia tabaci* systematics: how many species are there? J Integr Agric 11:176–186
8. Gilbertson RL, Batuman O, Webster CG et al (2015) Role of the insect supervectors *Bemisia tabaci* and *Frankliniella occidentalis* in the emergence and global spread of plant viruses. Annu Rev Virol 2:67–93
9. Hogenhout SA, Ammar ED, Whitfield AE et al (2008) Insect vector interactions with persistently transmitted viruses. Annu Rev Phytopathol 46:327–359
10. Czosnek H, Ghanim M (2002) The circulative pathway of begomoviruses in the whitefly vector *Bemisia tabaci* - insights from studies with *tomato yellow leaf curl virus*. Ann Appl Biol 140:215–231
11. Rosen R, Kanakala S, Kliot A et al (2015) Persistent, circulative transmission of begomoviruses by whitefly vectors. Curr Opin Virol 15: 1–8
12. Czosnek H, Hariton-Shalev A, Sobol I et al (2017) The incredible journey of begomoviruses in their whitefly vector. Viruses 9:273
13. Fiallo-Olivé E, Pan LL, Liu SS et al (2020) Transmission of begomoviruses and other whitefly-borne viruses: dependence on the vector species. Phytopathology 110:10–17
14. Li M, Hu J, Xu FC et al (2010) Transmission of *tomato yellow leaf curl virus* by two invasive biotypes and a Chinese indigenous biotype of the whitefly *Bemisia tabaci*. Int J Pest Manag 56:275–280
15. Wei J, Zhao JJ, Zhang T et al (2014) Specific cells in the primary salivary glands of the whitefly *Bemisia tabaci* control retention and transmission of begomoviruses. J Virol 88:13460–13468
16. Chi Y, Pan LL, Bouvaine S et al (2020) Differential transmission of *Sri Lankan cassava mosaic virus* by three cryptic species of the whitefly *Bemisia tabaci* complex. Virology 540:141–149
17. Ruan YM, Luan JB, Zang LS et al (2007) Observing and recording copulation events of

whiteflies on plants using a video camera. Entomol Exp Appl 124:229–233

18. Qin L, Wang J, Bing XL et al (2013) Identification of nine cryptic species of *Bemisia tabaci* (Hemiptera: Aleyrodidae) from China by using the mtCOI PCR-RFLP technique. Acta Entomol Sin 56:186–194
19. Czosnek H, Ghanim M (2002) The circulative pathway of begomoviruses in the whitefly vector *Bemisia tabaci*: insights from studies with *tomato yellow leaf curl virus*. Anna Appl Biol 140:215–231
20. Jiu M, Zhou XP, Liu SS (2006) Acquisition and transmission of two begomoviruses by the B and a non-B biotype of *Bemisia tabaci* from Zhejiang, China. J Phytopathol 154:587–591

Chapter 7

Mastrevirus Transmission by the Insect Vectors, Leafhoppers

Anders Kvarnheden, Elham Yazdkhasti, and Jim Nygren

Abstract

Mastreviruses are important pathogens on many crops and they are transmitted in a persistent manner by leafhoppers. For experimental studies on mastreviruses, transmission with leafhoppers remains as an important method for virus inoculation. Here, we describe a protocol for setting up a culture of the leafhopper vector *Psammotettix alienus* and efficient leafhopper-mediated transmission of wheat dwarf virus.

Key words Cicadellidae, Geminivirus, *Psammotettix*, Wheat, Wheat dwarf virus

1 Introduction

Mastreviruses (genus *Mastrevirus*; family *Geminiviridae*) cause disease in important crop plants, such as wheat (*Triticum aestivum*), barley (*Hordeum vulgare*), maize (*Zea mays*), and legumes [1, 2]. In the genus *Mastrevirus*, 45 species have been recognized by ICTV [3] with the most widely distributed mastreviruses probably being maize streak virus (MSV), wheat dwarf virus (WDV), and chickpea chlorotic dwarf virus (CpCDV). Initially, mastreviruses were found in Africa, Asia, Europe, and Oceania, but recently, there are also reports of new mastreviruses infecting maize in both South and North America [4, 5].

The only natural way of transmission of mastreviruses is by leafhoppers (family Cicadellidae) in a persistent manner [2]. The relation between mastrevirus and leafhopper vector is quite specific where virus isolates of a mastrevirus species are transmitted only by leafhoppers of a certain genus. WDV is transmitted by leafhoppers of the genus *Psammotettix* (Fig. 1), MSV by leafhoppers of the genus *Cicadulina* and CpCDV by leafhoppers of the species *Orosius albicinctus*. When acquired by the leafhopper, WDV has been

Francisco Murilo Zerbini et al. (eds.), *Geminiviruses: Methods and Protocols*, Methods in Molecular Biology, vol. 2912, https://doi.org/10.1007/978-1-0716-4454-6_7,

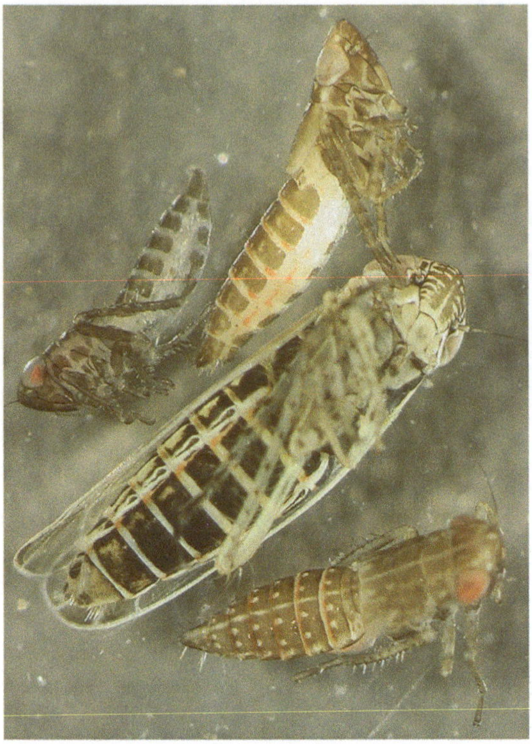

Fig. 1 One adult and three nymphs of the leafhopper *Psammotettix alienus*, which is a vector of wheat dwarf virus. (Photograph by Louis Vimarlund)

shown to induce cellular processes in the leafhopper enabling it to being retained [6].

Leafhoppers were used in the initial attempts to identify the cause of wheat dwarf disease [7–9]. Subsequently, transmission experiments with *P. alienus* have been carried out to determine the ability of WDV to infect different hosts, study host response to infection and identify resistance [10–14]. It has also been used to study the susceptibility of wheat plants of different age [15] as well as interactions between different strains of WDV and between WDV and barley yellow dwarf virus-PAV [16, 17]. In these experiments, *P. alienus* leafhoppers have been found to have a very high transmission rate of WDV for both nymphs and adults. A complication with leafhoppers is that they multiply only sexually and cultures of leafhoppers are more difficult to maintain than clonal cultures of aphids. For several mastreviruses, agroinoculation with infectious DNA constructs have been demonstrated as an efficient alternative to the use of leafhoppers [18–20]. However, in the case of WDV, the infection rate for infectious clones consistently has been rather low [21] and the use of leafhoppers still remains as the method of choice for most applications.

2 Materials

1. Sweep net connected to bottle.
2. Insect aspirator.
3. Falcon tubes.
4. Cages made on plant pots from metal wire, tape and nylon stockings (17 cm × 13 cm × 13 cm), net cages in plastic or wood (Fig. 2).
5. Magnifier glasses (10×) or stereomicroscope.
6. Seedlings of wheat and barley.
7. Greenhouse facilities.
8. Consumables and equipment for WDV testing using double antibody sandwich enzyme-linked immunosorbent assay (DAS-ELISA), PCR or quantitative PCR (qPCR).
9. Insecticide.

3 Methods

3.1 Establishment of a Leafhopper Culture

1. Collect leafhoppers from infested wheat field using sweep net with bottle (*see* **Note 1**).
2. Transfer leafhoppers from bottle into Falcon tubes using aspirator.
3. Transfer leafhoppers from tubes to young wheat seedlings. Keep seedlings and leafhoppers in small cages.
4. Using magnifier glass or stereomicroscope, select individuals of *P. alienus* and transfer to new plants (*see* **Notes 2** and **3**).
5. Test wheat plants exposed to *P. alienus* leafhoppers for WDV infection using DAS-ELISA, PCR or qPCR [10, 14].

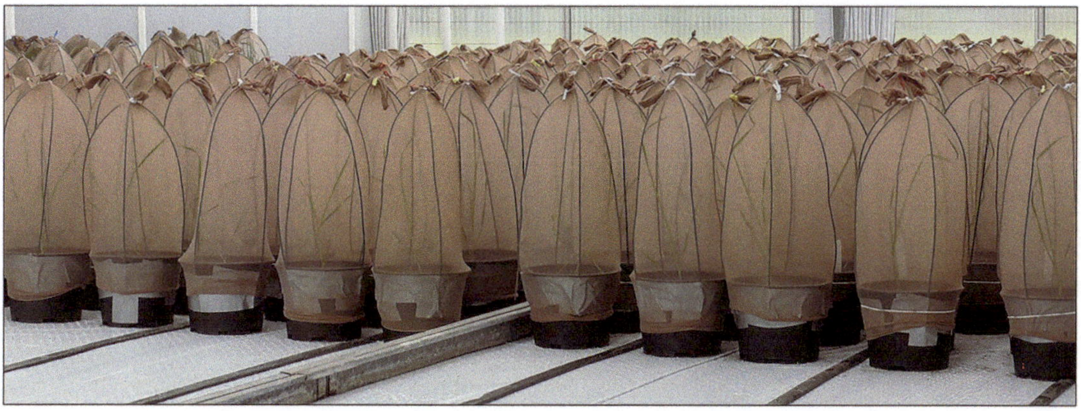

Fig. 2 Cages for transmission of wheat dwarf virus to wheat plants using the leafhopper *Psammotettix alienus*

6. For establishing a WDV-free culture, transfer and maintain leafhoppers on a nonhost. This can be barley for isolates of the WDV-E strain infecting wheat.

3.2 Maintenance of a Leafhopper Culture

1. If breeding successfully, the leafhoppers will lay eggs on the plants (*see* **Note 4**). Once nymphs appear, transfer them to new healthy plants (*see* **Note 5**).
2. For long-term maintenance, the culture can be kept in larger net cages with multiple plants.
3. Keep the cages in a greenhouse with 16/8 h day/night photoperiod and 20/18 °C day/night temperature (*see* **Notes 6** and **7**).
4. Replace old infected plants when they die with new healthy host plants (*see* **Note 8**).

3.3 Virus Transmission Using Leafhoppers

1. For virus acquisition, allow 3–5 leafhoppers (adults and/or nymphs) from a virus-free culture to feed for 7 days on WDV-infected plants (Fig. 3). Alternatively, take leafhoppers from a culture maintained on WDV-infected plants.
2. Transfer the leafhoppers from the source plants using an aspirator to the plants to be inoculated (*see* **Note 9**).
3. Count the leafhoppers during the inoculation period and replace with new ones to maintain the same number of insects.
4. After 7 days, remove the leafhoppers from the plants and treat the plants with an insecticide. The plants can now be kept outside of the cages.

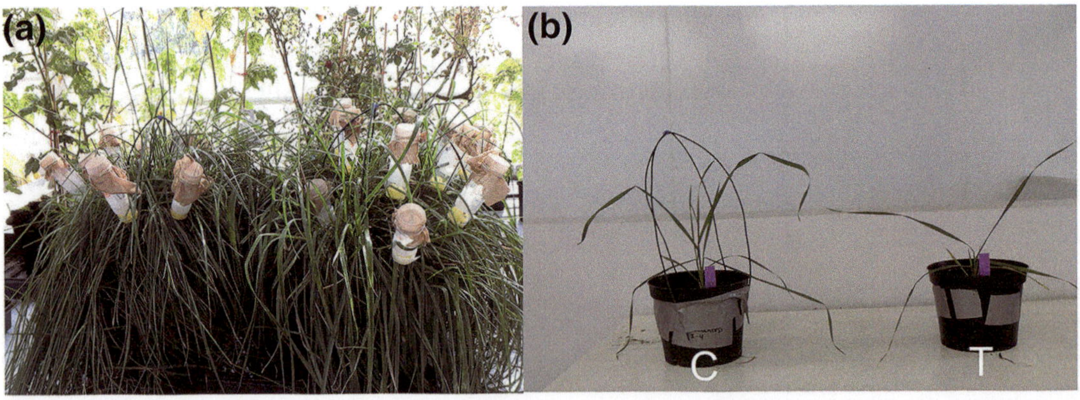

Fig. 3 Transmission of wheat dwarf virus (WDV) from ryegrass to wheat using viruliferous leafhoppers (*Psammotettix alienus*) and clip cages made of Falcon tubes. Panel **(a)** shows two plants of ryegrass (*Lolium perenne* and *L. multiflorum*) used as sources for WDV acquisition by leafhoppers. Panel **(b)** shows wheat plants at 23 days after exposure to leafhoppers. C, control plant exposed to leafhoppers without WDV; T, test plant exposed to leafhoppers with WDV (Reproduced from ref. 14 under the terms of Creative Commons Attribution License)

5. Monitor for symptoms of infection with WDV, such as yellowing and stunting. For young wheat plants, symptoms of infection are usually visible after 1 week.
6. Test for systemic infection in young leaves using DAS-ELISA, PCR or qPCR [10, 14] (*see* **Note 10**).

4 Notes

1. The levels of WDV-infected plants and *P. alienus* leafhoppers vary greatly between years. Some years, it can be difficult to find the leafhoppers in the fields.
2. There is competition between leafhoppers of different species. If other leafhoppers are contaminating the culture of *P. alienus*, they may take over. Therefore, it is important to check all leafhoppers when starting up the culture.
3. It is difficult to separate between individuals of different *Psammotettix* species. It can be done visually using taxonomic keys, by mating sound or molecular bar codes [22].
4. The leafhoppers place the eggs inside the leaves where they can be difficult to find.
5. When handling the insects, it is important to note that the leafhopper nymphs cannot fly, but jump.
6. The leafhoppers are sensitive to heat. During summer, the greenhouse should be well ventilated or cooled.
7. The leafhoppers may sense the different seasons outside and have difficulties in reproducing during winter.
8. Predators can pose a risk for the culture. It is important to inspect the culture frequently and eliminate spiders and other predators as soon as they appear.
9. The inoculation using viruliferous leafhoppers can be done either in a cage or using clip cages.
10. After transmission, leafhoppers can also be tested for WDV using PCR [14].

Acknowledgments

We would like to thank the late Professor Klas Lindsten for help establishing the technique. Financial support from Swedish Farmers' Foundation for Agricultural Research is acknowledged. Our research on WDV is part of the Euphresco network for phytosanitary research coordination and funding: "Diagnosis and epidemiology of viruses infecting cereal crops" (2021-A-374).

References

1. Kanakala S, Kuria P (2019) *Chickpea chlorotic dwarf virus*: an emerging monopartite dicot infecting mastrevirus. Viruses 11:5
2. Kvarnheden A, Lett J-M, Peterschmitt M (2016) Mastreviruses: tropical and temperate leafhopper-borne geminiviruses. In: Brown JK (ed) Vector-mediated transmission of plant pathogens. APS publications, St Paul, pp 231–241
3. Fiallo-Olivé E, Lett J-M, Martin DP, Roumagnac P, Varsani A, Zerbini FM, Navas-Castillo J, ICTV Report Consortium (2021) ICTV virus taxonomy profile: *Geminiviridae* 2021. J Gen Virol 102:001696
4. Fontenele RS, Alves-Freitas DMT, Silva PIT, Foresti J, Silva PR, Godinho MT, Varsani A, Ribeiro SG (2018) Discovery of the first maize-infecting mastrevirus in the Americas using a vector-enabled metagenomics approach. Arch Virol 163:263–267
5. Lappe RR, Elmore MG, Lozier ZR, Jander G, Miller WA, Whitham SA (2022) Metagenomic identification of novel viruses of maize and teosinte in North America. BMC Genomics 23:767
6. Wang H, Liu Y, Liu W, Wu K, Wang X (2022) F-actin dynamics in midgut cells enables virus persistence in vector insects. Mol Plant Pathol 23:1671–1685
7. Jungner J (1906) Die Zwergzikade (*Cicadula sexnotata* Fall.) und ihre Bekämpfung. DLG, Berlin
8. Lindsten K, Vacke J, Gerhardsson B (1970) A preliminary report on three cereal virus diseases new to Sweden spread by *Macrosteles* and *Psammotettix* leafhoppers. Natl Swedish Inst Plant Prot Contrib 14:175–180
9. Vacke J (1961) Wheat dwarf virus disease. Biol Plant (Praha) 3:228–233
10. Nygren J, Shad N, Kvarnheden A, Westerbergh A (2015) Variation in susceptibility to *Wheat dwarf virus* among wild and domesticated wheat. PLoS One 10:e0121580
11. Pfrieme AK, Ruckwied B, Habekuß A, Will T, Stahl A, Pillen K, Ordon F (2022) Identification and validation of quantitative trait loci for *wheat dwarf virus* resistance in wheat (*Triticum* spp.). Front Plant Sci 13:828639
12. Sharaf A, Nuc P, Ripl J, Alquicer G, Ibrahim E, Wang X, Maruthi MN, Kundu JK (2023) Transcriptome dynamics in *Triticum aestivum* genotypes associated with resistance against the wheat dwarf virus. Viruses 15:689
13. Vacke J (1972) Host plants range and symptoms of wheat dwarf virus. Ved Pr Výz Ústavú Rostl Výroby Praha-Ruzyn 17:151–162
14. Yazdkhasti E, Hopkins RJ, Kvarnheden A (2021) Reservoirs of plant virus disease: occurrence of wheat dwarf virus and barley/cereal yellow dwarf viruses in Sweden. Plant Pathol 70:1552–1561
15. Lindblad M, Sigvald R (2004) Temporal spread of wheat dwarf virus and mature plant resistance. Crop Protect 23:229–234
16. Abt I, Souquet M, Angot G, Mabon R, Dallot S, Thébaud G, Jacquot E (2020) Functional transcomplementation between wheat dwarf virus strains in wheat and barley. Viruses 12:34
17. Armand T, Souquet M, Korn L, Gauthier K, Jacquot E (2023) Asymmetric interactions between barley yellow dwarf virus-PAV and wheat dwarf virus in wheat. Front Plant Sci 14:1194622
18. Monjane AL, Dellicour S, Hartnady P, Oyeniran KA, Owor BE, Bezuidenhout M, Linderme D, Syed RA, Donaldson L, Murray S, Rybicki EP, Kvarnheden A, Yazdkhasti E, Lefeuvre P, Froissart R, Roumagnac P, Shepherd DN, Harkins GW, Suchard MA, Lemey P, Varsani A, Martin DP (2020) Symptom evolution following the emergence of maize streak virus. elife 9:e51984
19. Morris BA, Richardson KA, Haley A, Zhan X, Thomas JE (1992) The nucleotide sequence of the infectious cloned DNA component of tobacco yellow dwarf virus reveals features of geminiviruses infecting monocotyledonous plants. Virology 187:633–642
20. Shahmohammadi N, Dizadji A, Bihamta M, Kvarnheden A (2020) Diversity and occurrence of chickpea chlorotic dwarf virus on legumes from Iran. Plant Pathol 69:139–148
21. Ramsell JNE, Boulton MI, Martin DP, Valkonen JPT, Kvarnheden A (2009) Studies on the host range of the barley strain of *Wheat dwarf virus* using an agroinfectious viral clone. Plant Pathol 58:1161–1169
22. Abt I, Derlink M, Mabon R, Virant-Doberlet-M, Jacquot E (2018) Integrating multiple criteria for the characterization of *Psammotettix* populations in European cereal fields. Bull Entomol Res 108:185–202

Chapter 8

Transmission of Grabloviruses by Insect Vectors

Victoria J. Hoyle, Madison T. Flasco, and Marc Fuchs

Abstract

Among the three viruses of the genus *Grablovirus* in the plant virus family *Geminiviridae*, insect vector transmission is documented only for grapevine red blotch virus (GRBV), for which *Spissistilus festinus* (Hemiptera: Membracidae), the three-cornered alfalfa hopper, is identified as a vector. Transmission of GRBV by *S. festinus* is circulative, nonpropagative; it is also transstadial but neither transovarial, nor via seeds. Here, we thoroughly describe the *S. festinus*-mediated transmission process of GRBV with *Vitis* species, the natural hosts of the virus, and *Phaseolus vulgaris* plants, an experimental pseudo-systemic herbaceous host of the virus.

Key words Acquisition access period, Grapevine red blotch virus, Inoculation access period, *Medicago sativa*, *Phaseolus vulgaris*, Retention, Salivary glands, *Spissistilus festinus*, Transmission, *Vitis* spp.

1 Introduction

The genus *Grablovirus* was proposed in 2017 to accommodate the taxonomic classification of a few divergent virus species within the family *Geminiviridae* [1]. So far, three virus species are recognized in this genus: *Grapevine red blotch virus*, *Wild Vitis latent virus*, and *Prunus latent virus* with grapevine red blotch virus (GRBV), wild *Vitis* latent virus 1 (WvLV1), and *Prunus* geminivirus A (PrGVA) representing these species, respectively [2]. GRBV and WvLV1 infect *Vitis* spp. [3, 4] and PrGVA infects *Prunus* spp. [5]. Infectious clones of GRBV have been engineered and used to demonstrate red blotch disease causality [6] and transmission characteristics [7]. No infectious clones are available for WvLV1 and PrGVA.

Among the three grabloviruses reported so far, vector transmission has been documented only for GRBV with *Spissistilus festinus* (Say, 1830) (Hemiptera: Membracidae), the three-cornered alfalfa hopper [7–9]. No arthropod vectors are known or suspected for WvLV1 and PrGVA. Interestingly, GRBV infects all species of grapevines, including wine grape cultivars, interspecific

Francisco Murilo Zerbini et al. (eds.), *Geminiviruses: Methods and Protocols*, Methods in Molecular Biology, vol. 2912, https://doi.org/10.1007/978-1-0716-4454-6_8,

hybrids, table grapes, rootstocks, Muscadine grapes, and free-living vines in northern California and southern Oregon in the USA [10, 11]. The interconnectivity between wine grape cultivars and free-living vines for GRBV transmission was recently documented [9]. Transmission of GRBV by *S. festinus* is circulative, nonpropagative; it is also transstadial [7] but not transovarial [17]); nor does it occur via seeds [7]. Additionally, GRBV isolates belong to two distinct phylogenetic clades [12]; both of which are transmitted by *S. festinus* [7].

The transmission rate of GRBV by *S. festinus* from an infected wine grape cultivar to a healthy wine grape cultivar in the greenhouse is low (10–20%) [7, 9, 13] but substantially higher (77%) from infected free-living vines to healthy free-living vines [9]. Transmission also occurs from infected free-living vines to a wine grape cultivar (15%), and from an infected wine grape cultivar to healthy free-living vines (100%) [9]. Such distinct GRBV transmission rates depending on the virus donor or virus recipient plant suggest a preferential feeding behavior of *S. festinus* on different plant hosts, a feature that could result in variable virus acquisition and transmission efficiencies.

S. festinus is a vector of epidemiological relevance [8]. Spread occurs in the vineyard when GRBV-infected grapevines are asymptomatic and GRBV titer is not maximal [14], suggesting opportunistic GRBV—*S. festinus*—grapevine interactions, and a recent coevolution of this pathosystem. Here we thoroughly describe the transmission of GRBV by *S. festinus* with *Vitis* species, the natural hosts of the virus, in the laboratory and in the vineyard, and with *Phaseolus vulgaris* plants, an experimental pseudo-systemic herbaceous host of the virus, in the laboratory.

2 Materials

S. festinus specimens used in transmission assays are from colonies reared on alfalfa (*Medicago sativa* Galaxy 100 Brand, a blend of cultivars) or snap bean (*P. vulgaris* cv. Hystyle) in the laboratory. Choose the appropriate plant and other materials for select transmission assays to be carried out in the laboratory (Fig. 1) or in the vineyard (Fig. 4).

2.1 Plant Materials

1. Potted GRBV-infected grapevines (for example *Vitis vinifera* cv. "Cabernet franc") and excised leaves of GRBV-negative grapevines as virus donor and recipient tissue, respectively.
2. Potted GRBV-infected free-living grapevines (*Vitis californica* or hybrids of *V. californica* x *V. vinifera* or of *V. californica* x rootstocks) and excised leaves of GRBV-negative free-living grapevines as virus donor and recipient tissue, respectively.

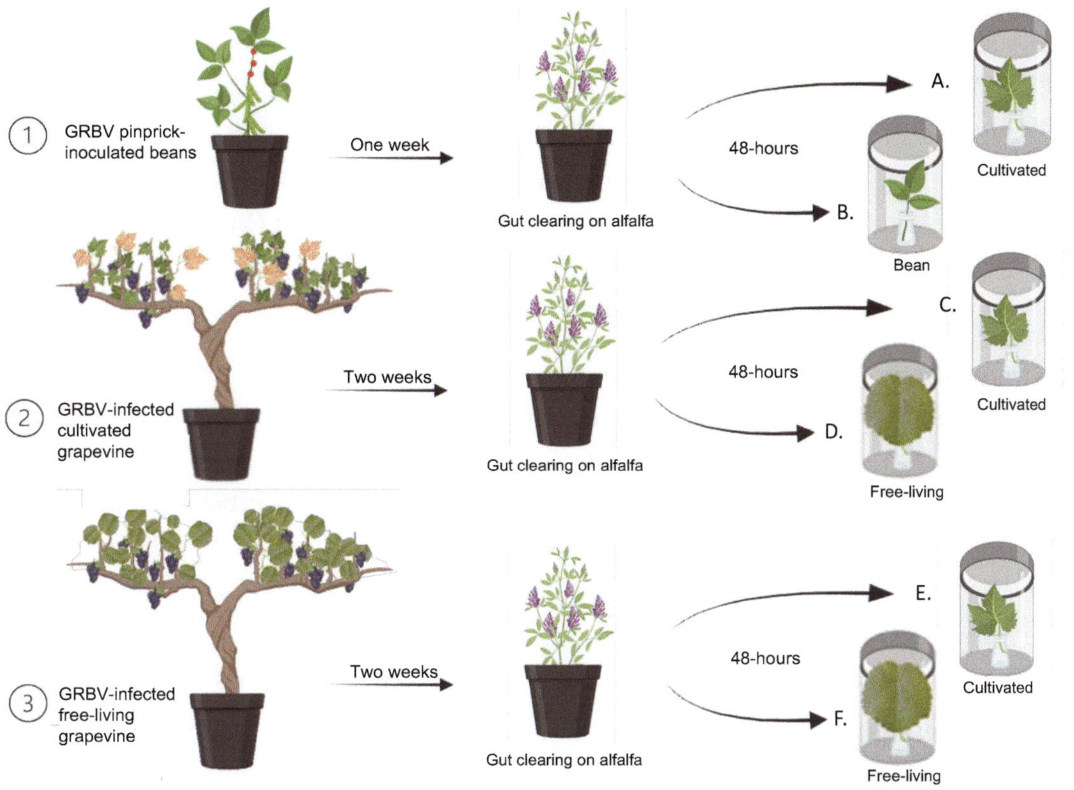

Fig. 1 Workflow for transmission assays in the greenhouse where GRBV-infected *Phaseolus vulgaris* are used as the donor and excised leaves of *Vitis vinifera* (A), or excised bean trifoliates (B) as the recipient. The second set of transmission assays relied on GRBV-infected *V. vinifera* grapevines as donor material and either healthy excised *V. vinifera* grape leaves (C) or healthy excised free-living grape leaves (D) as recipients. The final set of transmission assays used GRBV-infected free-living vines as donors and both healthy *V. vinifera* (E) and free-living (F) grape leaves as recipients

3. Potted GRBV-infected snap bean plants (*P. vulgaris* cv. Hystyle) and excised GRBV-negative snap bean leaves, as virus donor and recipient tissue, respectively.
4. Potted alfalfa plants (*M. sativa,* Galaxy 100 Brand, a blend of cultivars) for *S. festinus* gut clearing after the acquisition access period (AAP), and excised alfalfa shoots for *S. festinus* transport from the laboratory to the vineyard.

2.2 P. vulgaris *as Virus Donor Material*

1. Plates of Luria-Bertani medium supplemented with kanamycin containing cultures of agrobacteria carrying GRBV partial dimer clones for infection of snap bean plants via *Agrobacterium tumefaciens*-mediated inoculation.
2. Sterile dissecting needles.
3. Cheesecloth.
4. Twist ties.

2.3 Transmission Assays of GRBV in the Greenhouse

1. 20 mL collection glass vials.
2. Clear polypropylene 950 mL containers (Fabri-Kal).
3. Polypropylene donut lid carrying a nylon screen (BugDorm).
4. Parafilm.
5. Tape to secure collection glass vial to polypropylene container.
6. Insect cages for secondary containment (BugDorm).
7. Lunch trays for bottom of cages.
8. D-cell-powered aspirator and collection tubes (Gemplers).

2.4 Transmission Assays of GRBV in the Vineyard

1. 0.06 L deli containers (PlastiMade).
2. Clear polypropylene 950 mL containers (Fabri-Kal).
3. Polypropylene donut lid carrying a nylon screen (BugDorm).
4. D-cell-powered aspirator and collection tubes (Gemplers).
5. Insect sleeves (BugDorm).
6. Duct tape.
7. Binder clips.

2.5 Tissue Processing and GRBV Diagnostics

1. Sterile razor blades.
2. Weigh paper.
3. Bleach.
4. Sterile 2 mL microcentrifuge tubes.
5. Collection 1.2 mL polypropylene microtubes (racked, 10 × 96) and caps (120 × 8) (Qiagen).
6. Sterile 3 mm and 4.5 mm ball bearings.
7. MM300 TissueLyser.
8. H.P. Plant DNA Mini Kit for plant nucleic acid isolation.
9. MagMAX DNA Multi-Sample Ultra Kit from insect nucleic acid extraction.
10. Pairs of oligonucleotides for a GRBV diagnostic multiplex end-point PCR [12]:
    (a) CPfor 5′-AGCGGAAGCATGATTGAGACATTGACG-3′.
    (b) CPrev 5′-AACGTATGTCCACTTGCAGAAGCCGC-3′.
    (c) Repfor 5′- CAAGTCGTTGTAGATTGAGGACG TATTGG-3′.
    (d) Reprev 5′-AGCCACACCTACACGCCTTGCTCATC-3′.
    (e) 16Sfor 5′-TGCTTAACACATGCAAGTCGGA-3′.
    (f) 16Srev 5′-AGCCGTTTCCAGCTGTTGTTC-3′.
11. Reagents for end-point PCR.

12. Bio-Rad S1000 thermal cycler.
13. Electrophoresis system with gel casting.
14. Agarose.
15. GelRed.
16. Pairs of oligonucleotides for quantitative GRBV PCR [8, 15, 16]:
    (g) pREP3v 5′-ACATCTCTGGGYTTKGTGATATT-3′.
    (h) pREP4v5′-CTACACGCCTTGCTCATCTT-3′.
    (i) NADPfor 5′-GGTGTTGGTGTCTCCATAGTT-3′.
    (j) NADPrev 5′-CCTAGTTGCCTTGAGGTCTTT-3′.
    (k) T197for 5′-TGGGCAATTGGACGTTATTAG-3′.
    (l) T197rev 5′-GCCACGGTCTTGAACATAAAA-3′.
    (m) Sf18Sfor 5′-GTGAGGTCTTCGGACTGGTG-3′.
    (n) Sf18Srev 5″-GGTTCACCTACGGAAACCTTG-3′.
17. SYBR Green reagents for real-time PCR.
18. Bio-Rad CFX96 Touch Real-Time PCR Detection System.

3 Methods

3.1 Transmission of GRBV by S. festinus *Using Snap Bean in the Laboratory (Fig. 1)*

1. Sow seeds of *P. vulgaris* "Hystyle" and grow snap bean plants in the greenhouse at 22 ± 3 °C and a 16:8 h light:dark photoperiod.
2. Sow seeds of *M. sativa* (Galaxy 100 Brand, a blend of cultivars) and grow alfalfa plants in the greenhouse at 22 ± 3 °C and a 16: 8 h light:dark photoperiod.
3. Select 2- to 3-week-old snap bean plants for pinprick inoculation with a GRBV infectious clone after removing basal leaves, flowers, and pods (*see* **Note 1**).
4. Pinprick inoculate snap bean plants using sterile dissecting needles swiped through a solid culture of *A. tumefaciens*-carrying a partial dimer GRBV clone in 2- to 3-cm intervals beginning at the basal leaves' junction and continuing all the way up the plants and across the petiole and leaf junctions (Fig. 2) (*see* **Notes 2** and **3**).
5. Maintain inoculated snap bean plants in a BSL-2 greenhouse at 22 ± 3 °C and a 16:8 h light:dark photoperiod for at least 1 week to establish infection.
6. Remove any new growth on inoculated snap bean plants before adding *S. festinus* and wrap the uninoculated areas with cheesecloth, securing it with twist ties before adding *S. festinus* (Fig. 2) (*see* **Notes 3–5**).

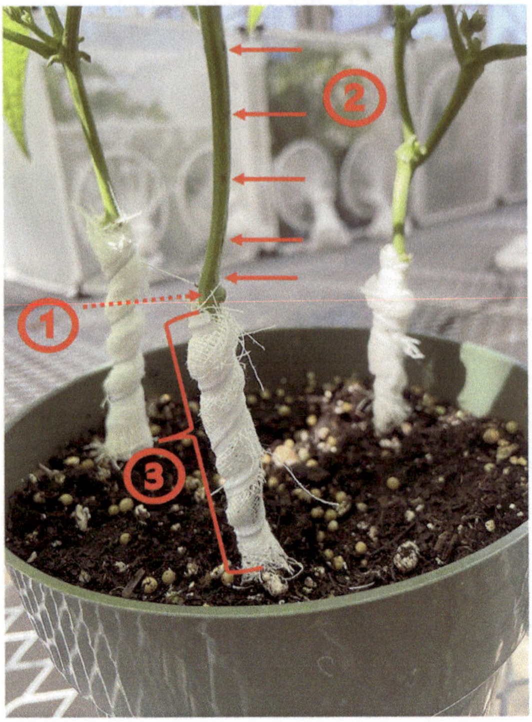

Fig. 2 Agroinoculation of *Phaseolus vulgaris* with an infectious GRBV clone starting at the basal leaf junction (1) and continuing upward throughout the plant tissue in 2–3 cm increments (2). The area below the basal leaf junction (1) is "mummified" using cheesecloth maintained with twist ties (3). New growth, flowers, and bean pods were removed prior to inoculation

7. Move inoculated snap bean plants into an insect cage.
8. Transfer adult *S. festinus* of mixed sex from a laboratory-maintained colony into cages with inoculated snap bean plants to feed for at least a 6-day AAP in the greenhouse at 22 ± 3 °C and a 16:8 h light:dark photoperiod (*see* **Note 6**).
9. Capture all *S. festinus* with a D-cell-powered aspirator after completion of the AAP, and transfer them to alfalfa plants, a nonhost of GRBV, for a 48-h gut clearing period in an insect cage in the greenhouse at 22 ± 3 °C and a 16:8 h light:dark photoperiod (*see* **Note 7**).
10. Fill a 20 mL glass collection vial with distilled water and cover by stretching parafilm on top of the vial and poking a small hole in the middle of the stretched parafilm (Fig. 3).
11. Create a detached leaf chamber by taping the bottom of the filled 20 mL glass collection vial to the bottom of a clear polypropylene 950 mL container (Fig. 3).
12. Repeat **steps 10** and **11** to create additional detached leaf chambers, as appropriate.

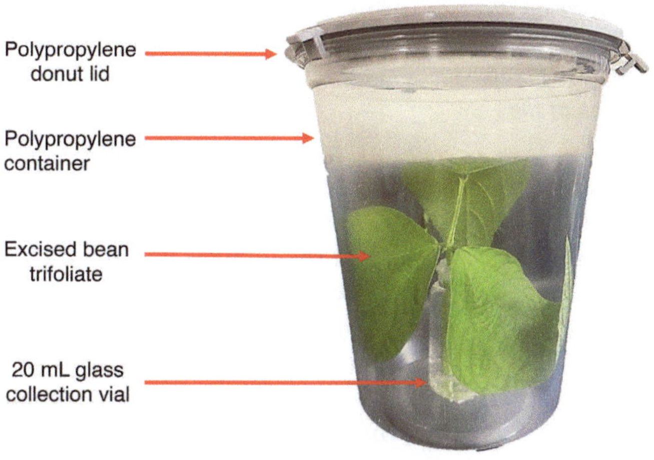

Fig. 3 Depiction of a detached leaf chamber and the necessary components denoted by arrows for use in transmission assays ofgrapevine red blotch virus by viruliferous *Spissistilus festinus*

13. Excise leaves of 3- to 4-week-old uninoculated snap bean plants and place them in parafilm-covered 20 mL collection vials containing distilled water through the poked hole, holding the petioles upright and submerged in water (Fig. 3) (*see* **Note 8**).
14. Transfer 5–8 *S. festinus* from alfalfa plants used for the gut clearing step onto each excised leaf from an uninoculated snap bean plant (**step 13**) in an insect cage to provide secondary containment.
15. Seal the detached leaf chamber with a polypropylene donut lid carrying a nylon screen and place it in a controlled environmental chamber 25 °C, 16:8 h light:dark photoperiod, and 80% relative humidity.
16. Transfer 5–8 *S. festinus* from the laboratory-maintained colony onto an excised leaf from an uninoculated 3- to 4-week-old snap bean plant (**step 13**) as negative controls, and seal with a polypropylene donut lid in a separate insect cage.
17. Refresh the water regularly in the 20 mL glass collection vials containing excised snap bean leaves (*see* **Note 9**) during a 4-day inoculation access period (IAP).
18. Capture all *S. festinus* using a D-cell-powered aspirator at the completion of the IAP for GRBV testing.
19. Maintain excised snap bean leaves in a controlled environmental chamber at 25 °C, 16:8 h light:dark photoperiod, and 80% relative humidity for 2 weeks.
20. Collect excised leaves and separate petioles and petiole-leaf junctions for GRBV testing.

3.2 Transmission of GRBV by S. festinus *from Snap Bean Plants to Grapevines in the Laboratory (Fig. 1)*

1. Grow hardwood cuttings of GRBV-negative *V. vinifera* and GRBV-infected free-living vines to maturity in the greenhouse at 22 ± 3 °C and a 16:8 h light:dark photoperiod.
2. Implement **steps 1–11** of Subheading 3.1, as described.
3. Excise individual leaves from *V. vinifera* or free-living vine and place them in a parafilm-covered 20 mL collection vial containing distilled water with a hole poked through the parafilm to hold the petioles upright and submerged in water (Fig. 3) (*see* **Note 8**).
4. Maintain the excised grapevine leaves in a clear polypropylene 950-mL container in a controlled environmental chamber 25 °C, 16:8 h light:dark photoperiod, and 80% relative humidity.
5. Transfer 5–8 *S. festinus* from the GRBV-infected snap beans onto an excised leaf of a GRBV-negative grapevine in an insect cage for secondary containment.
6. Seal the detached leaf chamber with a polypropylene donut lid carrying a nylon screen.
7. Transfer 5–8 *S. festinus* from the laboratory-maintained colony onto a GRBV-negative excised grapevine leaf as negative control in a separate insect cage.
8. Refresh the water regularly in the 20 mL glass collection vials during the 4-day IAP (*see* **Note 9**).
9. Capture *S. festinus* using a D-cell-powered aspirator at the completion of the IAP for GRBV testing, doing so in a separate insect cage to provide secondary containment.
10. Maintain excised grapevine leaves in a controlled environmental chamber 25 °C, 16:8 h light:dark photoperiod, and 80% relative humidity for an additional 2 weeks.
11. Collect excised leaves and separate petioles, mid-ribs, and secondary veins for GRBV testing.

3.3 Transmission of GRBV by S. festinus *from Grapevines to Grapevines in the Laboratory (Fig. 1)*

1. Grow hardwood cuttings of GRBV-infected *V. vinifera* and GRBV-infected free-living vines to maturity in the greenhouse at 22 ± 3 °C and a 16:8 h light:dark photoperiod.
2. Move GRBV-infected potted grapevine plants, i.e., *V. vinifera* or free-living vines, into an insect cage.
3. Transfer 15–20 *S. festinus* from the laboratory-maintained colony onto leaves of caged GRBV-infected grapevines and allow treehoppers to feed for 2–3 weeks in the greenhouse at 22 ± 3 °C and a 16:8 h light:dark photoperiod (*see* **Note 10**).
4. Capture *S. festinus* with a D-cell-powered aspirator and transfer them on alfalfa, a nonhost of GRBV, for a 48-h gut clearing period in the greenhouse at 22 ± 3 °C and a 16:8 h light:dark photoperiod (*see* **Note 7**).

5. Proceed with **steps 10** and **11** of Subheading 3.1 as described.
6. Excise individual grapevine leaves from GRBV-negative *V. vinifera* or free-living vine and place them in a parafilm-covered 20 mL collection vial containing sterile water with a hole poked through the parafilm to hold the petioles upright and submerged in water (*see* **Note 7**).
7. Maintain the excised grapevine leaves in a clear polypropylene 950 mL container sealed with a polypropylene donut lid carrying a nylon screen in a controlled environmental chamber 25 °C, 16:8 h light:dark photoperiod, and 80% relative humidity.
8. Transfer 5–8 *S. festinus* from alfalfa onto an excised grapevine leaf in an insect cage to provide secondary containment.
9. Transfer 5–8 *S. festinus* from the laboratory-maintained colony onto an excised grapevine leaf as negative control in a separate insect cage.
10. Refresh the water regularly in the glass collection vials during the 4-day IAP (*see* **Note 9**).
11. Capture *S. festinus* using a D-cell-powered aspirator for GRBV testing at the completion of the IAP.
12. Maintain excised grapevine leaves in a controlled environmental chamber 25 °C, 16:8 h light:dark photoperiod, and 80% relative humidity for 2 weeks.
13. Collect excised grapevine leaves, and separate petioles, mid-ribs, and secondary veins for GRBV testing.

3.4 Transmission of GRBV with S. festinus *in the Vineyard (Fig. 4)*

1. Punch tiny holes in the lid and cup of 0.06 L deli containers using a narrow screwdriver to ensure airflow.
2. Place alfalfa shoots at the bottom of the pre-punched deli containers (*see* **Note 11**).
3. Collect viruliferous *S. festinus* from **step 8** of Subheading 3.1 or **step 3** of Subheading 3.3 and transfer them into the pre-punched deli container, doing so in a separate insect cage for secondary containment.
4. Place the deli containers containing viruliferous *S. festinus* in a clear polypropylene 950 mL container.
5. Transport viruliferous *S. festinus* to a select GRBV-negative vineyard.
6. Choose leaves and petioles on individual grapevines in the select vineyard for exposure to viruliferous *S. festinus* (*see* **Note 12**).
7. Place an insect sleeve on the selected leaves and petioles (*see* **Note 13**).

8. Place the viruliferous *S. festinus* contained in a 0.06 L deli container inside the insect sleeve, making sure the lid is secure.
9. Secure the open end of the insect sleeve to the shoot of interest using duct tape (*see* **Note 14**) and to the trellis wire using a binder clip (*see* **Note 15**).
10. Manually release the viruliferous *S. festinus* by gently opening the lid of the 0.06 L deli container from the outside of the insect sleeve with your hands (*see* **Note 16**).
11. Repeat **steps** 7 and **8** on the same vine targeting different canopy levels and canes or on different vines (Fig. 4).
12. Maintain the viruliferous *S. festinus* for a 2-week IAP.
13. Take note of the number of alive and dead *S. festinus* after the desired 2-week IAP (*see* **Note 17**).
14. Manually remove the binder clip and duct tape on the end of the insect sleeve at the completion of the IAP, ensuring no gaps between the sleeve and the petiole, and no damage to the inoculated tissue.
15. Collect live *S. festinus* by slowly loosening the insect sleeve and placing the collection tube of a D-cell-powered aspirator inside the sleeve.
16. Repeat the *S. festinus* collection process ensuring all treehoppers are collected without damaging the leaf or petiole.
17. Transfer captured *S. festinus* from the aspirator container to a 50 mL conical tube for GRBV testing.
18. Collect inoculated grapevine leaves that exhibit extensive *S. festinus* feeding damage or signs of oviposition for GRBV testing (*see* **Notes 18** and **19**).
19. Repeat **step 19** in subsequent visits to the vineyard until the end of the growing season to collect all remaining tissue exposed to viruliferous *S. festinus*.
20. Separately process the petiole and leaf tissues from the collected grapevine leaves for GRBV testing.

3.5 Testing of Plant Material and S. festinus for GRBV by PCR

1. Process snap bean and grapevine tissues on a weigh paper using a sterile razor blade, dipped in bleach between samples, and store plant fragments (approximately 100 mg) in labelled 2 mL sterile microfuge tubes containing one or two sterile 4.5 mm ball bearings which were either dipped into liquid nitrogen or stored at −20 °C for at least 24 h.
2. Homogenize the plant material using a TissueLyser at 30 Hz for 90 s.
3. Extract nucleic acids from the plant homogenates using the H.P. Plant DNA Mini Kit or the Mag MAX-96 A1/ND Isolation Kit on a KingFisher instrument.

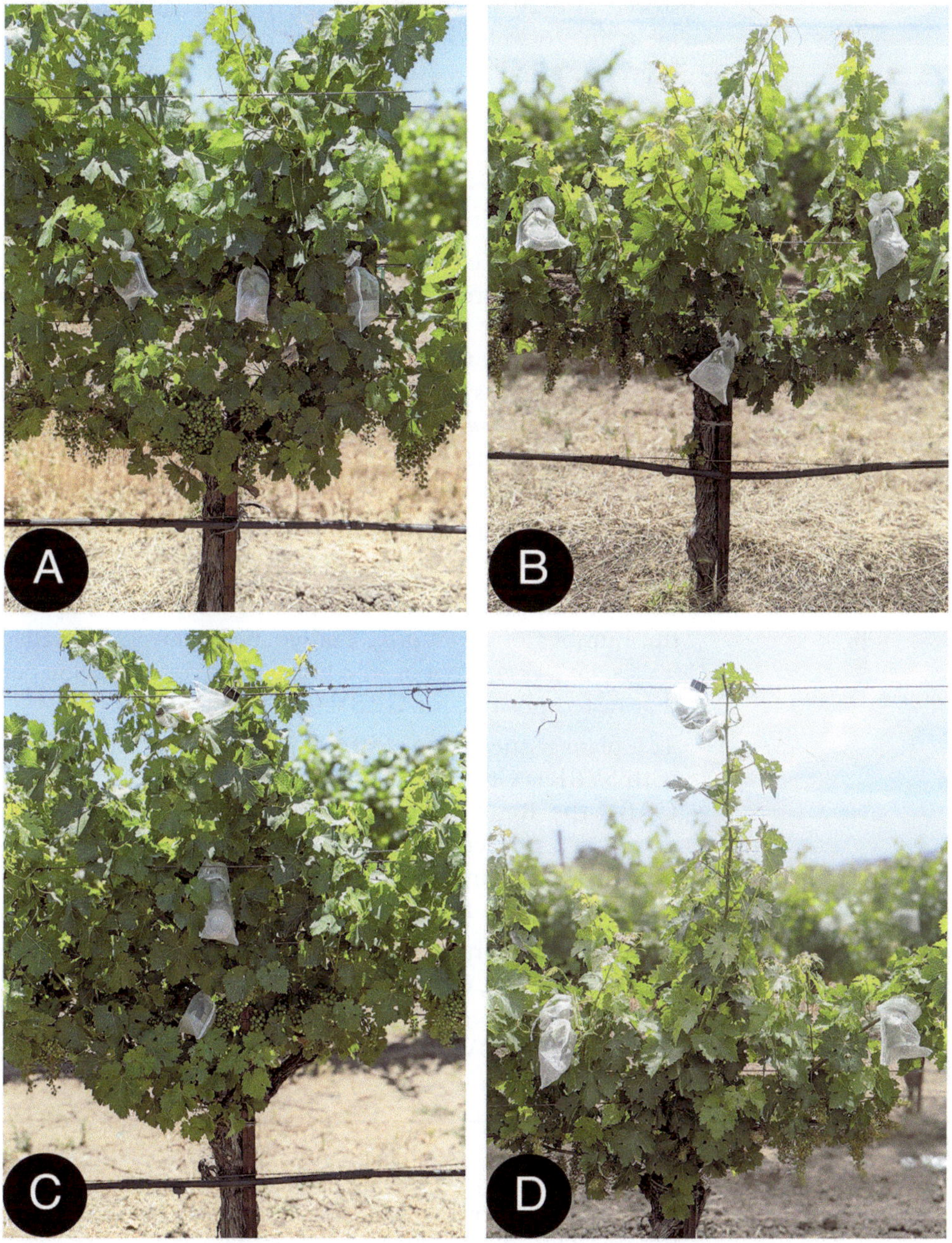

Fig. 4 Lollipop sleeve configurations used in transmission assays of grapevine red blotch virus in the vineyard in which single grapevine leaf petioles were exposed to two viruliferous *Spissistilus festinus*. (**a**) A middle-middle-middle sleeve configuration. (**b**) A bottom-middle-middle sleeve configuration. (**c**) A top-middle-bottom sleeve configuration. (**d**) A middle-top-middle sleeve configuration

4. Place individual *S. festinus* captured during the transmission assays in the laboratory or in the vineyard in labelled sterile 2 mL microfuge tubes containing one or two sterile 4.5 mm ball bearings which were either dipped into liquid nitrogen or

stored at −20 °C for at least 24 h. Alternatively, place specimens in 96-well sampling plates containing one 3 mm ball bearings stored at −20 °C for at least 24 h.

5. Homogenize the *S. festinus* specimens using a TissueLyser at 30 Hz for 90 s.
6. Extract nucleic acids from *S. festinus* using the MagMAX DNA Multi-Sample Ultra Kit on a KingFisher instrument.
7. Run a multiplex end-point PCR to determine the presence of GRBV using primers a and b designed in the open reading frame coding for the GRBV coat protein (CP), primers c and d designed in the GRBV replication-associated proteins (RepA), as well as primers e and f for *Vitis* tissues [15], primers k and l for *P. vulgaris* tissues [9], or primers m and n for *S. festinus* specimens [8]. *See* Subheading 2.5, **item 10** for the primer composition.
8. Visualize DNA amplicons by agarose gel electrophoresis and UV illumination after staining with GelRed.
9. Analyze and interpret the end-point PCR results and calculate the number of *S. festinus*, excised bean leaves, excised grape leaves, i.e., *V. vinifera* or free-living vines, or grapevine petioles that tested positive for GRBV.
10. Test plant tissues and *S. festinus* specimens for GRBV by qPCR with SYBR® Green reagents, primers g and h designed in the GRBV the RepA coding region, and selective housekeeping genes, i.e., primers i and j for grape [15], primers k and l for bean [9], and primers m and n for *S. festinus* [8]. *See* Subheading 2.5, **item 16** for the primer composition.
11. Analyze and interpret the qPCR results and calculate the number of *S. festinus*, excised bean leaves, excised grape leaves, i.e., *V. vinifera* or free-living vines, or grapevine petioles that tested positive for GRBV.

4 Notes

1. New growth, flowers and bean pods can be removed using fingers. This will facilitate the allocation of resources to tissue that will sustain GRBV replication and movement.
2. Make sure the needle depth is sufficient to reach the phloem, i.e., the preferred plant tissue localization of GRBV, but not so deep that it punctures through the plant material.
3. Bean is a pseudo-systemic host of GRBV, thus sustaining a limited long-distance virus movement. This is why multiple pinpricks throughout the plants' stem and petioles are necessary [7].

4. Remove new growth, flowers, and bean pods using fingers to reduce any feeding on uninoculated tissue by *S. festinus*, thus increasing the rate of GRBV acquisition.
5. Female *S. festinus* tend to oviposit lower in the canopy and near the soil line (V. Hoyle and M. Flasco, personal observations). Wrapping the uninoculated area below the basal leaf junction forces female treehoppers to remain higher in the leaf canopy, improving the rate of GRBV acquisition.
6. Use younger *S. festinus* males or females to maximize the duration of the experiments.
7. A 48-h gut clearing period on alfalfa, a nonhost of GRBV, is used to eliminate most virions from the mouth parts and gut of the treehoppers, and thus, irrevocably assess acquisition of GRBV in the salivary glands.
8. Cut off a small fragment from the bottom of the petiole at an angle using a sterile razor blade prior to submerging the petioles in water to assist water uptake to leaves. Keep petiole bottoms as negative control for GRBV testing by PCR.
9. Place the detached leaf chambers in a secondary cage for the water refreshing step to catch treehoppers that might escape and then return them to their designated chamber. Use a 2 mL plastic pipettor to drip water into glass collection vials by placing the pipette tip against the petiole right above the parafilm entry site. Reduce the stretching of the parafilm when refreshing water in vials, otherwise *S. festinus* will move below the parafilm, increasing their potential for drowning.
10. A high rate of *S. festinus* mortality can be expected when plant hosts used in transmission assays, i.e., grapevines, differ from the rearing plant hosts, i.e., snap bean or alfalfa. For this reason, the use of more *S. festinus* is recommended when *V. vinifera* and free-living grapes are used as virus donor plants in transmission assays.
11. Supplement deli containers with a small collection of alfalfa shoots for *S. festinus* feeding, thus, increasing treehopper survival for up to 24 h.
12. Due to the added weight of the insect sleeve and deli container, it is important to select fully emerged leaves with strong petioles for inoculation.
13. The insect sleeve configuration requires two viruliferous *S. festinus* and is referred to as a lollipop configuration [8].
14. Tear the piece of duct tape in half lengthwise prior to securing the insect sleeve to the petiole to ensure no damage is done to the petiole and *S. festinus* have access to as much tissue as possible. The duct tape should be tight enough to ensure no insect escape while also not being overly restrictive.

15. Binder clips relieve the pressure on the inoculated petiole. Any portion of the insect sleeve can be secured so long as manipulating the petiole to the nearest wire does further increase physical stress.
16. Due to wind and vineyard maintenance, it is not uncommon for the lids to fall back on the cups of the deli container, often trapping viruliferous *S. festinus* inside. Fully separating the two components of the container helps alleviate this possibility.
17. It is essential to understand the location and proportion of live *S. festinus* prior to collection. This ensures all specimens are retrieved for subsequent GRBV testing.
18. Balancing the IAP to allow for sufficient feeding without extensive feeding damage is required for successful transmission. Two weeks is an adequate IAP on *Vitis* species.
19. Collecting grapevine leaves only with signs of oviposition or extensive feeding damage ensures inoculated tissue can remain on the vine as long as possible. Collections should aim to obtain inoculated tissue just before leaf drop, assuming the tissue quality is retained for subsequent extraction and testing.

Acknowledgments

This research was funded by the California Department of Food and Agriculture, Pierce Disease's Control Program (19-0262-000-SA, 20-0264-000-SA, 21-267-000-SA, 22-0551-000-SA, and 23-0390-000-SA), USDA-NIFA-AFRI (2023-67011-40492), USDA-NIFA Federal Capacity Funds, and Cornell AgriTech Venture Funds.

References

1. Varsani A, Roumagnac P, Fuchs M, Navas-Castillo J, Moriones E, Idris A, Briddon RW, Rivera-Bustamante R, Zerbini FM, Martin DP (2017) *Capulavirus* and *Grablovirus*: two new genera in the family *Geminiviridae*. Arch Virol 162:1819–1831
2. Fiallo-Olivé E, Lett J-M, Martin DP, Roumagnac P, Varsani A, Zerbini FM, Navas-Castillo J (2021) ICTV virus taxonomy profile: *Geminiviridae*. J Gen Virol 102:001696
3. Cieniewicz E, Thompson JR, McLane H, Perry KL, Dangl GS, Corbett Q, Martinson T, Wise A, Wallis A, O'Connell J, Dunst R, Cox K, Fuchs M (2018) Prevalence and genetic diversity of grabloviruses in free-living *Vitis* spp. Plant Dis 102:2308–2316
4. Perry KL, McLane H, Hyder MZ, Dangl GS, Thompson JR, Fuchs MF (2016) Grapevine red blotch-associated virus is present in free-living *Vitis* sp. proximal to cultivated grapevines. Phytopathology 106:663–670
5. Alabi OJ, Westrick NM, Golino D (2018) Prunus geminivirus A: a novel grablovirus infecting *Prunus* spp. Plant Dis 102:1246–1253
6. Yepes LM, Cieniewicz E, Krenz B, McLane H, Thompson JR, Perry KL, Fuchs M (2018) Causative role of grapevine red blotch virus in red blotch disease. Phytopathology 108:902–909
7. Flasco M, Hoyle V, Cieniewicz E, Roy B, McLane H, Perry KL, Loeb G, Nault B, Heck M, Fuchs M (2021) Grapevine red

blotch virus is transmitted by the three-cornered alfalfa hopper in a circulative, nonpropagative mode with unique attributes. Phytopathology 111:1851–1861

8. Flasco MT, Hoyle V, Cieniewicz EJ, Loeb G, McLane H, Perry K, Fuchs M (2023a) The three-cornered alfalfa hopper, *Spissistilus festinus*, is a vector of grapevine red blotch virus in vineyards. Viruses 15:927
9. Hoyle V, Flasco MT, Choi J, Cieniewicz EJ, McLane H, Perry K, Dangl G, Al Rwahnih M, Heck M, Loeb G, Fuchs MF (2022) Transmission of grapevine red blotch virus by *Spissistilus festinus* (Say, 1830) (Hemiptera: Membracidae) between free-living vines and *Vitis vinifera* 'Cabernet franc'. Viruses 14:1156
10. Cieniewicz E, Perry K, Fuchs M (2017) Grapevine red blotch: molecular biology of the virus and management of the disease. In: Meng B, Martelli GP, Golino DA, Fuchs M (eds) Grapevine viruses: molecular biology, diagnostics and management. Springer, Cham, Switzerland pp 303–314
11. Krenz B, Fuchs M, Thompson JR (2023) Grapevine red blotch disease: a comprehensive Q&A guide. PLOS Path 19:e1011671
12. Krenz B, Thompson JR, McLane HL, Fuchs M, Perry KL (2014) Grapevine red blotch-associated virus is widespread in the United States. Phytopathology 104:1232–1240
13. Bahder BW, Zalom FG, Jayanth M, Sudarshana MR (2016) Phylogeny of geminivirus coat protein sequences and digital PCR aid in identifying *Spissistilus festinus* as a vector of grapevine red blotch-associated virus. Phytopathology 106:1223–1230
14. Flasco M, Hoyle V, Powell G, Seiter J, Wise A, Cieniewicz EJ, Fuchs M (2024) Seasonal variation in grapevine red blotch virus titer in relation to disease symptom expression in vineyards. Phytobiomes 8:192-200
15. Setiono FJ, Chatterjee D, Fuchs M, Perry KL, Thompson JR (2018) The distribution and ability to detect grapevine red blotch virus in its host depends on time of sampling and tissue type. Plant Dis 102:2187–2193
16. Thibivilliers S, Joshi T, Campbell KB, Scheffler B, Xu D, Cooper B, Nguyen HT, Stacey G (2009) Generation of *Phaseolus vulgaris* ESTs and investigation of their regulation upon *Uromyces appendiculatus* infection. BMC Plant Biol 9:1–13
17. Hoyle VJ, Shultz M, McGinnity Schneider EJ., Roy BG, Fuchs M (2024) Lack of vertical transmission of grapevine red blotch virus by *Spissistilus festinus* but sex-associated differences in horizontal transmission. Insects 15:1014

Chapter 9

Sequence Demarcation Tool (SDT), a Free User-Friendly Computer Program Using Pairwise Genetic Identity Calculations to Classify Nucleotide or Amino Acid Sequences

Brejnev Muhizi Muhire, Philippe Roumagnac, Arvind Varsani, and Darren Patrick Martin

Abstract

Sequence Demarcation Tool (SDT) is a free user-friendly computer program that has been adopted by many geminivirologists as a means of robustly and reproducibly using pairwise genetic identity calculations to classify geminivirus whole genome sequences. As input SDT takes unaligned sequences and it outputs publication quality pairwise identity plots and color-coded distance matrices. Whereas the distance plots are useful for guiding the establishment of strain, species or genus demarcation thresholds that will yield minimal classification conflicts, the distance matrices aid the classification of sequences according to the taxonomic demarcation criteria of the International Committee on Taxonomy of Viruses. Accordingly, over the past 10 years, SDT has been extensively used for the establishment of new genera in the family *Geminiviridae* and for the classification of hundreds of new species within individual geminivirus genera.

Key words Classification, Virus sequence

1 Introduction

Complete or partial sequences of viral genomes have now become the most accessible form of data for viral analyses. The ongoing expansion of geminivirus whole genome and genome component sequence datasets requires consistent and relatively easy to apply comparative genomics techniques for determining either where newly determined geminivirus sequences fit into the existing classification hierarchy of genera, species, strains or subtypes or whether it is necessary to tentatively classify newly determined sequences as members of new geminivirus subtypes, strains, species or genera.

Several computational tools have been developed for the purpose of consistently calculating frequency distribution of pairwise

Francisco Murilo Zerbini et al. (eds.), *Geminiviruses: Methods and Protocols*, Methods in Molecular Biology, vol. 2912,
https://doi.org/10.1007/978-1-0716-4454-6_9,

sequence divergence so as to establish reasonable pairwise sequence identity thresholds enabling both refinements of the boundaries of hundreds of existing geminivirus species [1, 2], and to simplify the proposal of new geminivirus species and/or genera [3]. The main utility of these tools for the wider virology community is to ensure the objective and accurate classification of the large numbers of new complete virus genome or genome component sequences that are deposited into public databases each year.

The computational tool that is currently most widely used for this purpose within the geminivirus community is Sequence Demarcation Tool (SDT) [4]. SDT can be used either as a component of sequence analysis pipelines or as a stand-alone program with a user-friendly graphical interface that is currently Windows OS specific. It enables classification of virus sequences based on pairwise alignment and sequence identity calculations [4]. SDT is functionally similar to tools such as PASC (PAirwise Sequence Comparison [5]), the MegAlign clustal algorithm (DNAstar [6]), and DEmARC (DivErsity pArtitioning by hieRarchical Clustering [7]). Whereas DEmARC and the MegAlign clustal algorithm focus on classifications of sequences using pairwise identities calculated from multiple sequence alignments, PASC and SDT focus on achieving this using pairwise alignments.

Basically, SDT aligns all possible pairs of sequences using MUSCLE [8], ClustalW2 [9] or MAFFT [10], calculates Needleman-Wunsch (NW) [11] pairwise alignment-based genetic identity scores for each pair and uses a rooted neighbor-joining phylogenetic tree to cluster closely related sequences based on these identity scores. Further, SDT produces publication quality color-coded pairwise-identity matrices with sequences ordered according to their degrees of phylogenetic relatedness.

Over the past 10 years since its publication, SDT has been extensively used for the establishment of new genera in the family *Geminiviridae* [3] and for the classification of hundreds of new species within individual geminivirus genera [1, 2]. Besides its use by geminivirologists, SDT has also been helpful for classifying viruses in a significant number of virus families such as the *Anelloviridae* [12], *Circoviridae* [13], *Nanoviridae* [14], *Polyomaviridae* [15], and *Rhabdoviridae* [16].

2 Materials

2.1 Operating System

While the graphical user interface version of SDT (SDTv1.2) is a free Windows-based program. Command-line versions are also available for Linux (SDT_Linux) and MacOS (SDT_MacOS), and a parallel message passing interface-based version for Linux (SDTMPI_Linux) can be used on high performance computing clusters.

2.2 Download and Installation

1. The program can be downloaded from http://web.cbio.uct.ac.za/SDT.
2. Download the SDTv1.2_setup.exe file.
3. Run the SDTv1.2_setup.exe file as administrator, i.e., right-click and choose the "run as administrator" menu option that appears.
4. Follow the instructions of the setup program and use the default installation directory "C:\SDTv1.2".
5. The program folder SDTv1.2 contains the following:
   - A bin directory containing the following programs: MUSCLE [8], ClustalW2 [9] or MAFFT [10], and Neighbor (http://evolution.genetics.washington.edu/phylip.html).
   - A tmp directory that is used to store temporary files (*see* **Note 1**).
   - The executable SDTv1.2.exe which is the main program.
   - A README file which contains these instructions.
   - A FASTA file, test.fas, and a .SDT file, test.sdt, to test the program.
   - Two SDT files: mastrevirus_references.sdt and mastrevirus_references.fas used previously for classification of new mastreviruses.
   - Program configuration files: sdt.in, ST5UNST.txt and SDTv1.exe.manifest.
6. To start an analysis double-click the SDTv1.2.exe file and, when the program has launched (Fig. 1a), drag and either (i) drop on the main screen a fasta-formated file containing the sequences to be analyzed (*see* **Note 2**) or (ii) click on the "Open" menu on the top left side of the program window and select the FASTA file you want to analyze (*see* **Note 3**).
7. Select the alignment program you want to use.
8. Click the Run button.
9. When the run has completed the results can be saved in .SDT file format by clicking on the "Save" menu item.

The "Open" menu item can be used to load .SDT files containing past analysis results. Once a past analysis is loaded from a .SDT file the "Append" menu item can be used to load a FASTA file containing one or more additional sequences which will then all be compared both to each other and the sequences represented in the .SDT file.

The graphical outputs of SDT can be copied to the clipboard so that they can be pasted directly into programs such as PowerPoint or Word.

3 Methods

3.1 The SDT Main Menu

1. The Open menu (Fig. 1a) enables loading of input files (Fig. 1b), which the program will detect either as FASTA files (in which case the user is prompted to choose an alignment program to use for pairwise identity score calculation), or SDT files (in which case the program will give an option to append one or more sequences in FASTA format). Then, choose the alignment program (Fig. 1c), including MUSCLE, ClustalW2 or MAFFT programs. Pressing the "Run" command button initiates pairwise sequence alignment, the calculation of pairwise identity scores and the display of these scores in the form of a color-coded matrix. The checkbox at the bottom (by default checked) can be used to display the sequences ordered by phylogenetic relatedness (if the box is checked) or in their input orders (if the box is left unchecked, Fig. 1d).
2. The Save menu can be used to save various analysis results in a variety of formats after an analysis has completed.

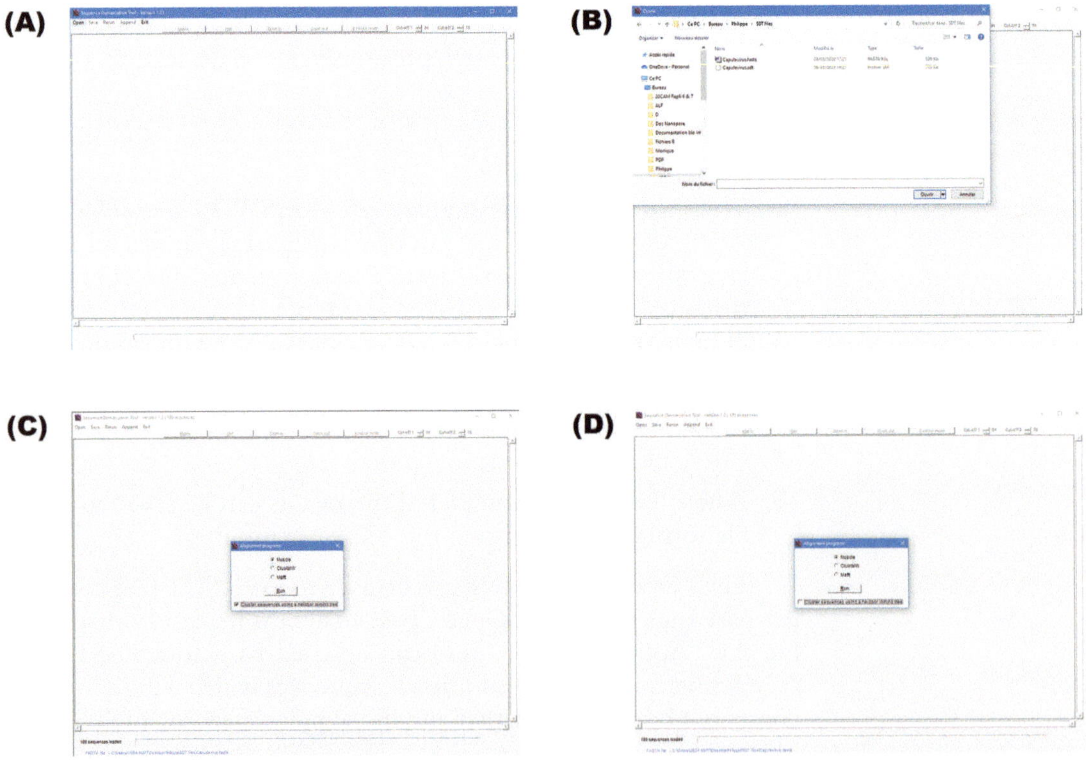

Fig. 1 (**a**) First window when the program is launched. (**b**) Choose a file (.sdt or .fasta) after having clicked on the Open command button. (**c**) Small window for selection of sequence alignment program after having clicked on the Run command button. (**d**) Uncheck the checkbox at the bottom if you do not want to display the sequences ordered by phylogenetic relatedness

3. The Rerun menu can be used to run the analysis on the loaded alignment using a different alignment program.
4. The Append menu can be used to add sequences to a loaded SDT file.
5. The Exit menu can be used to terminate the program.

3.2 SDT Main Command Buttons

1. Pressing the "Matrix" command button will result in a color-coded matrix (*see* **Note 4**) being displayed (Fig. 2a). Pressing the "Plot" command button will result in a distribution of pairwise identity scores being plotted (Fig. 2b).
2. The "Zoom in" and "Zoom out" command buttons can be used to enlarge or reduce the sizes of plot and matrix images.
3. The "Three color mode" command button allows switching between "full color spectrum" mode and the "three colors" mode (Fig. 2c) for the color-coded matrix representation of identity scores.
4. In "three colors mode" a discontinuous range of red, green and blue shades can be used to differentiate pairwise identity scores above and below two user defined threshold values. In Fig. 2b one cut-off value is set to 95% and the other to 84%. Such cut-offs might represent species or strain demarcation thresholds.

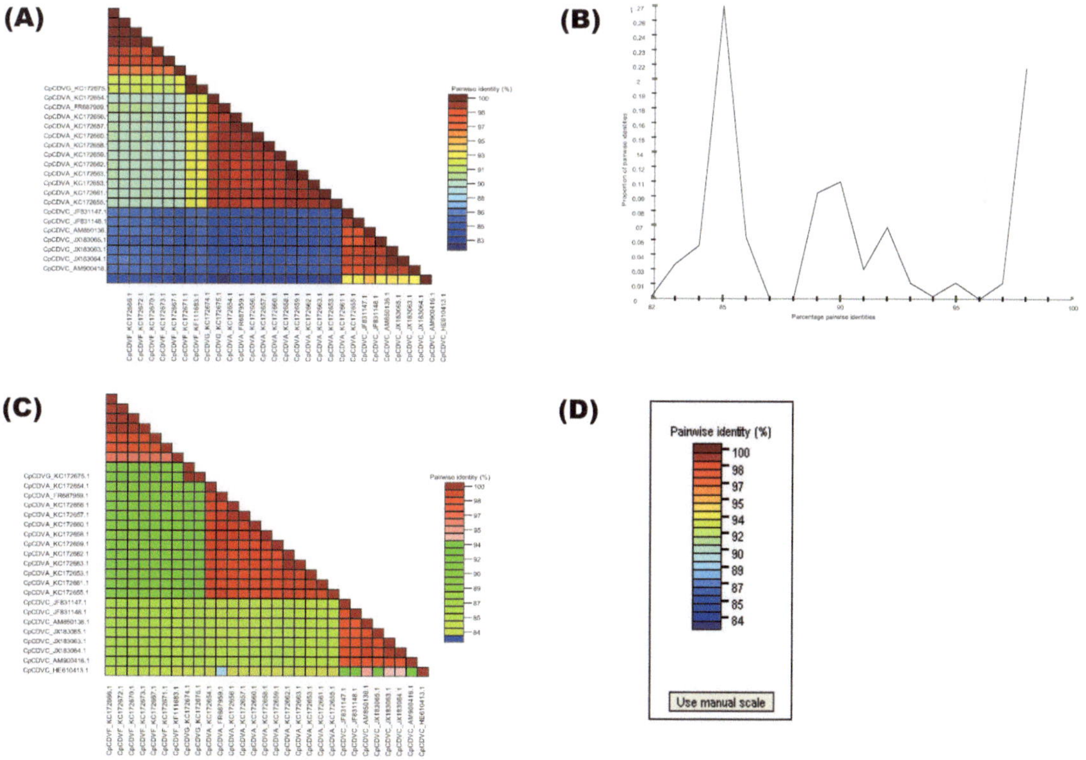

Fig. 2 (**a**) 2D color-coded matrix. (**b**) A plot displaying the distribution of pairwise identity scores. (**c**) 2D "three colors mode" coded matrix. (**d**) Command button to adjust color scale

5. The "Up" and "Down" buttons allow for adjustment of the two demarcation cut-offs when displaying matrices three color mode.
6. The "Use manual scale" command button (Fig. 2d) allows changing the color scale used in pairwise identities matrix.

3.3 Submenus

1. The "Save SDT file" submenu (Fig. 3a) can be used to save the sequence analysis results and the pairwise identity scores into a . SDT file for future analyses. This saves time in that the program will then not need to recalculate pairwise identity scores that have already been calculated. New sequences or even whole alignments can be appended to old. SDT datasets are analyzed much more quickly than if the entire dataset was analyzed from scratch.
2. The "Save identity scores" submenu (Fig. 3b) can be used to save sequence identity scores in a spreadsheet-readable text file format as either a single column (Fig. 3c) or a matrix (i.e., multiple columns; Fig. 3d).
3. The "Save matrix picture" submenu (Fig. 3e) can be used to save a 2D color-coded graphical image of the matrix as either an .EMF (enhanced meta file, vector graphic format that is good for rescaling) or a .BMP (bitmap graphic format that is not good for rescaling).

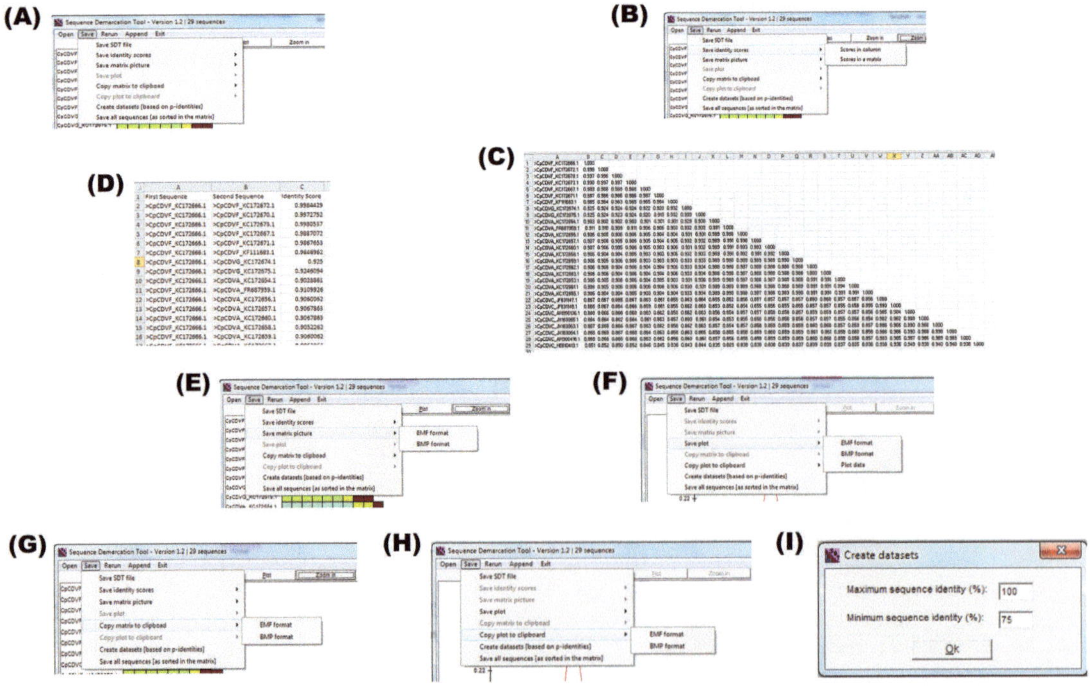

Fig. 3 (**a**) Save SDT file submenu. (**b**) Save identity scores submenu. (**c**) Column format. (**d**) Matrix format, (**e**) Save matrix picture submenu. (**f**) Save plot submenu. (**g**) Copy matrix to clipboard submenu. (**h**) Copy plot to clipboard submenu. (**i**) Small window for choosing the range of identities

4. The "Save plot" submenu (Fig. 3f) can be used to save the pairwise identity distribution plot in either .EMF or .BMP formats, or as a spreadsheet-readable list of the data used to produce the plot.
5. The "Copy matrix to clipboard" submenus (Fig. 3g) can be used to copy the matrix to the clipboard in either .EMF or . BMP formats so that it can be pasted into another program such as Microsoft Word, Powerpoint or any other graphical editor such as Adobe Illustrator.
6. The "Copy plot to clipboard" submenus (Fig. 3h) can be used to copy the plot image in either .EMF or .BMP formats to the clipboard so that it can be pasted into another program such as Word or Powerpoint.
7. The "Create datasets [based on p-identities]" submenu (Fig. 3i) can be used to objectively create datasets of sequences sharing a desired level of diversity/similarity to suite further genome evolution analyses such as inference of patterns of natural selection or the identification of conserved genomic secondary structures [17, 18]. After the sequence identity scores have been computed, a user must enter a maximum and minimum identity percentage in the "create datasets" window (Fig. 3i). The program will then partition the input sequence dataset into sets of nonoverlapping sequence files, with each file containing only sequence pairs with identities that are within the user-specified range.
8. "Save all sequences [as sorted in the Matrix]" submenu can be used to create a dataset of all sequences arranged as they appear in the matrix after clustering using a neighbor-joining tree.

4 Notes

1. At the end of every run the program saves all the output files into the tmp folder which a user can then manually retrieve if, for example, either the user forgets to save the analysis results before quitting, or the program unexpectedly crashes at the end of a run (this will occasionally happen if the dataset being analyzed is very large). The files stored in the tmp folder will all be overwritten during the next run of the program.
2. Large datasets containing 1000 sequences that are each ~2800 nt long will take approximately 3 days to analyze. In such cases (and even for much larger datasets) SDTMPI, a parallelized version of SDT, could be used. SDTMPI only calculates a matrix of pairwise identity scores but does not produce either the graphical identity score matrix or the pairwise identity score distribution plots. Given access to a

computer cluster with several processors, SDT produces a completed pairwise identity score matrix approximately 19–38 times quicker than SDT when running on 20–40 cores respectively (SDTMPI is available at http://web.cbio.uct.ac.za/SDT).

3. A user must ensure that the new sequences start at the same position as the sequences already loaded.
4. SDT does not display a color-coded matrix for datasets containing more than 500 sequences. It does, however, allow users to save the matrix to a file in either .BMP or .EMF formats.

References

1. Brown JK, Zerbini FM, Navas-Castillo J, Moriones E, Ramos-Sobrinho R, Silva JC, Fiallo-Olive E, Briddon RW, Hernandez-Zepeda C, Idris A, Malathi VG, Martin DP, Rivera-Bustamante R, Ueda S, Varsani A (2015) Revision of *Begomovirus* taxonomy based on pairwise sequence comparisons. Arch Virol 160:1593–1619
2. Muhire B, Martin DP, Brown JK, Navas-Castillo J, Moriones E, Zerbini FM, Rivera-Bustamante R, Malathi VG, Briddon RW, Varsani A (2013) A genome-wide pairwise-identity-based proposal for the classification of viruses in the genus *Mastrevirus* (family *Geminiviridae*). Arch Virol 158:1411–1424
3. Roumagnac P, Lett JM, Fiallo-Olivé E, Navas-Castillo J, Zerbini FM, Martin DP, Varsani A (2021) Establishment of five new genera in the family *Geminiviridae*: *Citlodavirus*, *Maldovirus*, *Mulcrilevirus*, *Opunvirus*, and *Topilevirus*. Arch Virol 167:695–710
4. Muhire BM, Varsani A, Martin DP (2014) SDT: a virus classification tool based on pairwise sequence alignment and identity calculation. PLoS One 9:e108277
5. Bao Y, Chetvernin V, Tatusova T (2012) PAirwise sequence comparison (PASC) and its application in the classification of filoviruses. Viruses 4:1318–1327
6. Fauquet CM, Stanley J (2003) Geminivirus classification and nomenclature: Progress and problems. Ann Appl Biol 142:165–189
7. Lauber C, Gorbalenya AE (2012) Partitioning the genetic diversity of a virus family: approach and evaluation through a case study of picornaviruses. J Virol 86:3890–3904
8. Edgar RC (2004) MUSCLE: multiple sequence alignment with high accuracy and high throughput. Nucleic Acids Res 32:1792–1797
9. Larkin MA, Blackshields G, Brown NP, Chenna R, McGettigan PA, McWilliam H, Valentin F, Wallace IM, Wilm A, Lopez R, Thompson JD, Gibson TJ, Higgins DG (2007) Clustal W and Clustal X version 2.0. Bioinformatics 23:2947–2948
10. Katoh K, Standley DM (2013) MAFFT multiple sequence alignment software version 7: improvements in performance and usability. Mol Biol Evol 30:772–780
11. Needleman SB, Wunsch CD (1970) A general method applicable to the search for similarities in the amino acid sequence of two proteins. J Mol Biol 48:443–453
12. Wang X, Chen X, Song X, Cao L, Yang S, Shen Q, Ji L, Lu X, Zhang W (2023) Identification of novel anelloviruses in the blood of giant panda (*Ailuropoda melanoleuca*). Comp Immun Microbiol Inf Dis 100:102038
13. Morandini V, Dugger KM, Ballard G, Elrod M, Schmidt A, Ruoppolo V, Lescroël A, Jongsomjit D, Massaro M, Pennycook J, Kooyman GL, Schmidlin K, Kraberger S, Ainley DG, Varsani A (2019) Identification of a novel Adélie penguin circovirus at Cape Crozier (Ross Island, Antarctica). Viruses 11:1088
14. Vetten HJ, Knierim D, Rakoski MS, Menzel W, Maiss E, Gronenborn B, Winter S, Krenz B (2019) Identification of a novel nanovirus in parsley. Arch Virol 164:1883–1887
15. Abrantes J, Varsani A, Pereira P, Maia C, Farias I, Veríssimo A, Neves F (2023) Identification and characterization of a polyomavirus in the thornback skate (*Raja clavata*). Virol J 20:190
16. Bejerman N, Dietzgen RG, Debat H (2022) Unlocking the hidden genetic diversity of varicosaviruses, the neglected plant rhabdoviruses. Pathogens 11:1127

17. Muhire BM, Golden M, Murrell B, Lefeuvre P, Lett JM, Gray A, Poon AY, Ngandu NK, Semegni Y, Tanov EP, Monjane AL, Harkins GW, Varsani A, Shepherd DN, Martin DP (2013) Evidence of pervasive biologically functional secondary structures within the genomes of eukaryotic single-stranded DNA viruses. J Virol 8:1972–1989

18. Stenzel T, Piasecki T, Chrząstek K, Julian L, Muhire BM, Golden M, Martin DP, Varsani A (2014) Pigeon circoviruses display patterns of recombination, genomic secondary structure and selection similar to those of beak and feather disease viruses. J Gen Virol 95:1338–1351

Chapter 10

Phylogenetic Analysis of Geminiviruses

Roberto Ramos-Sobrinho

Abstract

Members of the family *Geminiviridae* have single-stranded (ss), circular DNA genomes that are encapsidated into non-enveloped quasi-icosahedral twinned (geminate) particles, causing yield losses in several economically important crops worldwide. Sequence-based approaches used for molecular characterization of *Geminiviridae* genomes, associated with powerful bioinformatic tools, provided a better picture about the true extent of the *Geminiviridae* species diversity. This chapter describes procedures to reconstruct *Geminiviridae* phylogenetic relationships based on coat protein (CP) and replication-associated protein (Rep) amino acid sequences and full-length nucleotide genomes using both maximum likelihood (ML) and Bayesian inference (BI) approaches. Although topological incongruences can be observed among the ML phylogenetic trees for CP, Rep, and genome sequences, suggesting inter-genera recombination, *Geminiviridae* exemplar viruses predominantly cluster according to the genera recognized by the International Committee on Taxonomy of Viruses.

Key words Plant viruses, ssDNA, *Geminiviridae*, Molecular phylogeny, Maximum likelihood, Bayesian inference

1 Introduction

The family *Geminiviridae* includes plant viruses with single-stranded (ss), circular DNA genomes of 2.5–5.2 kb in length, which are encapsidated into non-enveloped quasi-icosahedral twinned (geminate) particles. Geminiviruses infect a wide range of noncultivated and cultivated plants in tropical and subtropical regions worldwide, affecting crops of great socioeconomical importance [1]. Currently, 520 geminivirus species are officially recognized by the International Committee on Taxonomy of Viruses (ICTV; ictv.global/report/geminiviridae), classified into 14 genera (*Becurtovirus*, *Begomovirus*, *Capulavirus*, *Citlodavirus*, *Curtovirus*, *Eragrovirus*, *Grablovirus*, *Maldovirus*, *Mastrevirus*, *Mulcrilevirus*, *Opunvirus*, *Topilevirus*, *Topocuvirus*, and *Turncurtovirus*) based on host range, insect vector, genome organization, and phylogenetic relationships [1]. Most geminiviruses are transmitted by insects

Francisco Murilo Zerbini et al. (eds.), *Geminiviruses: Methods and Protocols*, Methods in Molecular Biology, vol. 2912,
https://doi.org/10.1007/978-1-0716-4454-6_10,

from at least four homopteran groups, including whiteflies (*Begomovirus*), leafhoppers (*Becurtovirus*, *Curtovirus*, *Mastrevirus*, *Mulcrilevirus*, and *Turncurtovirus*), aphids (*Capulavirus*), and treehoppers (*Grablovirus* and *Topocuvirus*), while no insect vector is known, thus far, for members of the genera *Citlodavirus*, *Eragrovirus*, *Maldovirus*, *Opunvirus*, and *Topilevirus* [1].

The genus *Begomovirus* is the largest geminivirus group, being comprised by 445 species infecting dicotyledonous hosts and are naturally transmitted by whiteflies of the *Bemisia tabaci* cryptic species complex [2]. Members of the genus *Begomovirus* can be either mono- or bipartite (genomic components commonly referred to as DNA-A and DNA-B), whereas the viruses classified into the other 13 genera have only one ssDNA molecule [1, 2]. The second largest group is the genus *Mastrevirus*, with 45 species that infect mostly monocotyledonous and some dicotyledonous plants and are transmitted by different leafhopper species [1, 3], followed by the genera *Capulavirus* ($n = 4$), *Citlodavirus* ($n = 4$), *Becurtovirus* ($n = 3$), *Curtovirus* ($n = 3$), *Grablovirus* ($n = 3$), *Maldovirus* ($n = 3$), *Turncurtovirus* ($n = 3$), *Mulcrilevirus* ($n = 2$), *Topilevirus* ($n = 2$), *Opunvirus* ($n = 1$), *Eragrovirus* ($n = 1$), and *Topocuvirus* ($n = 1$) (ictv.global/report/geminiviridae).

The increasing number of geminivirus genomes described and publicly available in genetic sequence databases has been greatly impacted by studies employing sequence-independent approaches such as rolling circle amplification (RCA) [4–8], and more recently, high-throughput sequencing (HTS) techniques [9–13]. These approaches have also yielded a better understanding about the true extent of plant virus diversity, including *Geminiviridae*, within both managed and natural environments [9, 11, 14–16]. Amongst the *Geminiviridae*-encoded proteins, the coat protein (CP) and replication-associated protein (Rep) seem to be the only coding regions conserved across members into this family and, therefore, have been largely used to reconstruct their phylogenetic relationships [5, 8, 11–13, 17–19].

In the present chapter, the current list of exemplar viruses for each *Geminiviridae* species was obtained from the Virus Metadata Resource (VMR) at the ICTV repository (ictv.global/vmr), and the GenBank accession numbers from reference sequences (RefSeqs) were used to retrieve full-length genomes from the nonredundant NCBI database (ncbi.nlm.nih.gov/genbank/). The nucleotide sequences were manually edited to start at the nicking site in the conserved nonanucleotide at the viral replication origin (TAATATT//AC and TAAGATT//CC). Further, the open reading frames (ORFs) for both CP (V1/AV1) and Rep (C1/AC1/C1:C2) were obtained from each geminivirus isolate and translated into amino acid sequences using Geneious v.8.1.9 (geneious.com). Multiple nucleotide (DNA-A) and amino acid (CP, Rep, and concatenated CP-Rep) sequence alignments were obtained using the MUSCLE algorithm [20], and manually adjusted in MEGA v.11 [21]. The phylogenetic relationship of *Geminiviridae* species based on the complete genome, CP, Rep, and concatenated CP-Rep datasets was reconstructed using 1000 ultrafast bootstrap replicates [22] implemented in IQ-TREE [23]. Protocols to reconstruct ML phylogenetic trees in PAUP v.4 [24] and RAxML v.8 [25], and BI phylogenies using MrBayes v.3.2.6 [26] through the CIPRES web portal [27] are also described. The best-fit nucleotide and amino acid substitution models were determined using IQ-TREE, but methods to perform this analysis in jModelTest v2.1.10 (github.com/ddarriba/jmodeltest2/releases/tag/v2.1.10r20160303), MrModeltest v2 (github.com/nylander/MrModeltest2), and ProtTest v3.4.2 (github.com/ddarriba/prottest3/releases) are shown. The trees were edited in FigTree v.1.4 (ztree.bio.ed.ac.uk/software/figtree) and Inkscape (https://inkscape.org/pt/).

2 Materials

1. List of exemplar viruses (Virus Metadata Resource—VMR) available at the International Committee on Taxonomy of Viruses (ICTV) webpage (ictv.global/vmr).
2. List of GenBank accession numbers for *Geminiviridae* reference sequences (RefSeqs) included in the VMR spreadsheet.
3. *Geminiviridae* reference sequences available at the NCBI-GenBank database (ncbi.nlm.nih.gov/genbank/).
4. Multiple sequence alignments in different formats such as FASTA, MEGA, PHYLIP, and NEXUS.
5. MEGA v.11 program [21], a tool package for conducting automatic and manual sequence alignment, inferring phylogenetic trees, and others. Available at megasoftware.net.
6. Geneious package (geneious.com). This is a commercially available program, but a free trial can be requested.
7. MUSCLE algorithm [20] for sequence alignment (implemented in both MEGA v.11 and Geneious).
8. IQ-TREE v2 software [23], an open-source software under the GNU-GPL for selecting nucleotide and amino acid substitution models and constructing ML phylogenies. Freely available at iqtree.org/#download.
9. jModelTest v2 software, a commonly used tool to carry out statistical selection of best-fit substitution models for nucleotide sequence data. Available at github.com/ddarriba/jmodeltest2/releases/tag/v2.1.10r20160303.

10. MrModeltest v.2 [28], a largely used tool to perform statistical selection of best-fit substitution models for nucleotide sequence data. Available at github.com/nylander/MrModeltest2.
11. Command Prompt, a command line interpreter application available in most Windows operating systems.
12. Notepad application available in most Windows operating systems.
13. PDF reader, a software used to open and view Portable Document Format (PDF) files.
14. Java application (java.com), which is a widely used object-oriented programming language and software platform that runs sequence analysis and phylogenetic tree editing programs.
15. ProtTest v.3 program, a tool to perform statistical selection of best-fit substitution models for amino acid sequence data. Available at github.com/ddarriba/prottest3/releases.
16. PAUP v.4.0b8 package [24], a program to reconstruct ML phylogenetic trees. Available at phylosolutions.com/paup-test/.
17. RAxML v.8 [25], a program to reconstruct ML-based phylogenetic trees employing a fast-bootstrap approach. Available at github.com/stamatak/standard-RAxML/tree/master.
18. MrBayes v.3 software [26], largely used to reconstruct phylogenetic trees employing a Bayesian Inference method. Available at nbisweden.github.io/MrBayes/download.html.
19. FigTree v.1, a well-known graphical viewer tool used for editing phylogenetic trees. Available at github.com/rambaut/figtree/.
20. Inkscape v.1, a freely available (inkscape.org/pt/) program for creating and editing vector images.

3 Methods

3.1 Building a *Geminiviridae* Dataset

1. Download the updated list of exemplar viruses from the Virus Metadata Resource (VMR) at the ICTV webpage (ictv.global/vmr). The spreadsheet is comprised by a list of species from all viral groups accepted by the ICTV.
2. Search for *Geminiviridae*. You will find columns containing several information such as family (here, *Geminiviridae*), genera, species, GenBank accession numbers, acronyms, and others.
3. In the VMR spreadsheet, search for the GenBank accession numbers of Reference Sequences (RefSeqs). In this chapter,

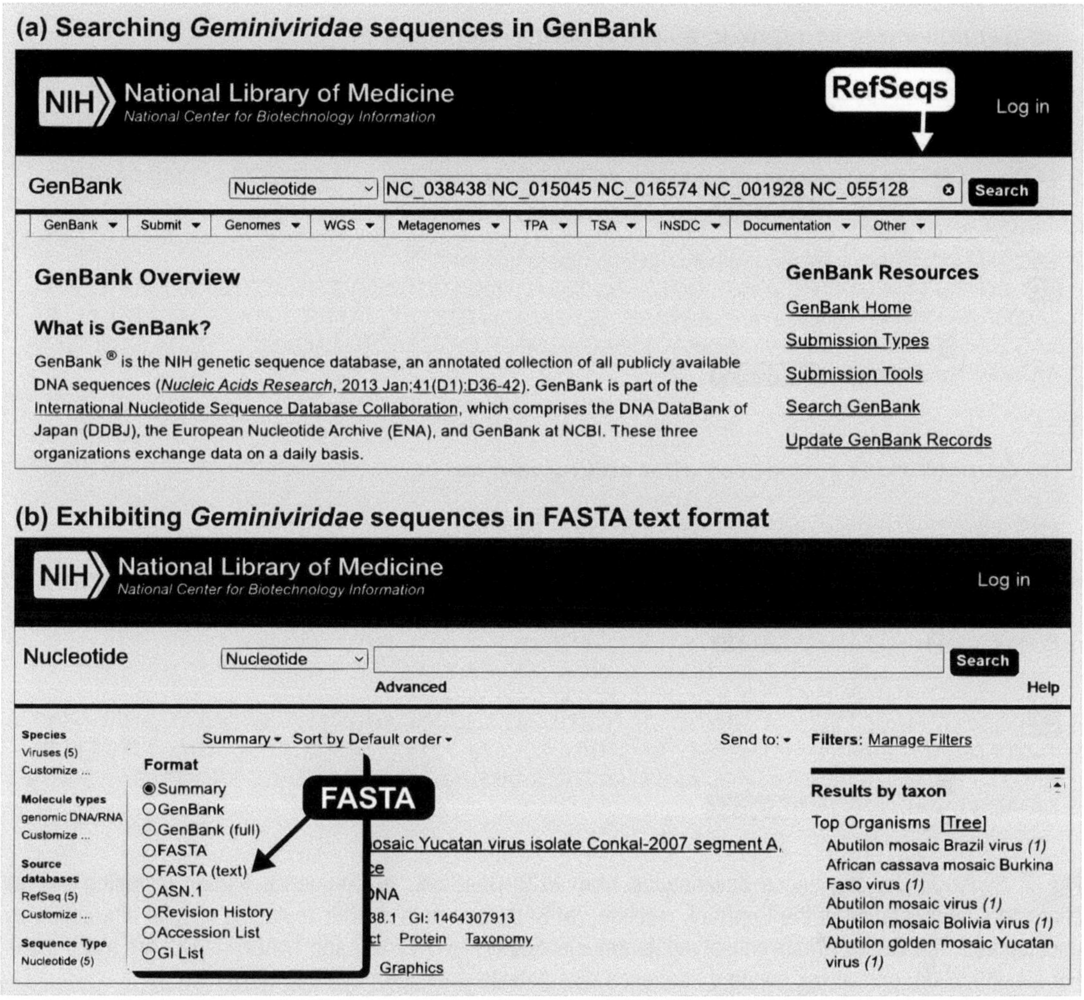

Fig. 1 GenBank website overview: (**a**) Searching for reference sequences (RefSeqs) of *Geminiviridae*; (**b**) Displaying *Geminiviridae* RefSeqs in FASTA format

most *Geminiviridae* RefSeqs were used to reconstruct the ML phylogenetic trees for members into this family. Due to the high number of species, especially in the genera *Begomovirus* and *Mastrevirus*, representative species and/or isolates can be selected for your analysis.

4. Download the *Geminiviridae* RefSeqs (full-length sequences) from GenBank (ncbi.nlm.nih.gov/genbank/). You can Copy the GenBank accession numbers directly from the VMR spreadsheet and Paste in the Search tile at the GenBank website (Fig. 1a). For *Begomovirus*, only DNA-A components were used here. After you click on Search, the list of sequences will be shown. Then, go to the Summary tile and click on FASTA

(a) *Geminiviridae* sequences as presented in GenBank

```
>NC_000882.1 Pepper leaf curl virus, complete genome
ACCGGATGGCCGCGATTTTTTTTCAAGTGGTCCCCCCGCGTGCGCTGGACCAATCATAACCATCCC
TCAAAGCTTGCATGCCTGCAGGTTATCCCATCAAAACGTGGTCCCCAAGTACTTACATCAAAACATG
TGGGATC...TTTATATGGAGACCCAATGGCATTATTGTAATTATGGAAAAGTACTTTAATTCAAATACCC
AAAGCGGCCATCCGTATAATATT

>NC_010417.1 Beet curly top Iran virus-[K], complete genome
CCCCGCGTTTACCTTTCCACGTGGCGTATGCTGAGTGGGCGGACGGTTGAGTGGGGAACACGCTT
TACTTTAAATTAAAGTAAAGTAGCACTAAGTGGGACCCACTTTTTTTATTTCTTTAAAGACTTTCTTTTT
AAGTCTT...TATGAGAGGAAGAGGAACTTAAGAGGAATGAGGAACTGAAGAGGGAGGTAGAGGGATA
AATAGGTAAACGCGGATAAGATT
```

(b) *Geminiviridae* sequences after editing names

```
>NC_000882_1_Pepper_leaf_curl_virus_complete_genome
ACCGGATGGCCGCGATTTTTTTTCAAGTGGTCCCCCCGCGTGCGCTGGACCAATCATAACCATCCC
TCAAAGCTTGCATGCCTGCAGGTTATCCCATCAAAACGTGGTCCCCAAGTACTTACATCAAAACATG
TGGGATC...TTTATATGGAGACCCAATGGCATTATTGTAATTATGGAAAAGTACTTTAATTCAAATACCC
AAAGCGGCCATCCGTATAATATT

>NC_010417_1_Beet_curly_top_Iran_virus_K_complete_genome
CCCCGCGTTTACCTTTCCACGTGGCGTATGCTGAGTGGGCGGACGGTTGAGTGGGGAACACGCTT
TACTTTAAATTAAAGTAAAGTAGCACTAAGTGGGACCCACTTTTTTTATTTCTTTAAAGACTTTCTTTTT
AAGTCTT...TATGAGAGGAAGAGGAACTTAAGAGGAATGAGGAACTGAAGAGGGAGGTAGAGGGATA
AATAGGTAAACGCGGATAAGATT
```

Fig. 2 *Geminiviridae* sequences downloaded from NCBI-GenBank: (**a**) Sequence names including special characters as presented in the GenBank website; (**b**) Sequence names after replacing special characters by underscores. The *Geminiviridae* conserved nonanucleotides (TAATATT//AC and TAAGATT//CC) are highlighted. For simplification, part of the genome sequence was deleted (indicated by three dots)

(text) (a new window will be opened containing the sequence information in FASTA format) (Fig. 1b).

5. Copy all sequences and paste into a Notepad file. Go to File → Save (select the folder directory), type the file name using FASTA extension (FileName.fas or FileName.fasta), change the file type to All files, and click on Save. This allows you to easily open the sequence file in MEGA by double clicking on it. The name of each FASTA sequence is preceded by the symbol >. You must avoid Space and special characters (such as "‘, .; /: -) in the sequence name as they will create error warnings when running the phylogenetic analysis. The most appropriated solution is to replace them with an underscore (Fig. 2a). Also, shorter names like Accession Number followed by Virus Acronym should be used (>NC_000882_PepLCV instead of >NC_000882_1_Pepper_leaf_curl_virus_complete_genomes; Fig. 2b).

6. In MEGA, visually check each sequence to guarantee they start at the nicking site in the conserved nonanucleotide at the viral replication origin (TAATATT//AC or TAAGATT//CC), where AC or CC are the first two positions of the *Geminiviridae* genomes (Fig. 3). Manually edit when it is needed, so all sequences start at AC or CC and end with TAATATT or TAAGATT (Fig. 3).
7. Go to the tile Data → Export alignment → FASTA Format, select the file directory and save it as FileName.fas or FileName.fasta (for example, geminiviridae.fas or geminiviridae.fasta).
8. The sequence file is now ready to prepare multiple nucleotide sequence alignments for complete genomes of *Geminiviridae.*
9. The *Geminiviridae* genome dataset can be used to retrieve ORFs V1/AV1=CP and C1/AC1/C1:C2 = Rep using Geneious (geneious.com) or any commercially/freely available program for sequence analysis that has an ORF finder tool implemented. Once the ORFs are recovered, create a FASTA file for each CP and Rep datasets (for example, cp.fas and rep.fas). It is important to make sure the CP and Rep sequences from a same exemplar virus (RefSeq) have identical names as it will allow the concatenation of these two genomic regions after translation to amino acid sequences and alignment (Fig. 4).

3.2 Creating Multiple Sequence Alignments for Nucleotide Sequences

1. Open the *Geminiviridae* genome dataset previously saved in FASTA format. In the main window of MEGA, click on the tile File → Open a File/Session and search for the directory where the FASTA file is located (select your file and open it). A window with the message Analyze or Align file? will pop-up (click on Align and the nucleotide sequences will be shown).
2. Click on the tile Alignment → Align by Muscle and a new window with the message Nothing selected for alignment. Select all? will pop-up (click on OK). Then, a new window for editing the Muscle parameters will be opened (click on OK and the Muscle algorithm will carry out the sequence alignment using standard parameters).
3. Visually check the whole alignment once it is done (manually edit it if needed). You will notice the program adds some gaps, represented by the character -, to the aligned sequences (gaps are added to optimize the alignment of homolog sites).
4. You have to save the *Geminiviridae* sequence alignment using both FASTA and MEGA formats.
5. Go to the tile Data → Export alignment → FASTA Format. Select the file directory and save it as FileName.fas (here, geminiviridae_align.fas).

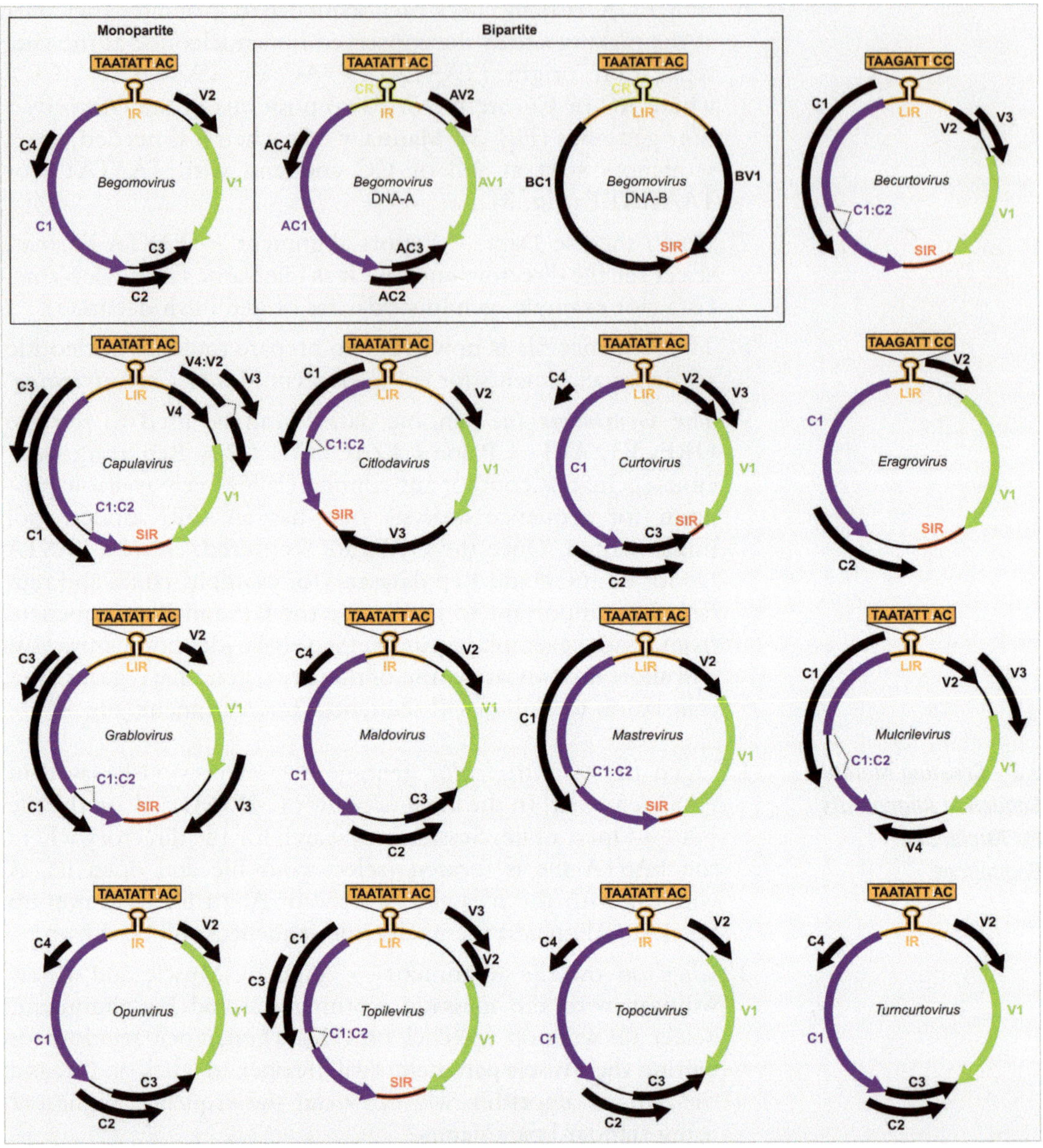

Fig. 3 Typical genome organization of viruses included into the family *Geminiviridae*. The open reading frames (ORFs) encoded on both viral (V) and complementary (C) strands are shown. V1/AV1 = coat protein (CP); V2/AV2 = movement protein (MP, absent in New World begomoviruses) or putative MP; V3 = putative MP or putative regulatory (regulatory in *Curtovirus*); V4 = unknown; C1/AC1/C1:C2 = replication-associated protein (Rep); C2/AC2 = transcriptional activator protein (TrAP), RNA-silencing suppressor (ss) or putative TrAP/ss; C3/AC3 = replication enhancer protein (Ren); C4/AC4 = silencing suppressor (ss) or putative ss; BV1 = nuclear shuttle protein (NSP); BC1 = MP; IR = intergenic region; CR = common region; LIR = long intergenic region; and SIR = short intergenic region. The conserved nonanucleotides at the origin of virion strand replication are highlighted in orange boxes. The proteins shared by all geminiviruses, and largely used to reconstruct the phylogenetic relationship among these viruses, are indicated in dark green (CP) and purple (Rep)

(a) Sequence names in the amino acid data set of *Geminiviridae* CP

```
>NC_000882_1_Pepper_leaf_curl_virus_complete_genome
MSKRPADIVISTPASKVRRRLNFDSPYVSRAAAPTVLVTNKRRSWANRTMYRKPRIYRMYKSPDVPRGC
EGPCKVQSYEQRHDVAHVGKVICVSDVTRGNGLTHRVGKGPVIKSVYVWGRIWMDEISSQESHQSVM
FFLVRDRRPFGTPQDFGQVFNMYDNEPSTATVKNDNRDRFQVLRRFQATVTGGQYASKEQAIVRKFMK
VNNHVTYNHQEAAKYDNHTENALLLYMACTHASNPVYATLKIRIYFYDSVQN

>NC_010417_1_Beet_curly_top_Iran_virus_K_complete_genome
MAVQSQKRKYTPPASWTRKRKTTGGRTVWKKYQWKRPVRSNRAVKLKMYDDMLGASGVGSTISNDG
MITMLNNYVQGIGDSQRSNNLTVTRHLKFDMSLMASGAFWASPNYMTQYHWVIVDRDVGSTFPTQLST
IFDIPTGGQAMPSTYRIRRDANERFIVKKKWQTHLMSTGTDYGGKQTYKAPSMPNYKKAMNINIRNINVK
TLWKDTGGGKYEDVKENAILYVVVNDNTDNTNMYATLFGNCRAYFY
```

(b) Sequence names in the amino acid data set of *Geminiviridae* Rep

```
>NC_000882_1_Pepper_leaf_curl_virus_complete_genome
MAPPKNLRINAKNYFLTYPHCSLTKEEALSQIQAIETPTIKLFIRICRELHEDGTPHLHILIQFEGKFQCKNP
RFFDLTSPTRSAHFHPNIQGAKSSTDVKEYIAKNGDVLDHGVFQIDGRSARGGCQSANDAYAEALNSGT
KASALAILKEEAPKDYILQFHNLNSNLDKIFSLRIEMYISPFLVSFDQVQRNLNEWVAANVVKPARPLRPISI
VVEGDSRTGKTMWARSLGPHNYLCGHLDLSPKVYNNDPWYNVIDDVDPHYLKHFKEFMGAQRDWQS
NTKYGKPVQIKGGIPTIFLCNPGPHSSYKEFLEEEKNTALKNWALKNAIFVTIEGPLFSGSHQGATQNRQ
EDN

>NC_010417_1_Beet_curly_top_Iran_virus_K_complete_genome
MPRAPNRNRPTPNQPGYLRFQKKNAFLTYSQIGGDFKDYIFEKLKTLLESYVILSLAVSLEHHQPTEEQP
EGGFHTHCIIQCDKKLDVNGNLFFNIILPDGRTIHPRIDGLNAPKRAFEYITKEDTSPRTFGELRLGGRSP
NSIGNSNVEWRRILDSSNTKEEFFSNIRESCPTDFVLRWPSILSFANNHFRPVVQPYTPRWTEFSRLPD
TIKEWAEQNIYFVSSDCLHYEICENCRGAILQDRQMTLEEYFHLDRLSGDLACSEDTNVLNLSRSQTTD
QSDQEVSTYADPPEQERPSGQDL
```

Fig. 4 The sequences belonging to a same *Geminiviridae* exemplar virus have identical names in both (**a**) coat protein (CP) and (**b**) replication-associated protein (Rep) datasets, which can be used to concatenate both datasets using bioinformatic packages such as Geneious and MEGA

6. Then, click on Data → Export alignment → MEGA Format. Select the file directory and save it as FileName.meg (here, geminiviridae_align.meg).
7. The files with multiple nucleotide sequence alignments are ready to be used in the following steps of the phylogenetic analysis.

3.3 Creating Multiple Sequence Alignments for Amino Acid Sequences

1. Open the FASTA file containing the CP-encoding nucleotide sequences previously retrieved from the *Geminiviridae* genome dataset. In MEGA, click on the tile File → Open a File/Session and search for the directory where the FASTA file is located (select your file and open it). A window with the message Analyze or Align file? will pop-up (click on Align and the nucleotide sequences will be shown).

2. The ORF nucleotide sequences must be translated to amino acid sequences before performing the alignment using Muscle. Click on Data → Translate/Untranslate and a new window with the message The current Genetic Code is: Standard. Is this correct? will be shown (click on Yes). Then, you will notice the nucleotide sequences will be translated to the encoded protein sequences.
3. Click on Alignment → Align by Muscle and a new window with the message Nothing selected for alignment. Select all? will pop-up (click on OK). Then, a new window for editing the Muscle parameters is opened (click on OK to carry out the sequence alignment using standard parameters of the Muscle algorithm).
4. Visually check the whole alignment once it is done (manually edit it whether needed). As mentioned above, the program adds some gaps, represented by the character -, to the aligned sequences to optimize the alignment of homolog sites. Save the *Geminiviridae* CP sequence alignment using FASTA and MEGA formats.
5. Go to the tile Data → Export alignment → FASTA Format. Select the file directory and save it as FileName.fas (here, cp_align.fas).
6. Then, click on Data → Export alignment → MEGA Format. Select the file directory and save it as FileName.meg (here, cp_align.meg).
7. Repeat **steps 1–6** using the Rep-encoding sequences.
8. Both CP and Rep files with multiple amino acid sequence alignments are ready to be used in the following steps of the phylogenetic analysis.

3.4 Saving the Alignment Files in Different Formats

1. Different packages for sequence analysis can be used to save nucleotide and amino acid alignments. Both MEGA and Geneious are reported here.
2. In MEGA, click on the tile File → Open a File/Session and search for the directory where the alignment file, previously saved in MEGA format, is located (select your file and open it). You will notice two new tiles (TA and Close Data) appear in the MEGA main window. Click on TA (stands for Sequence Data Explorer) and the sequence alignment will be shown in a new window.
3. On this new window, the nucleotide sites similar to the consensus sequence, determined by MEGA, are presented as a special character (dot). To show the actual sequences, clink on TA (in this window, it stands for Use Identical Symbol) and dots will be automatically replaced by the actual viral sequences. The alignment is now ready to be saved in different formats.

4. Click on the tile Data → Export Data to show the window Sequence Data Export Options. Go to the tile Format, select the PHYLIP format and click on OK (search for the appropriated folder directory and save it as FileName.phy).
5. Repeat **step 4** to save the sequence alignment in a NEXUS format. Select the option Nexus (PAUP 3.0/MacClade) and click on OK (search for the folder directory and save it as FileName.nex or FileName.nexus). In this chapter, the files were named as geminiviridae_align.phy, geminiviridae_align.nex, cp_align.phy, cp_align.nex, rep_align.phy, and rep_align.nex.
6. The PHYLIP and NEXUS alignment files are ready to be used in the following steps of the phylogenetic analysis. It is important to note that MEGA limits the number of characters for sequence names when exporting alignment data to PHYLIP (10 characters) or NEXUS (32 characters) (*see* **Note 1**).
7. In Geneious, go to the tile File → Import → From File and search for the FASTA file containing the sequence alignment (select it and click on Import). A new window will pop-up and you must choose between Nucleotide sequences or Protein sequences for *Geminiviridae* genomes and CP and Rep sequences, respectively (click on OK). Alternatively, you can just drag the FASTA file from your computer folder to the Geneious main window and it will be automatically uploaded.
8. Select the alignment just added to Geneious and go to File → Export → Selected Documents (a new window will be opened). Search for the folder directory, select the PHYLIP format, type the file name as FileName.phy and click on Export → Proceed. In the new window, select the option Relaxed Phylip—Full length names followed by a single space and click on OK (this option will not limit the number of characters for sequence names).
9. To save the alignment data in a NEXUS format, repeat **step 8** but selecting NEXUS format. Go to the tile File → Export → Selected Documents (a new window will be opened). Search for the appropriated folder directory, select the NEXUS format, type the file name as FileName.nex and click on Export → Proceed. In the new window, select the options Export without metacomments and Replace these characters in names with underscore: spaces or –:,;()’ and click on OK.
10. The PHYLIP and NEXUS alignment files are ready to be used in the following steps of the phylogenetic analysis, with no limitation in the number of characters for sequence names (*see* **Note 1**).

3.5 Selecting the Best-Fit Substitution Models Using IQ-TREE

1. The procedure described here is for selecting the best-fit substitution model using the IQ-TREE v2 software (iqtree.org/). Other programs such as jModelTest (github.com/ddarriba/jmodeltest2/releases/tag/v2.1.10r20160303) and MEGA can perform the same type of analysis (*see* **Note 2**). However, IQ-TREE is faster than both jModelTest and MEGA, being also freely available at the IQ-TREE web server (iqtree.cibiv.univie.ac.at/).
2. Create a folder for each sequence dataset into your preferred directory and add the *Geminiviridae* alignment files (complete genomes, CP, and Rep) in PHYLIP format (in this chapter, geminiviridae_align.phy, cp_align.phy, and rep_align.phy).
3. Open the Command Prompt under Windows. You can use the Windows search tool by typing CMD, and the Command Prompt will be shown (click on it to open).
4. On the Command Prompt, type the whole path to the IQ-TREE bin folder. Search for it in the unzipped IQ-TREE folder, Right-Click on the bin folder to Copy it as a path and Paste in the Command Prompt main window followed by \iqtree2 (path to the IQ-TREE bin folder\iqtree2). Here, the command used was C:\Users\UENF\Downloads\iqtree-2.2.2.6-Windows\iqtree-2.2.2.6-Windows\bin\iqtree2.
5. Type the command -s (add Space) followed by the path to the PHYLIP file containing the sequence alignment (path to the PHYLIP file folder\FileName.phy). This command allows iqtree2 to read the input file (nucleotide or amino acid sequence alignments).
6. Type the command -m MF to search for the best substitution model (or -m TESTONLY to test the models resembling jModelTest/ProtTest).
7. Type the command -redo to overwrite all previous output files.
8. The entire command line must be path to the IQ-TREE bin folder\iqtree2 -s path to the PHYLIP file folder\FileName.phy -m MF -redo. Here, the following command was used for the complete genome dataset: C:\Users\UENF\Downloads\iqtree-2.2.2.6-Windows\iqtree-2.2.2.6-Windows\bin\iqtree2 -s C:\Users\UENF\Downloads\Geminiviridae\geminiviridae_align.phy -m MF -redo. The command lines for all datasets are shown in Fig. 5a.
9. Press ENTER to perform the analysis. An IQ-TREE report (FileName.iqtree), Tree used for ModelFinder (FileName.treefile), and Screen log file (FileName.log) will be created in the folder where the PHYLIP file is located. IQ-TREE will test all

(a) Command template

Path to the IQ-TREE bin folder\iqtree2 -s Path to the PHYLIP file folder\FileName.phy -m MF -redo

This chapter

Geminiviridae genomes

C:\Users\UENF\Downloads\iqtree-2.2.2.6-Windows\iqtree-2.2.2.6-Windows\bin\iqtree2 -s C:\Users\UENF\Downloads\Geminiviridae\geminiviridae_align.phy -m MF -redo

Geminiviridae CP

C:\Users\UENF\Downloads\iqtree-2.2.2.6-Windows\iqtree-2.2.2.6-Windows\bin\iqtree2 -s C:\Users\UENF\Downloads\Geminiviridae\CP\cp_align.phy -m MF -redo

Geminiviridae Rep

C:\Users\UENF\Downloads\iqtree-2.2.2.6-Windows\iqtree-2.2.2.6-Windows\bin\iqtree2 -s C:\Users\UENF\Downloads\Geminiviridae\REP\rep_align.phy -m MF -redo

(b) IQ-TREE report log

SEQUENCE ALIGNMENT

Input data: 492 sequences with 9453 nucleotide sites
Number of constant sites: 2045 (= 21.6333% of all sites)
Number of invariant (constant or ambiguous constant) sites: 2045 (= 21.6333% of all sites)
Number of parsimony informative sites: 5468
Number of distinct site patterns: 7635

ModelFinder

Best-fit model according to BIC: GTR+F+I+G4

List of models sorted by BIC scores:

Fig. 5 Selecting the best-fit substitution model in IQ-TREE v.2. (**a**) Command line to run IQ-TREE from a Command Prompt; (**b**) IQ-TREE log file showing the best-fit nucleotide substitution model for *Geminiviridae* complete genomes

possible substitution models and find the best-fit substitution model to your dataset (*see* **Note 3**).

10. Once the analysis is done, open the IQ-TREE report (FileName.iqtree) using notepad (or any other text editing program) and search for the best-fit model according to BIC (the best fit-model chosen by IQ-TREE v2 is shown right next to it). For example, Best-fit model according to BIC: GTR + F + I + G4 (Fig. 5b).
11. Repeat **steps 2–10** to choose the best-fit amino acid substitution models for both CP and Rep amino acid datasets.
12. The best-fit models used here were as follows: complete genomes (GTR + F + I + G4), CP (LG + F + I + G4), and Rep (LG + G4) (*see* **Note 4**).

3.6 Selecting the Best-Fit Nucleotide Substitution Model Using jModelTest

1. Create a folder into your preferred directory and add the aligned *Geminiviridae* complete genome file in FASTA, PHYLIP, or NEXUS format.
2. Open jModelTest under Windows (double click on it to open the GUI version).
3. Go to the tile File → Load DNA alignment. Search for the folder directory, select the alignment file in one of the formats mentioned above and click on Open (if the file is correct, the log printed to the jModelTest v2 main window will show the following message: Reading data file "FileName.phy"...OK at

the bottom (also, the number of sequences and sites in the alignment are shown). For example, Reading data file "geminiviridae_align.phy"...OK → number of sequences: 492 → number of sites: 9453 for the *Geminiviridae* genome dataset analyzed here.

4. Go to the tile Analysis → Compute likelihood scores (click on Compute likelihood). A new window will pop-up showing the number of models being tested and the analysis status.
5. Once the likelihood calculation is done, you can choose the best-fit substitution model using Akaike Information Criterion (AIC) or Bayesian Information Criterion (BIC).
6. For AIC analysis, go to the tile Analysis → Do AIC calculation, mark the option Write PAUP* block and click on Do AIC calculation.
7. For BIC analysis, go to Analysis → Do BIC calculation, mark the option Write PAUP* block and click on Do BIC calculation.
8. The results for both AIC- and BIC-based best-fit substitution models will be shown on the main log window. To save it, go to Edit → Save console (a new window will be opened). Search for the folder directory and save it as FileName.out (you can open this file using notepad). Alternatively, you can save it as a PDF file using the tile Edit → Print console (a new window will be opened). Search for the folder directory and save it as FileName.pdf (you can open this file using a PDF reader).
9. Open the file you just saved and search for AKAIKE INFORMATION CRITERION (AIC) or BAYESIAN INFORMATION CRITERION (BIC). The message Model selected: → Model = 'best-fit substitution model' appears right below the title of the analysis performed (AIC or BIC). For example, Model selected: → Model = GTR + I + G and Model selected: → Model = TIM2 + I + G for AIC and BIC, respectively (Fig. 6).
10. Finally, a PAUP command block is written for each AIC and BIC criteria, which can be used to reconstruct ML phylogenetic trees using PAUP. In the output file, search for Tree for the best AIC model = or Tree for the best BIC model =, and you will find the PAUP command block right above the searched term. The PAUP command block is written as BEGIN PAUP; best-fit substitution model calculated for your dataset; END;. For example, BEGIN PAUP; Lset base = (0.3770 0.2256 0.1758) nst = 6 rmat = (3.4617 5.1753 3.5827 0.4632 15.2906) rates = gamma shape = 0.7160 ncat = 4 pinvar = 0.1540; END; and BEGIN PAUP; Lset base = (0.3770 0.2229 0.1763) nst = 6 rmat = (4.8624 7.1220 4.8624 1.0000 21.1384)

```
Best-fit nucleotide substitution model by AIC

---------------------------------------------------------------
*                                                             *
*        AKAIKE INFORMATION CRITERION (AIC)                   *
*                                                             *
---------------------------------------------------------------

Model selected:
  Model = GTR+I+G

...

PAUP* Commands Block:
 If you want to load the selected model and associated estimates in PAUP*,
 attach the next block of commands after the data in your PAUP file:

...

BEGIN PAUP;
Lset base=(0.3770 0.2256 0.1758) nst=6 rmat=(3.4617 5.1753 3.5827 0.4632 15.2906) rates=gamma shape=0.7160 ncat=4 pinvar=0.1540;
END;
```

Fig. 6 Selecting the best-fit substitution model using Akaike Information Criterion (AIC) in jModelTest v.2. The log printed to the jModelTest console shows both the selected model and the PAUP command block (highlighted in bold)

rates = gamma shape = 0.7170 ncat = 4 pinvar = 0.1550; END;, for AIC and BIC criterion, respectively (Fig. 6; *see* **Note 5**).

3.7 Selecting the Best-Fit Nucleotide Substitution Model Using MrModelTest

1. Create a folder into an appropriated directory and add the aligned *Geminiviridae* complete genome file in NEXUS format. Also, add the following files to the folder: MrModelblock.nex, mrmodeltest.exe (github.com/nylander/MrModeltest2), and win-paup4b10-console.exe (phylosolutions.com/paup-test/).
2. Open the executable program win-paup4b10-console.exe by double clicking on it under Windows.
3. Type execute FileName.nex (press Enter). Here, execute geminiviridae_align.nex (if the file is processed correctly, the message Processing of file "geminiviridae_align.nex" completed appears at the bottom of the PAUP window).
4. Type execute mrmodelblock.nex (this NEXUS file contains a command block used, by PAUP, to calculate the likelihood of the models being tested). Once the analysis is done, the files model.scores and modelfit will be saved to your folder (close the PAUP window).
5. Open the Command Prompt under Windows. You can use the Windows search tool and type CMD, and the Command Prompt will be shown (click on it to open).
6. Change the Command Prompt directory to the folder where your model.scores and mrmodeltest.exe files are located by typing cd (add Space) 'folder path'. Here, cd C:\Users\UENF

```
Best-fit nucleotide substitution model by AIC

--------------------------------------------------------------------------------
*                                                                              *
*          AKAIKE INFORMATION CRITERION (AIC)                                  *
*                                                                              *
--------------------------------------------------------------------------------

Model selected: GTR+I+G

...

PAUP* Commands Block: If you want to implement the previous estimates as likelihod settings in PAUP*, attach the next block of commands
after the data in your PAUP file:

...

BEGIN PAUP;
Lset Base=(0.3770 0.2256 0.1758) Nst=6 TRatio=1.0500 Rates=gamma Shape=0.7160 Pinvar=0.1540;
END;

...

MrBayes Commands Block: If you want to implement a "best" model in MrBayes, attach the next block of commands after the data in your
NEXUS file:

...

BEGIN MRBAYES;
Lset nst=6 rates=invgamma;
Prset statefreqpr=dirichlet(1,1,1,1);
END;
```

Fig. 7 Selecting the best-fit nucleotide substitution model using Akaike Information Criterion (AIC) in ModelTest v.2. The program's log printed to the output file shows the selected model and PAUP and MrBayes command blocks (highlighted in bold)

\Downloads\Geminiviridae (you can right-click on your folder to Copy it as a path and Paste in the Command Prompt). Press Enter and the directory will be changed. Type dir and press Enter and the files inside your folder will be listed on the Command Prompt console.

7. Type mrmodeltest.exe <mrmodel.scores> FileName.out (press Enter). Here, mrmodeltest.exe <mrmodel.scores> geminiviridae.out (this command will select the best-fit substitution model based on the likelihood values saved in the mrmodel. scores file).
8. This analysis is quickly performed, and the message Program is done appears on the Command Prompt window (close it). A new file (FileName.out) will be saved to your folder (here, geminiviridae.out).
9. Open this file using notepad and search for AKAIKE INFORMATION CRITERION (AIC) (the best-fit model information will be right below). For example, AKAIKE INFORMATION CRITERION (AIC) → Model selected: GTR + I + G (Fig. 7).

10. The mrmodeltest.exe program writes both PAUP and MrBayes command blocks to the output file, which can be used to reconstruct ML and Bayesian phylogenetic trees using PAUP and MrBayes, respectively.
11. In the output file, search for PAUP* Commands Block: or MrBayes Commands Block: and you will find the PAUP and MrBayes command blocks right below the searched term. The PAUP command block is written as BEGIN PAUP; best-fit substitution model calculated for your dataset; END;. For example, BEGIN PAUP; Lset Base = (0.3770 0.2256 0.1758) Nst = 6 TRatio = 1.0500 Rates = gamma Shape = 0.7160 Pinvar = 0.1540; END;. The MrBayes command block is written as BEGIN MRBAYES; best-fit substitution model calculated for your dataset; END;. For example, BEGIN MRBAYES; Lset nst = 6 rates = invgamma; Prset statefreqpr = dirichlet [1]; END; (Fig. 7).

3.8 Selecting the Best-Fit Amino Acid Substitution Model Using ProtTest

1. Create a folder for each sequence dataset into your preferred directory and add the *Geminiviridae* alignment files for CP and Rep amino acid sequences in FASTA, PHYLIP, or NEXUS format.
2. To open the graphical interface (GUI version) of ProtTest v.3 (github.com/ddarriba/prottest3/releases) under Windows, open the Command Prompt by typing CMD in the Windows search tool, and the Command Prompt will be shown (click on it to open).
3. Change the Command Prompt directory to the folder where ProtTest java executable (prottest-3.4.2.jar) is located by typing cd 'folder path'. Here, cd C:\Users\UENF\Downloads \prottest-3.4.2–20,160,508\prottest-3.4.2 (you can right-click on your folder to Copy it as a path and Paste in the Command Prompt window). Press Enter and the directory will be changed. Type dir and press Enter and the files inside your folder will be listed on the Command Prompt window (you must see the file runXProtTestHPC is this list).
4. Type runXProtTestHPC and press Enter (the graphical interface of ProtTest will be opened in a new window).
5. On ProtTest, go to the tile File → Load DNA alignment. Search for the folder directory where the CP or Rep alignment dataset is located, select the alignment file in one of the formats mentioned above and click on Open (if the file is correct, the log printed to the ProtTest main window will show the message Alignment contains 'number of sequences' sequences of length 'number of sites' at the bottom. Here, Alignment contains 492 sequences of length 383 for the CP dataset.

6. Go to the tile Analysis → Compute likelihood scores (click on Compute). A new window will pop-up showing the number of models being tested and the analysis status.
7. Once the calculation is done (information on date and time of run appears at the bottom of the ProtTest log window), you can choose the best-fit substitution model using Akaike Information Criterion (AIC) or Bayesian Information Criterion (BIC).
8. Go to Selection → Results and click on the tiles AIC or BIC to see the selection results. To export the results to the ProtTest log window, click on Export to main console (under the AIC or BIC tiles).
9. The results for both AIC and BIC best-fit models will be shown on the ProtTest main log window. To save it, go to the tile File → Print console (a new window will be opened). Search for the folder directory and save it as FileName.pdf (for example, cp.pdf). You can open this file using a PDF reader.
10. Open the PDF file you just saved and search for AKAIKE INFORMATION CRITERION or BAYESIAN INFORMATION CRITERION. The message Best model according to AIC: 'best-fit model selected by ProtTest' appears right below the title of the analysis performed (AIC or BIC). For example, AKAIKE INFORMATION CRITERION (AIC) → Best model according to AIC: LG + I + G + F or BAYESIAN INFORMATION CRITERION (BIC) → Best model according to BIC: LG + I + G + F, for the *Geminiviridae* CP amino acid dataset (Fig. 8).
11. Repeat **steps 2–10** to choose the best-fit amino acid substitution model for the *Geminiviridae* Rep dataset.
12. Finally, you can use these models to reconstruct ML phylogenetic trees based on amino acid sequence data.

3.9 Concatenating CP and Rep Sequence Alignment Data

1. Create a separate folder into your preferred directory and add the aligned CP and Rep amino acid sequences in FASTA format. Different programs such as MEGA, Geneious, SeqNinja, and Concatenator can be used to concatenate sequence data. Here, protocols for concatenating multiple amino acid sequence alignments of *Geminiviridae* CP and Rep are described for both Geneious and MEGA.
2. In Geneious, import both CP and Rep FASTA files by simply dragging them from your computer directory to the Geneious main window and they will be automatically uploaded.
3. Select both files and go to the tile Tools → Concatenate Sequences or Alignments. A new window will pop-up, allowing the modification of each dataset position by selecting the file

(a) Best-fit amino acid substitution model by AIC

```
************************************************************
          AKAIKE INFORMATION CRITERION
************************************************************

********************************************************************************
Best model according to AIC: LG+I+G+F
Confidence Interval: 100.0
********************************************************************************

...
```

(b) Best-fit amino acid substitution model by BIC

```
************************************************************
          BAYESIAN INFORMATION CRITERION
************************************************************

********************************************************************************
Best model according to BIC: LG+I+G+F
Confidence Interval: 100.0
********************************************************************************

...
```

Fig. 8 Selecting the best-fit amino acid substitution model using Akaike Information Criterion (AIC) and Bayesian Information Criterion (BIC) in ProtTest v.3. The program's log printed to the output file shows the models selected by AIC (**a**) and BIC (**b**), indicated in bold

and moving it by clicking on the tiles Move up or Move down. For example, *Geminiviridae* CP-Rep was comprised by 904 amino acid sites in length, where the concatenated data was arranged as follows: CP (positions 1–383) → Rep (positions 384–904). Remember, it is important that the CP and Rep sequences belonging to a same exemplar virus have identical names on both FASTA files (as indicated in Subheading 3.1).

4. Click on OK and a concatenated CP-Rep data file will be created to the Geneious main window. Select this file and export it using FASTA, PHYLIP, and NEXUS formats (*see* Subheadings 3.3 and 3.4).

5. Alternatively, in MEGA, go to the tile TA → Concatenate sequence alignments, select the folder where your CP and Rep alignments are located and click on Select folder. Then, select the data type of your input files (here, Protein Sequences) and click on OK. Similar to Geneious, it is crucial that the CP and Rep sequences belonging to a same exemplar virus have identical names on both FASTA files. In MEGA, the positioning of each dataset is determined by the alphabetical order

included in the name of the original FASTA files saved in your directory. For example, for cp_align.fas and rep_align.fas, the CP data will be placed before Rep and, therefore, you can modify each dataset position by renaming the files before concatenation.

6. You will notice two new tiles (TA and Close Data) appear in the MEGA main window. Click on TA (stands for Sequence Data Explorer) and the sequence alignment will be shown in a new window.
7. On this new window, the nucleotide sites similar to the consensus sequence, determined by MEGA, are presented as a special character (Dot). To show the actual sequences, clink on TA (it stands for Use Identical Symbol) and dots will automatically be replaced by the actual viral sequences. The *Geminiviridae* CP-Rep data was comprised by 904 amino acid sites in length, where the concatenated data was arranged as CP (positions 1–383) → Rep (positions 384–904). The concatenated alignment is now ready to be saved in MEGA, FASTA, PHYLIP, and NEXUS formats (*see* Subheadings 3.3 and 3.4).

3.10 Reconstructing ML Phylogenetic Trees Using IQ-TREE

1. The procedure described here is for reconstruction of maximum likelihood (ML) trees using IQ-TREE v.2 (iqtree.org/). Other programs such as RaxML and PAUP can also perform the same type of analysis. However, IQ-TREE uses an ultrafast bootstrap approach, which is faster than RaxML and PAUP, being a great tool to reconstruct ML phylogenies using large datasets such as *Geminiviridae*. IQ-TREE is freely available at the IQ-TREE web server (iqtree.cibiv.univie.ac.at/).
2. Open the Command Prompt under Windows. You can use the Windows search tool and type CMD, and the Command Prompt will be shown (click on it to open).
3. On the Command Prompt, type the whole path to the IQ-TREE bin folder. You can find it in the unzipped IQ-TREE folder, right-click on the bin folder to Copy it as a path and Paste in the Command Prompt followed by \iqtree2 (path to the bin folder\iqtree2). Here, the command used was: C:\Users\UENF\Downloads\iqtree-2.2.2.6-Windows\iqtree-2.2.2.6-Windows\bin\iqtree2.
4. Type the command -s (add Space) followed by the path to the PHYLIP file containing the sequence alignment (path to the PHYLIP file folder\FileName.phy). This command allows iqtree2 to read the input file (nucleotide or amino acid sequence alignments). For example, the command used for complete genomes of *Geminiviridae* was: -s C:\Users\UENF\Downloads\Geminiviridae\geminiviridae_align.phy.

Command template

Path to the bin folder\iqtree2 -s Path to the PHYLIP file folder\FileName.phy -m Best-fit model -B 1000 -T AUTO -alrt 1000 -redo

This chapter

Geminiviridae genomes

C:\Users\UENF\Downloads\iqtree-2.2.2.6-Windows\iqtree-2.2.2.6-Windows\bin\iqtree2 -s C:\Users\UENF\Downloads\Geminiviridae\geminiviridae_align.phy -m GTR+F+I+G4 -B 1000 -T AUTO -alrt 1000 -redo

Geminiviridae CP

C:\Users\UENF\Downloads\iqtree-2.2.2.6-Windows\iqtree-2.2.2.6-Windows\bin\iqtree2 -s C:\Users\UENF\Downloads\Geminiviridae\CP\cp_align.phy -m LG+F+I+G4 -B 1000 -T AUTO -alrt 1000 -redo

Geminiviridae Rep

C:\Users\UENF\Downloads\iqtree-2.2.2.6-Windows\iqtree-2.2.2.6-Windows\bin\iqtree2 -s C:\Users\UENF\Downloads\Geminiviridae\REP\rep_align.phy -m LG+G4 -B 1000 -T AUTO -alrt 1000 -redo

Fig. 9 Command line to run IQ-TREE v.2 from a Command Prompt when reconstructing maximum likelihood (ML) phylogenetic trees for *Geminiviridae* data

5. To set the substitution model, type the command -m followed by the best-fit model determined in Subheading 3.5 (*Geminiviridae* genome = GTR + F + I + G4).
6. Type the ultrafast bootstrap command -B 1000 (for 1000 ultrafast bootstrap replications).
7. You can ask IQ-TREE to select the best number of CPU THREADS by typing the command -T AUTO.
8. IQ-TREE also provides an implementation of the SH-like approximate likelihood ratio test. To perform this test, type the command -alrt 1000 (for 1000 ultrafast bootstrap replications).
9. Type the command -redo to overwrite all previous output files.
10. The entire command line must be path to the bin folder \iqtree2 -s path to the PHYLIP file folder\FileName.phy -m best-fit model -B 1000 -T AUTO -alrt 1000 -redo. Here, the following command was used for the *Geminiviridae* genome dataset: C:\Users\UENF\Downloads\iqtree-2.2.2.6-Windows \iqtree-2.2.2.6-Windows\bin\iqtree2 -s C:\Users\UENF \Downloads\Geminiviridae\geminiviridae_align.phy -m GTR +F+I+G4 -B 1000 -T AUTO -alrt 1000 -redo. The command lines for all datasets are shown in Fig. 9.
11. Press ENTER to perform the analysis. An IQ-TREE report (FileName.iqtree), Maximum-likelihood tree (FileName.treefile), and Likelihood distances (FileName.mldist) files will be created in the folder where the PHYLIP alignment is located. Further, the ultrafast bootstrap approximation results will be written to Split support values (FileName.splits.nex), Consensus tree (FileName.contree), and Screen log (FileName.log) files. These files will be saved to the same aforementioned folder. The CONTREE file contains the ML tree with bootstrap support values.

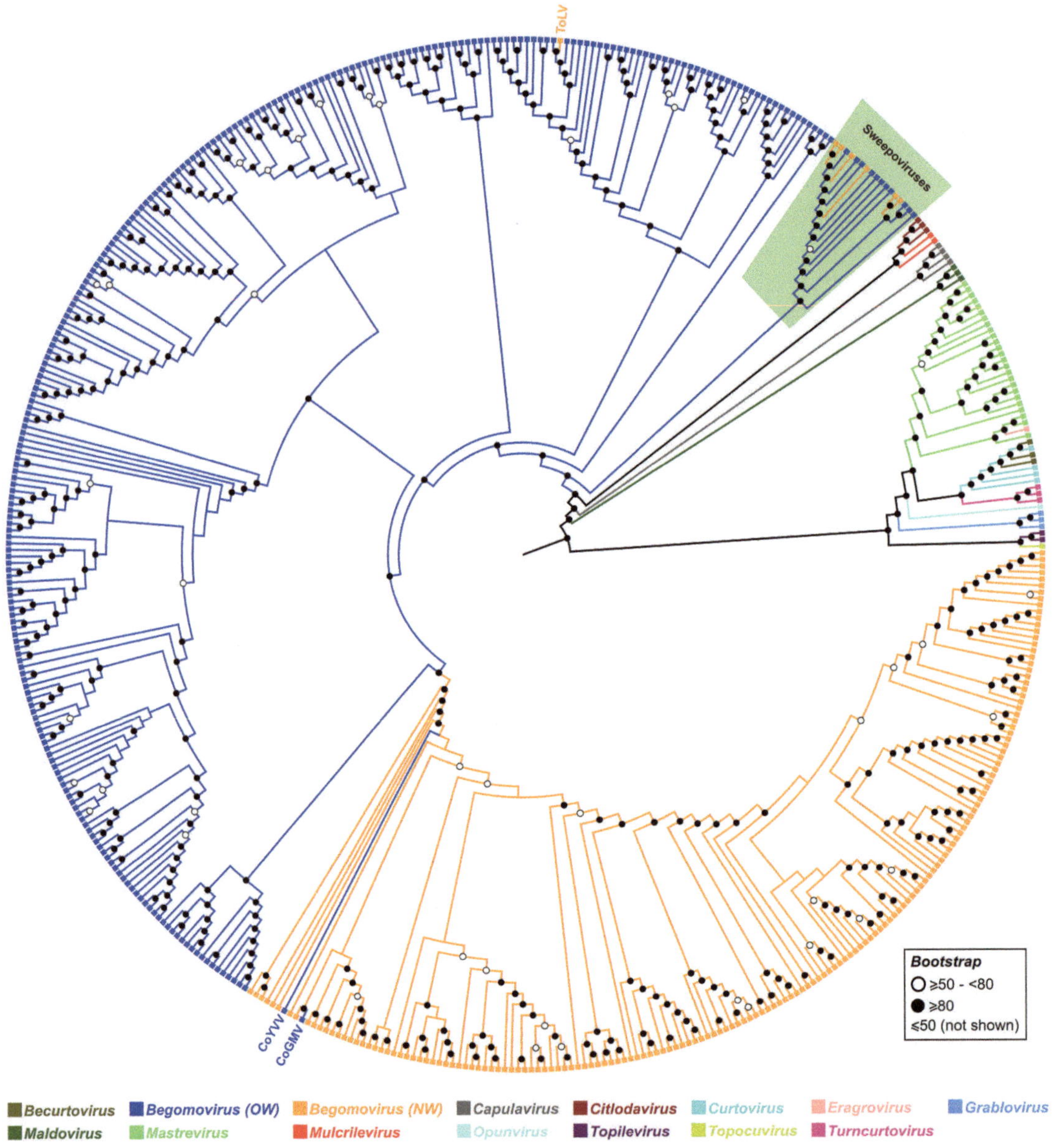

Fig. 10 Midpoint-rooted maximum likelihood (ML) phylogenetic tree based on coat protein (CP) amino acid sequences of exemplar viruses from *Geminiviridae* species. Bootstrap values ≥ 80 (filled circles) and between 50 and 80 (empty circles) are shown near to each branch node, while bootstraps <50 are not shown. CoYVV=corchorus yellow vein virus, CoGMV=corchorus golden mosaic virus, and ToLV=tomato latent virus

12. Repeat **steps 2–12** to reconstruct ML phylogenies to CP and Rep amino acid sequences.
13. The ML phylogenetic trees reconstructed based on CP, Rep, and complete genome sequences of *Geminiviridae* are shown in Figs. 10, 11, and 12, respectively.

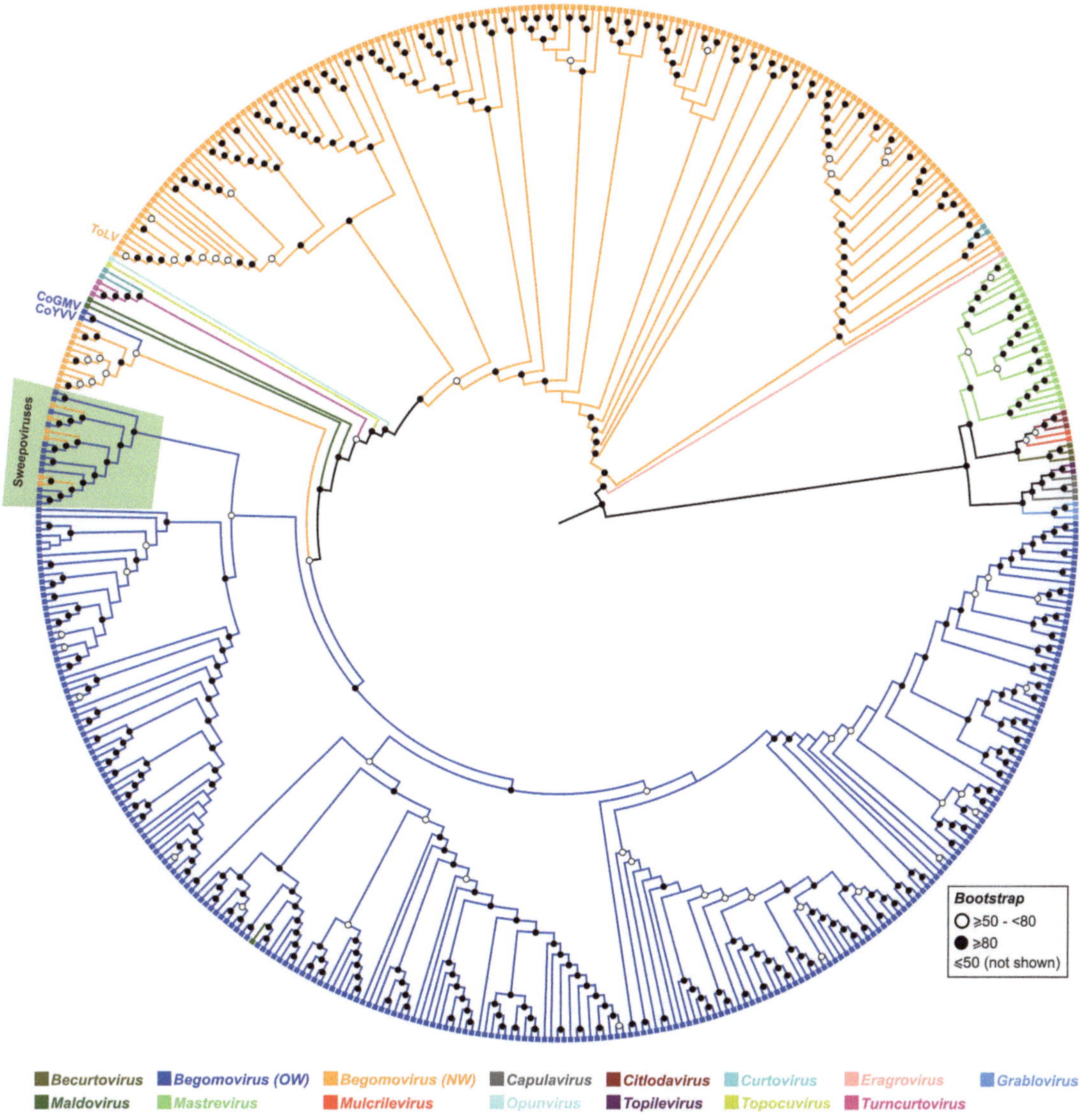

Fig. 11 Midpoint-rooted maximum likelihood (ML) phylogenetic tree based on replication-associated protein (Rep) amino acid sequences of exemplar viruses from *Geminiviridae* species. Bootstrap values ≥80 (filled circles) and between 50 and 80 (empty circles) are shown near to each branch node, while bootstraps <50 are not shown. CoYVV=corchorus yellow vein virus, CoGMV=corchorus golden mosaic virus, and ToLV=tomato latent virus

3.11 Reconstructing ML Phylogenetic Trees Based on Concatenated Amino Acid Data Using IQ-TREE

1. The procedure described here is for reconstruction of ML trees based on concatenated data using the IQ-TREE software (iqtree.org/). IQ-TREE uses an ultrafast bootstrap approach, which is a good solution when working with large datasets such as *Geminiviridae*.

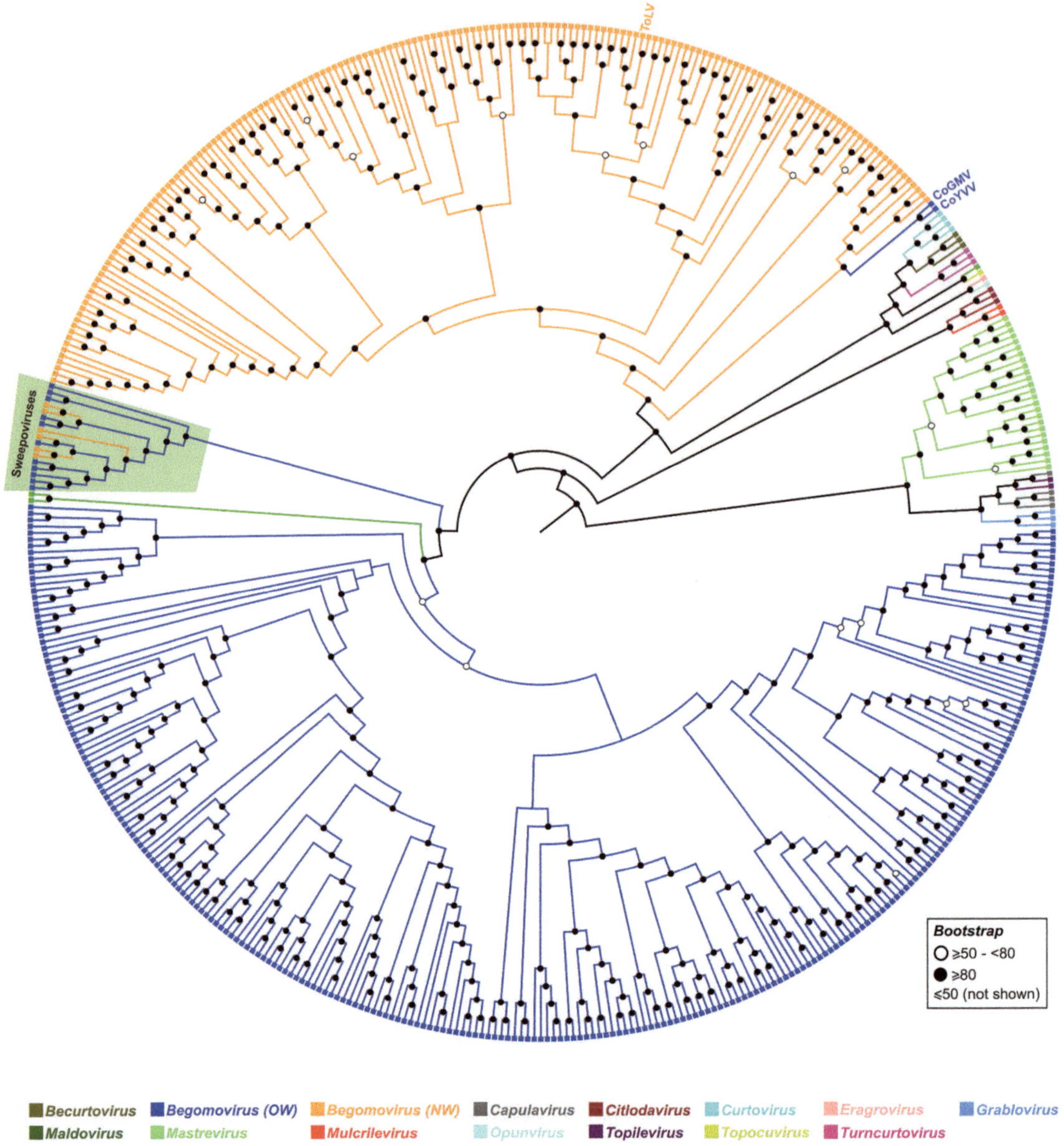

Fig. 12 Midpoint-rooted maximum likelihood (ML) phylogenetic tree based on complete genome nucleotide sequences of exemplar viruses from *Geminiviridae* species. Bootstrap values $\geq$80 (filled circles) and between 50 and 80 (empty circles) are shown near to each branch node, while bootstraps <50 are not shown. CoYVV=corchorus yellow vein virus, CoGMV=corchorus golden mosaic virus, and ToLV=tomato latent virus

2. Create a folder for the concatenated dataset into your preferred directory and add the alignment in PHYLIP format (here, merged amino acid data for CP and Rep).
3. Create a NEXUS file containing the partitioning command that will be used by IQ-TREE to determine specific substitution models for each genomic region/partition. Open a

(a) Command block template

```
#nexus
begin sets;
charset PartitionName1 = first nucleotide position-last nucleotide position;
charset PartitionName2 = first nucleotide position-last nucleotide position;
charpartition mine = substitution model:PartitionName1, substitution model:PartitionName2;
end;
```

This chapter
Geminiviridae CP-Rep

```
#nexus
begin sets;
charset CP = 1-383;
charset Rep = 384-904;
charpartition mine = LG+F+I+G4:CP, LG+G4:Rep;
end;
```

(b) Command template

```
Path to the bin folder\iqtree2 -s path to the PHYLIP file folder\FileName.phy -p Path to the NEXUS file folder\FileName.nex -B 1000 -T AUTO -alrt 1000 -redo
```

This chapter
Geminiviridae CP-Rep

```
C:\Users\UENF\Downloads\iqtree-2.2.2.6-Windows\iqtree-2.2.2.6-Windows\bin\iqtree2 -s C:\Users\UENF\Downloads\Geminiviridae\CP_Rep\concat_CP_Rep_aa_align.phy -
p C:\Users\UENF\Downloads\Geminiviridae\CP_Rep\part_cp_rep.nex -B 1000 -T AUTO -alrt 1000 -redo
```

Fig. 13 Reconstructing maximum likelihood (ML) phylogenetic trees in IQ-TREE v.2. (**a**) NEXUS command block to specify amino acid substitution models for each *Geminiviridae* CP and Rep partition; (**b**) Command line to run IQ-TREE from a Command Prompt when reconstructing ML trees for *Geminiviridae* concatenated data

notepad window by searching for it in the Windows search tool, and the application will be shown (click on it to open). Type the following information #nexus begin sets; charset PartitionName1 = first nucleotide position-last nucleotide position; charset PartitionName2 = first nucleotide position-last nucleotide position; charpartition mine = substitution model: PartitionName1, substitution model: PartitionName2; end;. In this chapter, the information for CP and Rep are as follows: #nexus begin sets; charset CP = 1–383; charset Rep = 384–904; charpartition mine = LG + F + I + G4:CP, LG + G4:Rep; end; (Fig. 13a) (*see* Subheadings 3.5 and 3.9 for selection of best-fit substitution models and data concatenation, respectively). Go to the tile File → Save, select the file directory (same folder where the PHYLIP file is located) and save it as FileName.nex (here, part_cp_rep.nex).

4. Open the Command Prompt under Windows. You can use the Windows search tool and type CMD, and the Command Prompt will be shown (click on it to open).
5. On the Command Prompt, type the whole path to the IQ-TREE v2 bin folder. You can find it in the unzipped IQ-TREE folder, right-click on the bin folder to Copy it as a path and Paste in the Command Prompt followed by \iqtree2 (path to the bin folder\iqtree2). Here, the command used was: C:\Users\UENF\Downloads\iqtree-2.2.2.6-Windows\iqtree-2.2.2.6-Windows\bin\iqtree2.

6. Type the command -s (add Space) followed by the path to the PHYLIP file containing the sequence alignment (path to the PHYLIP file folder\FileName.phy). This command allows iqtree2 to read the input file (nucleotide or amino acid sequence alignments). For example, the command used for *Geminiviridae* CP-Rep was: -s C:\Users\UENF\Downloads \Geminiviridae\CP_Rep\concat_CP_Rep_aa_align.phy.
7. Type the command -p followed by the path to the NEXUS file containing the best-fit substitution model information (path to the NEXUS file folder\FileName.nex). Here, the command used was: -p C:\Users\UENF\Downloads\Geminiviridae \CP_Rep\ part_cp_rep.nex.
8. Type the ultrafast bootstrap command -B 1000 (for 1000 ultrafast bootstrap replications).
9. You can ask IQ-TREE v2 to select the best number of CPU THREADS by typing the command -T AUTO.
10. IQ-TREE also provides an implementation of the SH-like approximate likelihood ratio test. To perform this test, type the command -alrt 1000 (for 1000 ultrafast bootstrap replications).
11. Type the command -redo to overwrite all previous output files.
12. The entire command line must be path to the bin folder\iqtree2 -s path to the PHYLIP file folder\FileName.phy -p path to the NEXUS file folder\FileName.nex -B 1000 -T AUTO -alrt 1000 -redo. Here, the following command was used: C:\Users\UENF \Downloads\iqtree-2.2.2.6-Windows\iqtree-2.2.2.6-Windows \bin\iqtree2 -s C:\Users\UENF\Downloads\Geminiviridae \CP_Rep\concat_CP_Rep_aa_align.phy -p C:\Users\UENF \Downloads\Geminiviridae\CP_Rep\part_cp_rep.nex -B 1000 -T AUTO -alrt 1000 -redo (Fig. 13b).
13. Press ENTER to perform the analysis. An IQ-TREE report (FileName.iqtree), Maximum-likelihood tree (FileName.treefile), and Likelihood distances (FileName.mldist) files will be created in the folder where the PHYLIP alignment is located. Further, the ultrafast bootstrap approximation results will be written to Split support values (FileName.splits.nex), Consensus tree (FileName.contree), and Screen log (FileName.log) files. These files will be saved to the same folder aforementioned. The CONTREE file contains the ML tree with bootstrap support values.
14. The ML phylogenetic tree reconstructed based on *Geminiviridae* CP-Rep merged data is shown in Fig. 14.

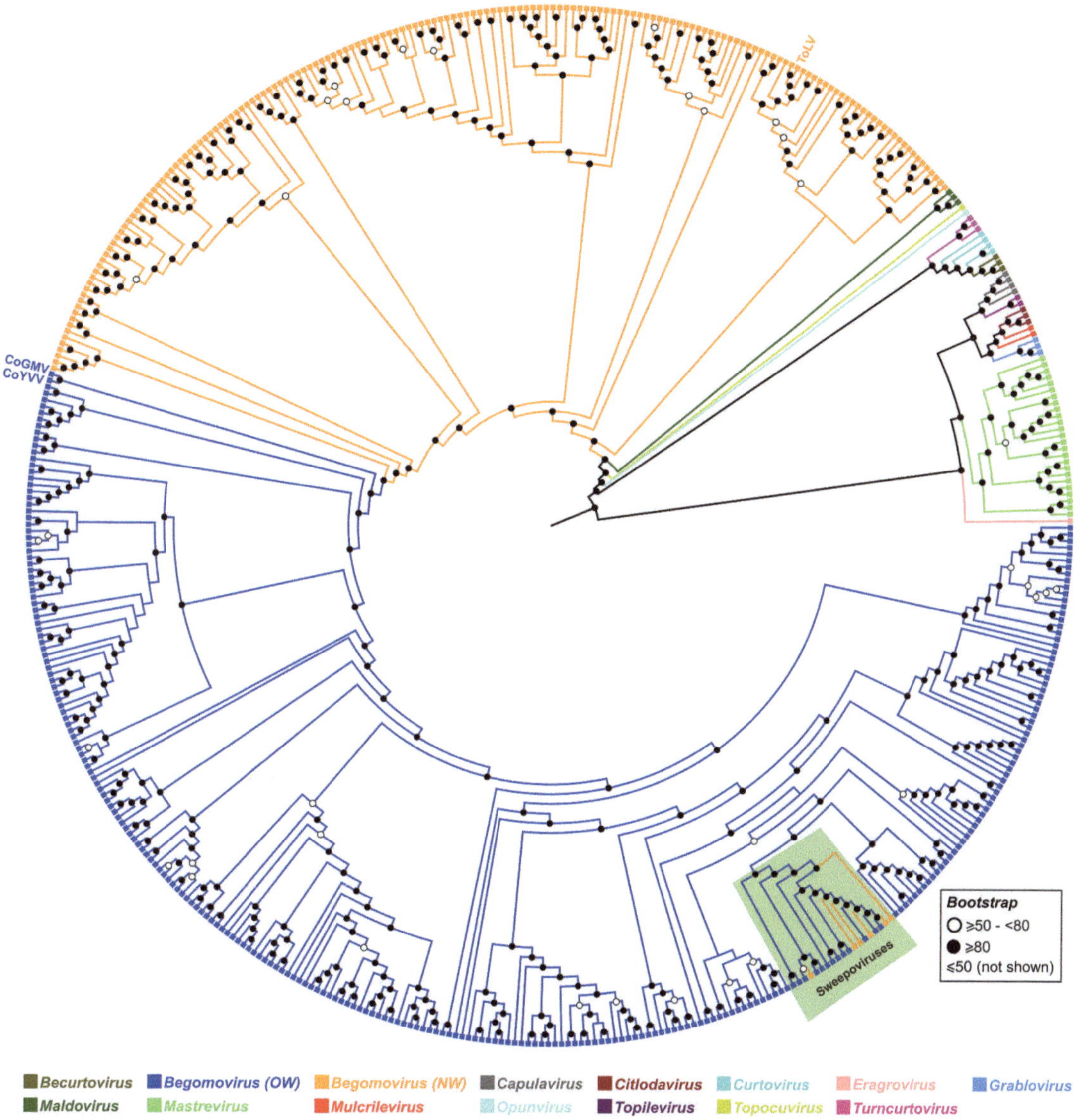

Fig. 14 Midpoint-rooted maximum likelihood (ML) phylogenetic tree based on concatenated amino acid sequences from coat protein (CP) and replication-associated protein (Rep) of exemplar viruses from *Geminiviridae* species. Bootstrap values ≥80 (filled circles) and between 50 and 80 (empty circles) are shown near to each branch node, while bootstraps <50 are not shown. CoYVV=corchorus yellow vein virus, CoGMV=corchorus golden mosaic virus, and ToLV=tomato latent virus

3.12 Reconstructing ML Phylogenetic Trees Using PAUP

1. This procedure is used to reconstruct ML trees using PAUP v.4. This program is largely used for inference of phylogenetic trees, but it is very time-consuming when using big datasets such as *Geminiviridae*. In this case, it is important to use high performance computers to run this analysis.
2. Create a folder into an appropriated directory and add the *Geminiviridae* complete genome alignment in NEXUS format

NEXUS file format template

```
#NEXUS
[ Title ]
begin data;
dimensions ntax=number of sequences nchar=number of sites;
format missing=? gap=- matchchar=. datatype=dna;

matrix
[!Domain=Data;]
...aligned sequence data...
;
end;
```

Example (*Geminiviridae* genomes)

```
#NEXUS
[ Title ]
begin data;
dimensions ntax=492 nchar=9453;
format missing=? gap=- matchchar=. datatype=dna;
matrix

[!Domain=Data;]
HQ113104_BCSMV_Australia_1999_Ma AC--------------------------CGCCCATCTTTAGCC...
JQ948061_PDSMV_Australia_2011_Ma AC--------------------------CGTCGCCCT-GCTTT...
...
;
end;
```

Fig. 15 Overview of a nucleotide sequence alignment in NEXUS format

(Fig. 15). Also, add the win-paup4b10-console.exe executable program. PAUP is also available in a GUI version (phylosolutions.com/paup-test/).

3. Open the NEXUS file (FileName.nex) using notepad and add the PAUP command block (*see* Subheadings 3.6 and 3.7) at the bottom of the file (also, add the command lines for ML search and bootstrap analysis right below it) (*see* **Note 6**). For example, BEGIN PAUP; log start file=FileName_screen.log replace=yes; Lset based on best-fit model selected in section 3.6; set criterion=Likelihood; hsearch start=NJ addseq=random nreps=1000; Savetree brlens=yes file=FileName.tre; set criterion=Likelihood; set maxtrees=100 increase=auto; Bootstrap brlens=yes Nreps=1000/start=NJ swap=NNI; Savetrees brlens=yes from=1 to=1000 savebootp=both maxdecimals=0 file=FileName_bootstrap.tre replace=yes; end;. For the *Geminiviridae* dataset used in the present chapter: BEGIN PAUP; log start file=geminiviridae_screen.log replace=yes; Lset base=(0.3770 0.2256 0.1758) nst=6

PAUP command block template

```
BEGIN PAUP;
log start file=FileName_screen.log replace=yes;
Lset based on best-fit model selected in section 3.6;
set criterion=Likelihood;
hsearch start=NJ addseq=random nreps=1000;
Savetree brlens=yes file=FileName.tre;
set criterion=Likelihood;
set maxtrees=100 increase=auto;
Bootstrap brlens=yes Nreps=1000/start=NJ swap=NNI;
Savetrees brlens=yes from=1 to=1000 savebootp=both maxdecimals=0 file=FileName_bootstrap.tre replace=yes;
end;
```

This chapter
Geminiviridae genomes

```
BEGIN PAUP;
log start file=geminiviridae_screen.log replace=yes;
Lset base=(0.3770 0.2256 0.1758) nst=6 rmat=(3.4617 5.1753 3.5827 0.4632 15.2906) rates=gamma shape=0.7160 ncat=4
pinvar=0.1540;
set criterion=Likelihood;
hsearch start=NJ addseq=random nreps=1000;
Savetree brlens=yes file=geminiviridae.tre;
set criterion=Likelihood;
set maxtrees=100 increase=auto;
Bootstrap brlens=yes Nreps=1000/start=NJ swap=NNI;
Savetrees brlens=yes from=1 to=1000 savebootp=both maxdecimals=0 file=geminiviridae_bootstrap.tre replace=yes;
end;
```

Fig. 16 PAUP command block for reconstruction of maximum likelihood (ML) phylogenetic trees

rmat=(3.4617 5.1753 3.5827 0.4632 15.2906) rates=gamma shape=0.7160 ncat=4 pinvar=0.1540; set criterion=Likelihood; hsearch start=NJ addseq=random nreps=1000; Savetree brlens=yes file=geminiviridae.tre; set criterion=Likelihood; set maxtrees=100 increase=auto; Bootstrap brlens=yes Nreps=1000/start=NJ swap=NNI; Savetrees brlens=yes from=1 to=1000 savebootp=both maxdecimals=0 file=geminiviridae_bootstrap.tre replace=yes; end; (Fig. 16).

4. Save the NEXUS file containing the PAUP command block and close it.
5. Open win-paup4b10-console.exe by double clicking on it under Windows.
6. Type execute FileName.nex (press Enter). Here, execute geminiviridae_align.nex. When the NEXUS file is processed correctly, a real-time log with the bootstrap information will be written to the PAUP main window. Also, the message Processing of file "geminiviridae_align.nex" completed appears at the bottom of the PAUP window. The log printed to the PAUP main window will be saved to the output FileName_screen.log (here, geminiviridae_screen.log).

7. The ML phylogenetic tree with bootstrap support values will the saved to FileName_bootstrap.tre (here, geminiviridae_-bootstrap.tre), which can be edited in programs such as FigTree.

3.13 Reconstructing ML Phylogenetic Trees Using RAxML

1. This procedure is used to reconstruct ML phylogenetic trees using a fast bootstrap approach in the RAxML v.8 program (github.com/stamatak/standard-RAxML/tree/master).
2. Create a folder into your preferred directory and add the *Geminiviridae* complete genome alignment in PHYLIP format. Also, add the raxmlHPC.exe executable program. RAxML does not offer many options for nucleotide and amino acid substitution models, and program developers recommend using GTR + G (General Time Reversible model of nucleotide substitution under the Gamma model of rate heterogeneity) for nucleotide sequences. Therefore, there is no need to calculate the best-fit substitution model when using RAxML to build ML phylogenies.
3. To perform a bootstrap (1000 replications) analysis and search for the best-scoring ML tree, first open the Command Prompt under Windows. You can use the Windows search tool and type CMD, and the Command Prompt will be shown (click on it to open).
4. Change the Command Prompt directory to the folder where your PHYLIP and raxmlHPC.exe files are located by typing cd 'folder path'. Here, cd C:\Users\UENF\Downloads\Geminiviridae (you can right-click on your folder to Copy it as a path and Paste in the Command Prompt). Press Enter and the directory will be changed. Type dir and press Enter to list the files inside your folder.
5. Then, type the command raxmlHPC -f a -x 12345 -p 12345 -N 1000 -m GTRGAMMA -s InputFileName.phy -n OutputFileName, where -f a (rapid bootstrap analysis and search for best-scoring ML tree), -x (rapid bootstrap random number seed), -p (parsimony random seed), -N (number of bootstrap replications), -m (substitution model), -s (PHYLIP file containing the aligned sequences), and -n (name for output files). In this chapter, the command used for *Geminiviridae* genome data was: raxmlHPC -f a -x 12345 -p 12345 -N 1000 -m GTRGAMMA -s geminiviridae_align.phy -n geminiviridae (press Enter) (Fig. 17). When the RAxML command and PHYLIP file are correctly set, a real-time log with the bootstrap replication number will be printed to the Command Prompt window. Then, best-scoring ML tree search starts with the message Starting ML search appearing in the Command Prompt window.

Command templates

Nucleotide sequences

```
raxmlHPC -f a -x 12345 -p 12345 -N 1000 -m GTRGAMMA -s InputFileName.phy -n OutputFileName
```

Amino acid sequences

```
raxmlHPC -f a -x 12345 -p 12345 -N 1000 -m PROTGAMMAAUTO -s InputFileName.phy -n OutputFileName
```

This chapter

Geminiviridae genomes

```
raxmlHPC -f a -x 12345 -p 12345 -N 1000 -m GTRGAMMA -s geminiviridae_align.phy -n geminiviridae
```

Geminiviridae CP

```
raxmlHPC -f a -x 12345 -p 12345 -N 1000 -m PROTGAMMAAUTO -s cp_align.phy -n cp
```

Geminiviridae Rep

```
raxmlHPC -f a -x 12345 -p 12345 -N 1000 -m PROTGAMMAAUTO -s rep_align.phy -n rep
```

Fig. 17 Command lines to run RAxML v.8 from a Command Prompt when reconstructing maximum likelihood (ML) phylogenetic trees for *Geminiviridae* complete genomes, coat protein (CP), and replication-associated protein (Rep) datasets

6. Once the ML search analysis is finished, several files containing the best tree (RAxML_bestTree.OutputFileName), all bootstrapped trees (RAxML_bootstrap.OutputFileName), best-scoring ML tree (RAxML_bestTree.OutputFileName), best-scoring ML tree with support values (RAxML_bipartitions.OutputFileName), and best-scoring ML tree with support values as branch labels (RAxML_bipartitionsBranchLabels.OutputFileName) are saved to your computer directory and the sentence Overall execution time for full ML analysis: is shown at the bottom of the Command Prompt window.
7. The ML phylogenetic tree containing the bootstrap support values is saved to RAxML_bipartitions.OutputFileName (here, RAxML_bipartitions.geminiviridae), which can be edited using FigTree.
8. When analyzing amino acid data, repeat **steps 2–7**, but using the following command: raxmlHPC -f a -x 12345 -p 12345 -N 1000 -m PROTGAMMAAUTO -s InputFileName.phy -n OutputFileName. In this case, the command -m PROTGAMMAAUTO will automatically determine which is the best-fit protein substitution model for your dataset.
9. In this chapter, the commands used for *Geminiviridae* CP and Rep datasets were: raxmlHPC -f a -x 12345 -p 12345 -N 1000 -m PROTGAMMAAUTO -s cp_align.phy -n cp, and raxmlHPC -f a -x 12345 -p 12345 -N 1000 -m PROTGAMMAAUTO -s rep_align.phy -n rep, respectively (Fig. 17). The ML phylogenetic trees containing the bootstrap support values were saved to RAxML_bipartitions.cp and RAxML_bipartitions.rep.

3.14 Reconstructing Bayesian Phylogenetic Trees Using MrBayes

1. This protocol can be used to reconstruct Bayesian Inference phylogenetic trees using MrBayes v. 3 (nbisweden.github.io/MrBayes/download.html). This program is largely used for inference of phylogenetic trees, being very time-consuming when using big datasets such as *Geminiviridae*. In this case, it is important to use parallel-processing, high performance computers to run this analysis.
2. Create a folder into your preferred directory and add the *Geminiviridae* alignment file (complete genomes) in NEXUS format. Also, add the mrbayes.exe executable program.
3. Open the alignment file (FileName.nex) using notepad and add the MrBayes command block (obtained in Subheading 3.7) at the bottom of the file. Further, add the command for Bayesian Inference analysis at the bottom of the NEXUS file. For example, BEGIN MRBAYES; autoclose = yes; best-fit substitution model calculated for your dataset; END; mcmc ngen = 10000000 samplefreq = 1000; sump nruns = 2 burnin = 2500; sumt nruns = 2 burnin = 2500; END; (*see* **Note 7**). For the *Geminiviridae* dataset used in the present chapter, BEGIN MRBAYES; autoclose = yes; Lset nst = 6 rates = invgamma; Prset statefreqpr = dirichlet(1,1,1,1); END; mcmc ngen = 10000000 samplefreq = 1000; sump nruns = 2 burnin = 2500; sumt nruns = 2 burnin = 2500; END; (Fig. 18).
4. Save the NEXUS file containing the MrBayes command block and close it.
5. Open mrbayes.exe by double clicking on it under Windows.
6. Type execute FileName.nex (press Enter). Here, execute geminiviridae_align.nex. When the NEXUS file is processed correctly, a real-time log with the MCMC generations and time remaining will be printed to the MrBayes main window.
7. The files FileName.p (parameters), FileName.t (trees), and FileName.con (parameters + trees) will be saved to your folder. Here, geminiviridae_align.p (parameters), geminiviridae_align.t (trees), geminiviridae_align.con (parameters + trees). The Bayesian phylogenetic tree with posterior probability values is in the file FileName.con (here, geminiviridae_align.con), therefore, use it to edit the tree in programs such as FigTree.
8. For reconstruction of Bayesian inference trees based on concatenated nucleotide sequences, you must select the best-fit substitution model for each dataset separately, and then, prepare the MrBayes command block for partitioned data as shown in Fig. 19.

MrBayes command block template

```
BEGIN MRBAYES;
autoclose=yes;
bLset based on best-fit model selected in section 3.7;
END;
mcmc ngen=10000000 samplefreq=1000; sump nruns=2 burnin=2500; sumt nruns=2 burnin=2500;
END;
```

This chapter
Geminiviridae genomes

```
BEGIN MRBAYES;
autoclose=yes;
Lset  nst=6  rates=invgamma;
Prset statefreqpr=dirichlet(1,1,1,1);
END;
mcmc ngen=10000000 samplefreq=1000; sump nruns=2 burnin=2500; sumt nruns=2 burnin=2500;
END;
```

Fig. 18 MrBayes v.3 command block for reconstruction of Bayesian inference phylogenetic trees

MrBayes command block template

Example for concatenated Geminiviridae CP and REP

```
BEGIN MRBAYES;
set autoclose=yes;
charset CP = 1-600;
charset Rep = 601-1680;
partition favored = 2: CP, Rep;
set partition = favored;
end;
BEGIN MRBAYES;
lset applyto=(1) nst=2   rates=gamma;
lset applyto=(2) nst=6   rates=invgamma;
BEGIN MRBAYES;
prset applyto=(1) statefreqpr=fixed(equal);
prset applyto=(2) statefreqpr=dirichlet(1,1,1,1);
end;
mcmc ngen=10000000 samplefreq=1000;sump nruns=2 burnin=2500; sumt nruns=2 burnin=2500;
end;
```

Fig. 19 MrBayes command block for reconstruction of Bayesian inference phylogenetic trees based on concatenated nucleotide sequence data

3.15 Editing Phylogenetic Trees in FigTree

1. The protocol described in this chapter aims to provide basic guidelines for editing phylogenetic trees using FigTree v.1 (github.com/rambaut/figtree/).
2. Open FigTree under Windows. You can use the Windows search tool and type FigTree, and the executable program will be shown (click on it to open).
3. On FigTree, go to the tile File → Open and search for the directory where the tree file is located (select your file and open it). For example, for the *Geminiviridae* ML trees reconstructed based on complete genomes, CP, and Rep data using IQ-TREE, the tree files were geminiviridae_align.contree, cp_align.contree, and rep_align.contree, respectively.
4. A new window to labeling the support values for the tree nodes (in this case, bootstrap values) will pop-up. You can keep it as label or rename to bootstrap (as done in this chapter) and click on OK (the tree will be uploaded to the main window of FigTree).
5. To change the thickness of the tree lines, go to the tile Appearance → Line Weight (here, it was moved up to 3; Figs. 10, 11, 12, and 14).
6. To add/modify a root to the phylogenetic tree, go to Trees → Root Tree → Rooting → Midpoint (you will notice the tree's topology will change automatically).
7. To edit the font type and size for the Operational Taxonomic Units (OTUs or isolates/sequences), go to Tip labels → Font (the window Setup color range will be opened). Select the desired font type and size and click on OK. In this chapter, tip labels were omitted due to the high number of OTUs (just uncheck the Tip labels box).
8. To add the bootstrap values to each tree node, check the Node labels box, and go to Node labels → Display, select the option bootstrap (or label if you decided to keep it when opening the tree file) and the values will be shown near to each tree node.
9. To edit the font type and size for the bootstrap values, go to Node labels → Font (the window Setup color range will be opened). Select the desired font type and size and click on OK. In this chapter, node labels or bootstrap values were represented by empty and filled circles as indicated in Figs. 10, 11, 12, and 14.
10. To change the OTUs color, select the tool Taxa at the top of the FigTree v1 main window, select the isolates you want to add a different color and click on the tile Color (select a color and click on OK). Repeat this step until all isolates have the appropriated color.

11. To change the color of the tree lines, select the tool Clade or Node at the top of the FigTree v1 main window, select the clade or node you want to add a different color and click on the tile Color (select a color and click on OK). Repeat this step until all lines have the appropriated color.
12. Finally, to change the layout of the phylogenetic tree, go to the tile Layout and select the type of tree topology (rectangular tree layout, polar tree layout or radial tree layout).
13. To export the phylogenetic tree using a vector format such as PDF, go to File → Export PDF. Select the file directory and save it as FileName.pdf (here, geminiviridae_align.pdf, cp_align.pdf, and rep_align.pdf). The files are now ready to be additionally edited using image editing programs such as Inkscape (inkscape.org/pt/).

3.16 IQ-TREE on a Web Server

1. The IQ-TREE v.2 software is freely available at the IQ-TREE web server (iqtree.cibiv.univie.ac.at/), HIV Sequence Database (hiv.lanl.gov/content/sequence/IQTREE/iqtree.html), and CIPRES web portal (phylo.org/portal2).
2. The procedure reported here provides basic guidelines to carry out ML analysis when reconstructing nucleotide- and amino acid-based phylogenetic trees using IQ-TREE on the IQ-TREE web server (iqtree.cibiv.univie.ac.at/).
3. Create a folder for each sequence dataset into your preferred directory and add the *Geminiviridae* alignment files (complete genomes, CP, and Rep) in PHYLIP format (this chapter, geminiviridae_align.phy, cp_align.phy, and rep_align.phy).
4. Open the IQ-TREE web server and go to the tile Alignment file → Browse (a new window will pop-up). Search for the directory you just created and select the PHYLIP file (for example, geminiviridae_align.phy). Click on OPEN to upload the file.
5. You can inform IQ-TREE the type of data by checking the appropriated box (go to Sequence type → DNA, Sequence type → Protein, or Sequence type → Codon). Additionally, you can just ask IQ-TREE to automatically detect the data type (Sequence type → Auto-detect).
6. To set the substitution model, IQ-TREE can automatically select the best-fit substitution model by going to the Substitution model and selecting the option Auto. Further, you can set the substitution model previously selected for each dataset in Subheading 3.5. Here, complete genomes (GTR + F + I + G4), CP (LG + F + I + G4), and Rep (LG + G4).

7. To set the branch support analysis, type the number of replications in the tile Number of bootstrap alignment (here, 1000 replications were used).
8. To perform the SH-like approximate likelihood ratio test, check the box YES on the tile SH-aLRT branch test, and type the number of replications in the tile #replicates (for example, 1000 replications).
9. Finally, type your email address in the tile Email (optional, to retrieve the results) and click on SUBMIT JOB. A notification will be sent to your email once the analysis is done, together with a link that can be used to retrieve the results.
10. A new window is opened once the job submission is successfully done. Click on OK and you will be redirected to a new webpage where the tiles Summary, Run Log, and Full results are shown for each analysis you have created.
11. To download the results, check the box of your analysis, located at the left side of the webpage, and click on DOWNLOAD SELECTED JOBS. Search for your folder directory and save it. The IQ-TREE report (FileName.iqtree), Maximum-likelihood tree (FileName.treefile), Consensus tree (FileName.contree), and Screen log file (FileName.log) can be found in the unzipped folder. The CONTREE file contains the ML tree with bootstrap support values.
12. Repeat **steps 3–12** to reconstruct ML phylogenies to CP and Rep amino acid sequences.
13. To perform a ML analysis for concatenated data, for example, CP-Rep dataset (*see* Subheadings 3.9 and 3.11), repeat **steps 3–12**. Additionally, upload the NEXUS file containing the partitioning command (*see* Subheading 3.11) by going to Partition file → Browse (a new window will pop-up). Search for the appropriated directory and select the NEXUS file. Click on OPEN to upload the file (type your email and submit the job).
14. The ML tree files are now ready to be viewed and edited in FigTree and Inkscape.

3.17 PAUP on a Web Server

1. The PAUP v.4 program is available at the CIPRES web portal (phylo.org/portal2), and the protocol described here provides basic guidelines to carry out ML analysis when reconstructing phylogenetic trees using PAUP on the CIPRES web portal.
2. Create a folder into your preferred directory and add the *Geminiviridae* alignment file (for example, complete genomes, CP, and Rep) in NEXUS format (this chapter, geminiviridae_align.nex, cp_align.nex, and rep_align.nex). The NEXUS alignment file must contain the PAUP command block for reconstruction of ML phylogenetic trees, as indicated in Subheadings 3.6, 3.7 and 3.8.

3. Open the CIPRES web portal and go to the tile Create New Folder (type the folder's label and click on Save). The new folder will contain two subfolders (Data and Tasks).
4. Click on the Data subfolder and go to the tile Upload data (a new window will pop-up). Then, go to Upload your files → Select files (select the NEXUS file in your folder directory and click on Open). To upload the file, click on Save.
5. Now, click on the subfolder Tasks and go to the tile Create new task (a new window will pop-up).
6. Select the input file (the NEXUS file you just uploaded to the Data subfolder). Go to Input → Select Input Data, check the box for the appropriated NEXUS file and click on Select data (you will be redirected to the tile Select tool).
7. Select the tool for your ML phylogenetic analysis by clicking on the appropriated program (here, PAUP on ACCESS 4.a168).
8. In the new window, go to Input parameters → 4 Parameter Sets (click to see the advanced parameters). Due to the fact that your NEXUS file already contains a PAUP command block, you just need to check the box My dataset has commands in a PAUP block*, set the number of hours you want your analysis to be run by typing it in the tile Maximum Hours to Run (click here for help setting this correctly)*. Additionally, set the likelihood criterion by selecting it in the tile Set the Optimality Criterion*, and click on Save Parameters.
9. Add a name to your analysis by typing it in the tile Description and click on Save and Run Task. Once the analysis is finished, the CIPRES web portal will send a notification to the email used for subscribing to the web portal.
10. Go to the CIPRES web portal, click on the subfolder Tasks and then click on the tile View Output (a new window with the results of your run will be shown).
11. The ML phylogenetic tree, including the bootstrap values, is saved to FileName.tre (for example, geminiviridae.tre) (click on Download to retrieve the tree).
12. The ML tree file is now ready to be viewed and edited in FigTree and Inkscape.

3.18 RaxML on a Web Server

1. The RAxML v.8 software is available at the CIPRES web portal (phylo.org/portal2), and the protocol described here provides basic guidelines to carry out ML analysis when reconstructing nucleotide- and amino acid-based phylogenetic trees using RAxML on the CIPRES web portal.
2. Create a folder into your preferred directory and add the *Geminiviridae* alignment files (for example, complete genomes, CP, and Rep) in PHYLIP format (this chapter, geminiviridae_align.phy, cp_align.phy, and rep_align.phy).

3. Open the CIPRES web portal and go to the tile Create New Folder (type the folder's label and click on Save). The new folder will contain two subfolders (Data and Tasks).
4. Click on the Data subfolder and go to the tile Upload data (a new window will pop-up). Then, go to Upload your files → Select files (select the PHYLIP file in your folder directory and click on Open). To upload the file, click on Save.
5. Now, click on the subfolder Tasks and go to the tile Create new task (a new window will pop-up).
6. Select the input file (the PHYLIP file you just uploaded to the Data subfolder). Go to Input → Select Input Data, check the box for the appropriated PHYLIP file and click on Select data (you will be redirected to the tile Select tool).
7. Select the tool for your ML phylogenetic analysis by clicking on the appropriated program (here, RAxML-HPC2 on ACCESS).
8. In the new window, go to Input parameters → 50 Parameter Sets (click to see the advanced parameters). Set the number of hours you want your analysis to be run by typing it in the tile Maximum Hours to Run (click here for help setting this correctly)*.
9. Type the number of sites of your alignment data in the tile Enter the number of patterns in your dataset (for example, for *Geminiviridae* complete genomes, the number of aligned sites was 9453).
10. Select the data type (nucleotide or protein) in the tile Please select the Data Type *.
11. In the tile Nucleic Acid Options → Choose model for bootstrapping phase, check the box GTRCAT or GTRGAMMA, when using nucleotide data. However, if you are analyzing protein data, go to Protein Analysis Options → Choose GAMMA or CAT model:, and check the box Protein GAMMA or Protein CAT.
12. Finally, go to Configure Bootstrapping, check the box Specify an Explicit Number of Bootstraps, and type the number of bootstrap replications in the tile Bootstrap iterations (for example, 1000 replications). Click on Save parameters.
13. Add a name to your analysis by typing it in the tile Description and click on Save and Run Task. Once the analysis is done, the CIPRES web portal will send a notification to the email used for subscribing to the web portal.
14. Go to the CIPRES web portal, click on the subfolder Tasks and then click on the tile View Output (a new window with the results of your run will be shown).

15. The best-scoring ML phylogenetic tree, including the bootstrap values, is saved to RAxML_bipartitions.result (click on Download to retrieve the tree).
16. The ML tree files are now ready to be viewed and edited in FigTree and Inkscape.

3.19 MrBayes on a Web Server

1. The MrBayes v.3 software is available at the CIPRES web portal (phylo.org/portal2), and the protocol described here provides basic guidelines to carry out Bayesian inference analysis when reconstructing nucleotide-based phylogenetic trees using MrBayes on the CIPRES web portal.
2. Create a folder into your preferred directory and add the *Geminiviridae* alignment file (for example, complete genomes) in NEXUS format (this chapter, geminiviridae_align.nex). The NEXUS alignment file must contain the MrBayes command block for reconstruction of Bayesian phylogenetic trees, as indicated in Subheading 3.14.
3. Open the CIPRES web portal and go to the tile Create New Folder (type the folder's label and click on Save). The new folder will contain two subfolders (Data and Tasks).
4. Click on the Data subfolder and go to the tile Upload data (a new window will pop-up). Then, go to Upload your files → Select files (select the NEXUS file in your folder directory and click on Open). To upload the file, click on Save.
5. Now, click on the subfolder Tasks and go to the tile Create new task (a new window will pop-up).
6. Select the input file (the NEXUS file you just uploaded to the Data subfolder). Go to Input → Select Input Data, check the box for the appropriated NEXUS file and click on Select data (you will be redirected to the tile Select tool).
7. Select the tool for your Bayesian phylogenetic analysis by clicking on the appropriated program (here, MrBayes on XSEDE 3.2.7a).
8. In the new window, go to Input parameters → 149 Parameter Sets (click to see the advanced parameters). Due to the fact that your NEXUS file already contains a MrBayes command block, you just need to check the box My Data Contains a MrBayes Data Block (CHECK THIS OR MrBayes BLOCK ENTRIES WILL BE OVERWRITTEN!!!)*, set the number of hours you want your analysis to be run by typing it in the tile Maximum Hours to Run (click here for help setting this correctly)*, and click on Save parameters.
9. Finally, add a name to your analysis by typing it in the tile Description and click on Save and Run Task. Once the analysis is completed, the CIPRES web portal will send a notification to the email used for subscribing to the web portal.

10. Go to the CIPRES web portal, click on the subfolder Tasks and then click on the tile View Output (a new window with the results of your run will be shown).
11. The majority-rule Bayesian phylogenetic tree, including the posterior probability values, is saved to infile.nex.con.tre (click on Download to retrieve the tree).
12. The Bayesian tree file is now ready to be viewed and edited in FigTree and Inkscape.

4 Notes

1. You must be aware that using an identical name for more than one sequence will create an error during the phylogenetic reconstruction analysis, which implicates in the program not being able to generate a tree file. To avoid this issue, you must always start the sequence names with the GenBank accession number (here, the RefSeq accession numbers that are usually comprised by nine characters). Alternatively, you can use other sequence analysis programs such as Geneious (geneious.com), which has an option (Relaxed Phylip—Full length names followed by a single space) to export the entire sequence name when exporting the alignment to PHYLIP and NEXUS formats.
2. ModelTest-NG v.0.1.7 (github.com/ddarriba/modeltest/releases) can be used to select best-fit substitution models for both nucleotide and amino acid datasets (as described in this chapter using MrModelTest, jModelTest, and ProtTest) and write PAUP and MrBayes command blocks for reconstruction of ML and Bayesian phylogenetic trees, respectively.
3. There is no need to inform the type of data (nucleotide or amino acid) you are using as it will be automatically detected by the IQ-TREE program, but this command is also available. Further, mixed data (nucleotide and amino acid sequences) can be used in IQ-TREE. In this case, independent PHYLIP files for each type of data, and a NEXUS files specifying the partitioning parameters are required.
4. GTR = General time reversible model; F = Empirical base frequencies; I=Invariable sites; G4 = Gamma rate heterogeneity; and LG = Improved general amino acid replacement matrix.
5. The selection of a substitution model is a very important step in molecular phylogenetics, especially due to the heterogeneity in genomic sequence data (sequence evolution is not homogeneous across sites and lineages). The Akaike Information Criterion (AIC) and the Bayesian Information Criterion (BIC) are

largely used approaches to select nucleotide and amino acid substitution models in phylogenetics.

6. BEGIN PAUP = PAUP block containing the command lines; AUTOCLOSE = YES to close the status window automatically after the run has ended; LOG START FILE = used to save the PAUP printed console to an output file; REPLACE = a previous output file will be automatically overwritten by the new data; LSET = command to set options for maximum likelihood analysis; NST = specifies the number of substitution types; RMATRIX = specifies the rate matrix; RATES = specifies a model of among-site rate variation (PAUP default assumes that all sites change at the same rate); SHAPE = specifies the shape of the gamma distribution used to accommodate among-site rate variation. NCAT = specifies the number of categories to divide the discrete approximation of the gamma distribution; PINVAR = specifies the proportion of invariable sites or the proportion of sites unable to accept substitutions; SET CRITERION = used to select the phylogenetic reconstruction approach; LIKELIHOOD = Maximum Likelihood; BOOTSTRAP NREPS = sets the number of bootstrap replication; SEARCH = HEURISTIC specifies the option for searching trees of each bootstrap replication; SWAP = specifies the algorithm used by branch-swapping; NNI = nearest-neighbor interchange; START = NJ used to obtain a starting tree for the maximum likelihood analysis; SAVETREES FILE = command to write trees currently in memory to a file; FROM = starting-tree-number specifies the number of the first tree to save; TO = ending-tree-number specifies the number of the last tree to save; SAVEBOOTP=BOTH to include bootstrap and jackknife proportions as branch lengths (BRLENS) and internal node labels (NODELABELS); MAXDECIMALS = specifies the maximum number of decimals stored in each tree description; BRLENS = the command YES will include the branch lengths to the bootstrap tree file.
7. BEGIN MRBAYES = MRBAYES block containing the command lines; AUTOCLOSE = YES to close the status window automatically after the run has ended; LSET = command to set options for Bayesian Inference analysis; NST = specifies the number of substitution types; RATES = specifies a model of among-site rate variation; PRSET = is used to define the prior probability distributions on the parameters of the model; MCMC = used to set the Bayesian analysis parameters; NGEN = sets the number of generations for which the analysis will be run; SAMPLEFREQ = specifies how often the chain is sampled; SUMP = command to summarize the sampled parameter values; SUMT = command to write output files such as summary statistics for the taxon bipartitions, tree with

clade credibility (posterior probability) values, and phylogram (if branch lengths have been saved); NRUNS = 2 sets two simultaneous, and completely independent, runs starting from different random trees; BURNIN = specifies the number of samples to be discarded before sampling of each step starts.

References

1. Fiallo-Olivé E, Lett JM, Martin DP, Roumagnac P, Varsani A, Zerbini FM, Navas-Castillo J (2021) ICTV virus taxonomy profile: *Geminiviridae*. J Gen Virol 102:001696
2. Brown JK, Zerbini FM, Navas-Castillo J, Moriones E, Ramos-Sobrinho R, Silva JC, Fiallo-Olivé E, Briddon RW, Hernández-Zepeda C, Idris A, Malathi VG, Martin DP, Rivera-Bustamante R, Ueda S, Varsani A (2015) Revision of *Begomovirus* taxonomy based on pairwise sequence comparisons. Arch Virol 160:1593–1619
3. Muhire B, Martin DP, Brown JK, Navas-Castillo J, Moriones E, Zerbini FM, Rivera-Bustamante R, Malathi VG, Briddon RW, Varsani A (2013) A genome-wide pairwise-identity-based proposal for the classification of viruses in the genus Mastrevirus (family Geminiviridae). Arch Virol 158:1411–1424
4. Inoue-Nagata AK, Albuquerque LC, Rocha WB, Nagata T (2004) A simple method for cloning the complete begomovirus genome using the bacteriophage phi29 DNA polymerase. J Virol Methods 116:209–211
5. Varsani A, Shepherd DN, Dent K, Monjane AL, Rybicki EP, Martin DP (2009) A highly divergent south African geminivirus species illuminates the ancient evolutionary history of this family. Virol J 6:36
6. Briddon RW, Heydarnejad J, Khosrowfar F, Massumi H, Martin DP, Varsani A (2010) Turnip curly top virus, a highly divergent geminivirus infecting turnip in Iran. Virus Res 152: 169–175
7. Bernardo P, Muhire B, François S, Deshoux M, Hartnady P, Farkas K, Kraberger S, Filloux D, Fernandez E, Galzi S, Ferdinand R, Granier M, Marais A, Monge Blasco P, Candresse T, Escriu F, Varsani A, Harkins GW, Martin DP, Roumagnac P (2016) Molecular characterization and prevalence of two capulaviruses: alfalfa leaf curl virus from France and Euphorbia caput-medusae latent virus from South Africa. Virology 493:142–153
8. Kamali M, Heydarnejad J, Massumi H, Kvarnheden A, Kraberger S, Varsani A (2015) Molecular diversity of turncurtoviruses in Iran. Arch Virol 161:551–561
9. Roossinck MJ, Martin DP, Roumagnac P (2015) Plant virus metagenomics: advances in virus discovery. Phytopathology 105:716–727
10. Roossinck MJ (2017) Deep sequencing for discovery and evolutionary analysis of plant viruses. Virus Res 239:82–86
11. Claverie S, Bernardo P, Kraberger S, Hartnady P, Lefeuvre P, Lett JM, Galzi S, Filloux D, Harkins GW, Varsani A, Martin DP, Roumagnac P (2018) From spatial metagenomics to molecular characterization of plant viruses: a geminivirus case study. Adv Virus Res 101:55–83
12. Fontenele RS, Abreu RA, Lamas NS, Alves-Freitas DMT, Vidal AH, Poppi el RR, Melo FL, Lacorte C, Martin DP, Campos MA, Varsani A, Ribeiro SG (2018) Passion fruit chlorotic mottle virus: molecular characterization of a new divergent geminivirus in Brazil. Viruses 10:169
13. Fontenele RS, Salywon AM, Majure LC, Cobb IN, Bhaskara A, Avalos-Calleros JA, Argüello-Astorga GR, Schmidlin K, Khalifeh A, Smith K, Schreck J, Lund MC, Köhler M, Wojciechowski MF, Hodgson WC, Puente-Martinez-R, Van Doorslaer K, Kumari S, Vernière C, Filloux D, Roumagnac P, Lefeuvre P, Ribeiro SG, Kraberger S, Martin DP, Varsani A (2020) A novel divergent geminivirus identified in asymptomatic New World Cactaceae plants. Viruses 12:398
14. Rocha CS, Castillo-Urquiza GP, Lima AT, Silva FN, Xavier CA, Hora-Júnior BT, Beserra-Júnior JE, Malta AW, Martin DP, Varsani A, Alfenas-Zerbini P, Mizubuti ES, Zerbini FM (2013) Brazilian begomovirus populations are highly recombinant, rapidly evolving, and segregated based on geographical location. J Virol 87:5784–5799
15. Bernardo P, Charles-Dominique T, Barakat M, Ortet P, Fernandez E, Filloux D, Hartnady P, Rebelo TA, Cousins SR, Mesleard F, Cohez D, Yavercovski N, Varsani A, Harkins GW, Peterschmitt M, Malmstrom CM, Martin DP, Roumagnac P (2018) Geometagenomics illuminates the impact of agriculture on the distribution and prevalence of plant viruses at the ecosystem scale. ISME J 12:173–184

16. Villamor DEV, Ho T, Al Rwahnih M, Martin RR, Tzanetakis IE (2019) High throughput sequencing for plant virus detection and discovery. Phytopathology 109:716–725
17. Liang P, Navarro B, Zhang Z, Wang H, Lu M, Xiao H, Wu Q, Zhou X, Di Serio F, Li S (2015) Identification and characterization of a novel geminivirus with a monopartite genome infecting apple trees. J Gen Virol 96:2411–2420
18. Roumagnac P, Granier M, Bernardo P, Deshoux M, Ferdinand R, Galzi S, Fernandez E, Julian C, Abt I, Filloux D, Mesléard F, Varsani A, Blanc S, Martin DP, Peterschmitt M (2015) Alfalfa leaf curl virus: an aphid-transmitted geminivirus. J Virol 89: 9683–9688
19. Al Rwahnih M, Alabi OJ, Westrick NM, Golino D (2018) Prunus geminivirus a: a novel grablovirus infecting *Prunus* spp. Plant Dis 102: 1246–1253
20. Edgar RC (2004) MUSCLE: multiple sequence alignment with high accuracy and high throughput. Nucleic Acids Res 32:1792–1797
21. Tamura K, Stecher G, Kumar S (2021) MEGA11: molecular evolutionary genetics analysis version 11. Mol Biol Evol 38:3022–3027
22. Hoang DT, Chernomor O, von Haeseler A, Minh BQ, Vinh LS (2018) UFBoot2: improving the ultrafast bootstrap approximation. Mol Biol Evol 35:518–522
23. Nguyen LT, Schmidt HA, von Haeseler A, Minh BQ (2015) IQ-TREE: a fast and effective stochastic algorithm for estimating maximum-likelihood phylogenies. Mol Biol Evol 32:268–274
24. Swofford DL (1998) PAUP*. Phylogenetic Analysis Using Parsimony (* and other methods). Version 4. Sinauer Associates, Sunderland, Massachusetts
25. Stamatakis A (2014) RAxML version 8: a tool for phylogenetic analysis and post-analysis of large phylogenies. Bioinformatics 30:1312–1313
26. Ronquist F, Teslenko M, van der Mark P, Ayres DL, Darling A, Höhna S, Larget B, Liu L, Suchard MA, Huelsenbeck JP (2012) MrBayes 3.2: efficient Bayesian phylogenetic inference and model choice across a large model space. Syst Biol 61:539–542
27. Miller MA, Pfeiffer W, Schwartz T (2010) Creating the CIPRES science gateway for inference of large phylogenetic trees. Gateway Computing Environments Workshop (GCE), New Orleans, LA, USA, pp 1–8
28. Nylander JAA (2004) MrModeltest version 2. Program distributed by the author. Evolutionary Biology Centre, Uppsala University, Uppsala

Chapter 11

Recombination Analysis of Geminiviruses Using Recombination Detection Program (RDP)

Alvin Crespo-Bellido, Darren Patrick Martin, and Siobain Duffy

Abstract

Geminiviruses are recombination-prone, and characterizing this evolutionary process within their genomes is a frequent goal of researchers. RDP is a stand-alone Windows program combining many algorithms that detect and characterize recombination. It has been widely used by the geminivirus community (and beyond). Here we describe the use of RDP4 and RDP5 for analysis of geminiviral nucleotide sequences including: (*i*) obtaining a reasonable dataset for analysis, (*ii*) making a credible multiple sequence alignment and (*iii*) analyzing an alignment with RDP on that alignment. RDP to both characterize recombination events and to produce statistically recombination-free datasets for other molecular evolution analyses.

Key words Recombination, Multiple sequence alignment, RDP5, Phylogenetics, Sub-alignment, Evolution, Horizontal gene transfer

1 Introduction

The detection of recombination within genetic and genomic data has been a high priority for evolutionary biologists. Not only is the horizontal transfer of genes among organisms of inherent interest, most models of molecular evolution (such as building phylogenetic trees) are compromised by recombination, so identifying it and eliminating it from datasets can improve the quality of downstream analyses [1, 2]. Within virology, one of the most widely used suites of tools for quantifying and understanding recombination is the aptly named Recombination Detection Program (RDP), which is currently in its fourth and fifth major release [3]. RDP brings together many separate algorithms to assess the evidence for recombination in a dataset—both an explicit timesaver, and RDP jointly considers data from the algorithms to help determine statistical support for a predicted recombination event. In this way, RDP is more than the sum of its parts, and its graphical interface has ensured it is more widely used than many of the component

Francisco Murilo Zerbini et al. (eds.), *Geminiviruses: Methods and Protocols*, Methods in Molecular Biology, vol. 2912, https://doi.org/10.1007/978-1-0716-4454-6_11,

algorithms would be if they were only supplied as code on public repositories. RDP runs natively on Windows, which can be emulated on other operating systems. Command line versions have also been developed for researchers eschewing a graphical interface and/or who want to implement RDP in pipelines—OpenRDP which implements many of the algorithms in RDP4, https://github.com/PoonLab/OpenRDP, and a command line version of RDP5 (RDP5CL) is distributed with RDP5 [3].

Within geminivirology, the adoption of RDP has been near universal as the author of the program (Darren Martin) has published widely on the molecular evolution of geminiviruses [4, 5]. In a world dominated by algorithms created for cellular organisms, and with virologists often unconsciously catering to RNA viruses, RDP is one of the only widely adopted tools that works from the default of geminivirus genomes. For instance, the default setting for the genomic architecture is circular, like geminiviruses. This isn't just a convenient default setting for the community, it means the recombination detection programs are coded to have the ability to check for recombination around the site of linearization needed to create alignments.

This chapter will explain how to use RDP (the stable version 4 [6] and continually improving version 5 [3]), which are both in widespread use, to analyze geminivirus nucleotide sequence data. RDP is commonly used to study the patterns of frequent recombination among geminiviruses (identifying breakpoints, which sequences are descended from a shared recombination event) and to eliminate detectably recombinant sequences from datasets to better suit the assumptions of phylogenetic tree reconstruction and other molecular evolutionary analyses.

2 Materials

2.1 Curating a Dataset

RDP4 can handle ~3000 geminiviral genomes in an analysis—though the larger the dataset, the longer the analysis will take. RDP5 accommodates larger datasets (up to 20,000 sequences [3]). Despite the large allowable dataset sizes, researchers should still exercise judgment in collating their datasets. Recombination detection relies on patterns of nucleotide differences in the dataset, so there is no value in including multiple identical sequences in the analysis. Statistically robust recombination detection is affected by the number of multiple comparisons made in the analysis, so including identical sequences will *harm* the analysis, by needlessly increasing the number of comparisons and reducing the sensitivity of the analyses.

Many times, researchers are interested in the recombination observed in their own dataset of field-collected sequences. Combining these with previously sequenced isolates of the same species from GenBank often makes sense because the field-collected isolates share ancestry with other isolates from the same species. Other researchers explicitly set out to examine recombination in a single group [7], or the evolution within a single species [5], which guides the choice of which GenBank sequences to use. Combining sequences from increasingly distantly related groups makes it difficult to get a good alignment of nucleotide sequences (see below) so there is an inherent trade-off in quality of dataset for an RDP analysis and including many sequences to serve as possible parental sequences for recombination events. The RDP manual recommends using another program coded by Darren Martin and his collaborators, the species demarcation tool SDT (http://web.cbio.uct.ac.za/~brejnev/, [8]), which can be used in tandem with RDP, to identify and use sequences that are >70% identical to one another. It is better to separately analyze groups of sequences that do not share at least 70% identity with each other (and the RDP manual cautions against including any sequence that has <60% identity to another in the dataset). SDT can also flag identical sequences for downsampling.

As all geminiviruses have relatively short genomes (<6 kb), the ability of RDP to handle very long sequences is of no consequence, though it allows the program to be used by all virologists and many studying cellular organisms. Recombination analyses are generally improved by using longer sequences, and the majority of RDP analyses published in the recent literature involve whole genome sequences [9–11]. Using shorter portions of the genome, such as just a single gene, may make it more difficult to detect recombination and make it impossible to detect both breakpoints for recombination events.

2.2 Alignment

Alignment is a key assumption for many molecular evolution analyses: specifically, it is important that your alignment reflects the real ancestry of sites in the aligned columns [12]. Getting the alignment right can take time, but achieving the best possible alignment will give your recombination detection the greatest chance of success and better reflect real evolutionary relationships. Computational algorithms for multiple sequence alignment abound, with variants of Clustal (http://www.clustal.org/ [13–15]), MUSCLE (https://www.drive5.com/muscle5/ [16]), and MAFFT (https://mafft.cbrc.jp/alignment/server/index.html [17]) being among the most widely used in virology. A google scholar search for "geminivirus alignment" and each of these algorithm names produced 3220 hits for Clustal—the oldest of these algorithms—1640 for MUSCLE and 653 for MAFFT. All of these algorithms will do a great job at aligning closely related sequences and will do a good job at aligning more distantly related sequences, though we authors tend to use MUSCLE or MAFFT. Very distantly related sequences are likely not best aligned with nucleotides (protein sequences would be better [18]), but those protein alignments would not be suitable for downstream analysis in RDP. However, aligning nucleotide sequences by an algorithm is not necessarily the end of the alignment process, and it is worthwhile to check alignments by eye to see if they can be improved. Often researchers run these alignment tools in a program that also supports manual changes to the alignment (e.g., Mega [19], Aliview [20], Geneious [21]). An alignment editor coded by the creators of RDP and distributed with the software (IMPALE, http://web.cbio.uct.ac.za/~arjun/) is also available. These programs also allow researchers to highlight a region of the alignment for realignment without realigning the entire dataset.

Alignment algorithms can handle the alignment of insertion/deletion mutations differently than humans would do by eye, and manual corrections to, or algorithmic realignment of, portions of alignments selected by the researcher should provide the best of both computational speed and a human's innate ability to sense patterns. Two examples of alignment correction that likely improve the likelihood of shared ancestry within each column of an alignment are shown in Fig. 1, on a small dataset of DNA-B sequences from Indian cassava mosaic virus (ICMV) and Sri Lankan cassava mosaic virus (SLCMV) sequences [7]. When the sequences are aligned with MUSCLE in Aliview, the patterns in panel 1A and 1C are produced, but manual tweaks to the alignment can increase the number of columns with only transition mutations in them (transitions are more common than transversions [22]) or otherwise move where a gap opens/ends to increase the identical nucleotides in the same alignment (Fig. 1b, d). Geminiviruses are capable of small and large insertion/deletion mutations, especially in non-coding regions [23–25], but the default parameters for alignment programs are not tuned for viral datasets and geminivirus alignments are worth checking for potential sites of manual improvement. For regions that appear to not be homologous (have different origins), the best thing to do for RDP analysis is to stagger them, introducing gaps for all of the sequences that fail to have a region homologous to each—computational alignment programs are not set up to do this, and you will likely have to move the sequence fragments yourself. Note that these necessary changes may expand the length of an alignment relative to the length of the nucleic acids used. For instance, in our recent work on cassava mosaic begomoviruses which have DNA-As with a maximum length of 2816, the alignment was 3149 bases long (https://zenodo.org/records/4029589). Alignment is somewhat

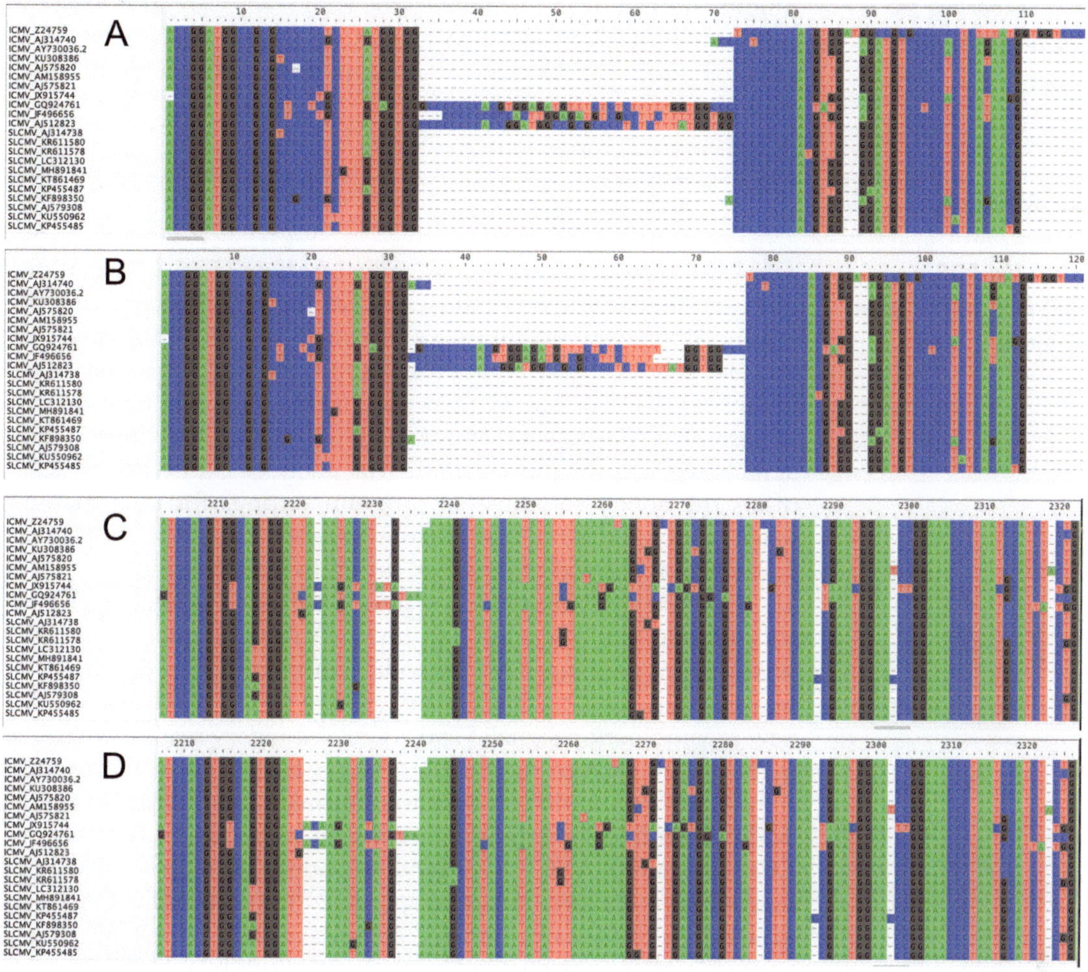

Fig. 1 A dataset of 11 ICMV and 11 SLCMV DNA-B segment sequences from GenBank, aligned by MUSCLE (**a**, **c**) and then with manual corrections (**b**, **d**). Aligned data available at https:/zenodo.org/records/3964977

subjective, where experienced researchers may produce slightly different alignments from the same dataset, but these subtle differences matter less than the overall importance of a well-aligned dataset.

Importantly, RDP5 can explicitly accommodate datasets that are concatenated (separate genomic regions entered as a single nucleotide sequence). This has long been done to test for reassortment (pseudorecombination) within bipartite begomoviruses in RDP, where the "recombination breakpoint" was calculated to be between the DNA-A and DNA-B segments if there had been reassortment among the segments [9, 26]. This round-about method works in RDP4, but RDP5 allows researchers use an exclamation point ("!") at the site of concatenation in the first sequence in an alignment (while being careful to not shift the sequences downstream out of alignment), to explicitly allow the program to differentiate between recombination and reassortment.

2.3 Exporting the Alignment to RDP

Alignments can be imported into the RDP5 software in the following formats: CLUSTAL, FASTA, GCG, GDE, MEGA, NEXUS, PHYLIP, and DNAMAN. Alignment viewers will export alignments in many of these formats.

3 Methods

3.1 The RDP Interface and Program Settings

The RDP software has a user-friendly interface (Fig. 2) that allows the user to easily modify analyses and directly interact with the results. While viral evolutionary biologists are often frustrated by the fact that many computational tools are fine-tuned for other organisms, RDP default settings are entirely appropriate for analysis of geminiviral sequences, and it is advisable that RDP be run with default settings for most geminivirus datasets. Nonetheless, RDP offers the ability to adjust all program settings for each method when searching for recombination signals using the "Options" command at the top of the main program window (Fig. 2).

The user can select which methods are used to detect recombination under the "General" tab in the "Analyze Sequences Using:" section after pressing the "Options" command (Fig. 3). Methods may be used for a "primary scan" (where the methods explore for new recombination signals) and/or a "secondary scan" (where the methods are used to examine sequences for which recombination signals are already detected by the "primary scan"-enabled methods). Generally, the default primary scan selections of RDP, GENECONV, and MAXCHI are recommended for a good balance of detection power, accuracy, and speed [27]. The BOOTSCAN and SISCAN methods are used for secondary scan by default, but a primary scan may be enabled for these methods by selecting the left box beside the method name (albeit at the cost of potentially much

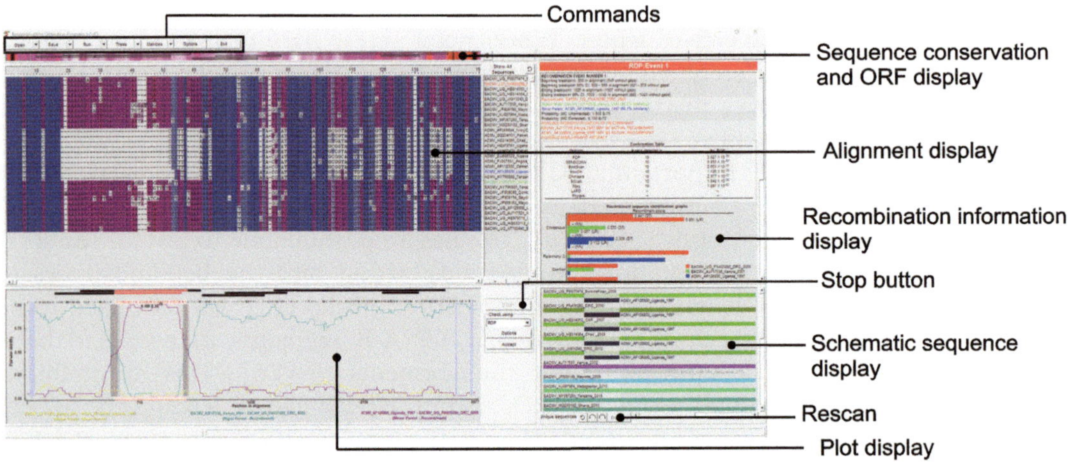

Fig. 2 RDP5 graphical interface

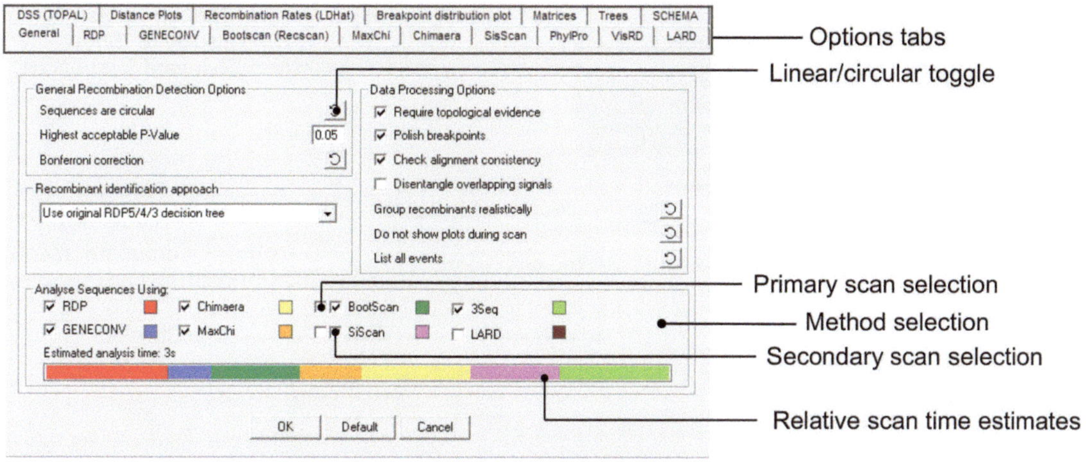

Fig. 3 General settings tab of the Options window

slower run times). Similarly, you may also enable the LARD method for secondary scan but note that this should only be done for very small datasets (<20 sequences) given that it is significantly slower than all the other methods. Indeed, LARD is one recombination detection algorithm that we run independently from RDP on large datasets [7]. Since the 3SEQ, RDP, GENECONV, MAXCHI or CHIMAERA methods are very fast, they are always used in secondary scans of recombination signals detected by other methods. When analyzing a large sequence dataset, it might be preferable to explore for recombination signals using the fast methods and then use the slower methods to validate the results. To assess whether certain selections are computationally feasible, a rough estimate of the expected analysis run time is displayed at the bottom of the "Options" window.

While often not necessary and unadvisable to beginners, you may also change method-specific settings by clicking on a particular method tab in the "Options" window. In general, the only settings that should ever be changed from their default values are window and step sizes, and the optimal sizes will vary for different methods and datasets. General rules on adjusting specific methods settings may be found in the RDP5 user manual (http://web.cbio.uct.ac.za/~darren/rdp.html).

As an example, we present an analysis of an alignment of isolates of two cassava mosaic begomovirus species—African cassava mosaic virus (ACMV) and East African cassava mosaic virus (EACMV)—and include representatives of the EACMV recombinant strain EACMV-Uganda (EACMV-Ug) which descended from a recombination event between ACMV and EACMV, and has been associated with a severe cassava mosaic disease pandemic in cassava across sub-Saharan Africa [28]. The alignment is available at https://zenodo.org/records/10498957 and the data in Figs. 4 and 5 are from this dataset.

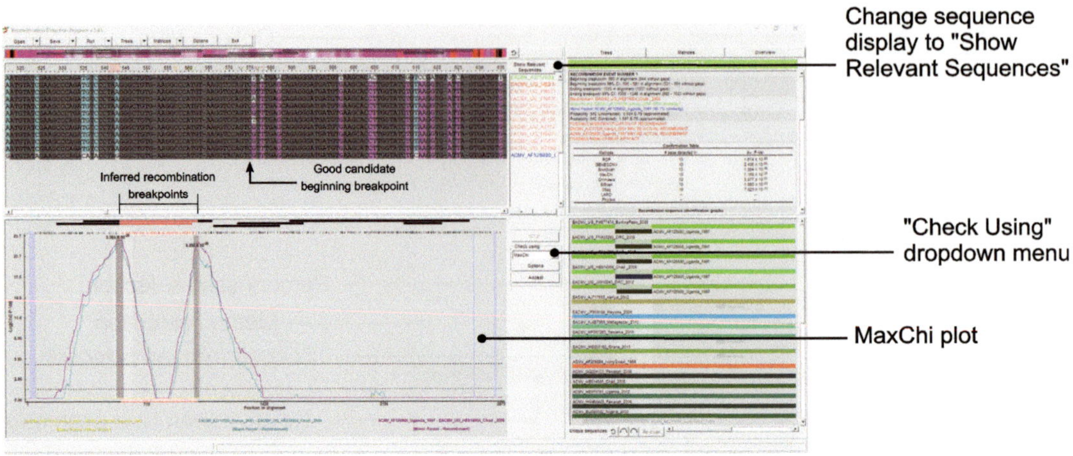

Fig. 4 Cross-checking inferred recombination breakpoints

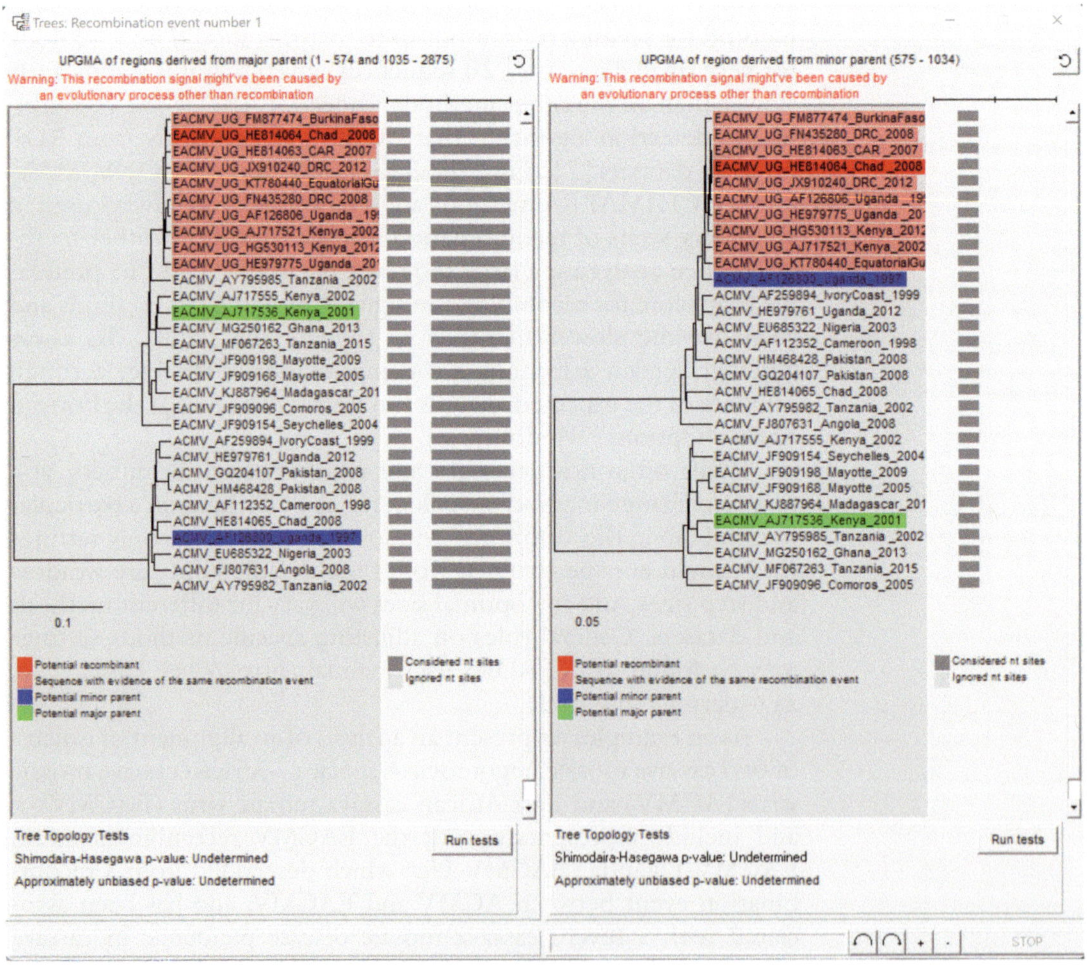

Fig. 5 Phylogenetic tree of regions corresponding to the major (left) and minor (right) parents inferred from recombination event 1

3.2 Exploratory Analysis

Once you have loaded your sequence alignment in the RDP software and selected all the desired program settings, you can start the analysis by pressing the "Run" button in the Commands section of the main window (Fig. 2). The software will then search for recombination signals within the alignment and characterize unique recombination events that generated the signals with the selected methods. The analysis may be stopped at any time using the "STOP" button in the graphical interface.

After the initial scan has been completed, the output will reflect a preliminary hypothesis of the recombination history of your dataset. The main output is found in the "Recombination information display" and will include: the position of putative recombination breakpoints, names of sequences within the dataset that are most similar to the parents of the putative recombinant sequence, an approximate probability that the recombination signal is a result of convergent evolution and not recombination, and the number of sequences in the dataset with similar recombination signals displayed in the recombination table (Fig. 2). Most importantly, this window will display warnings of potential issues and uncertainties in the analysis in capitalized red letters. These warnings are most applicable to the details of the recombination events, not the presence or absence of recombination. Therefore, the next step you take in the analysis will depend on your motivation for running the recombination analysis: if the detailed information about recombination events matter or not.

3.3 Generating Recombination-Free Datasets

If your goal is to generate a dataset that is statistically recombination-free for downstream analyses, then you may do so by clicking on the "Save" command dropdown button or right-clicking on the sequence display and selecting the desired option (Fig. 2). Options include generating alignments with recombinant sequences removed, alignments with only the recombinant fragments removed (and "masked" with alignment gaps), distributed alignments where the recombinant sequences are split up into separate regions, and alignments split into multiple sub-alignments at identified breakpoints. If you would like to be conservative in a downstream phylogenetic analysis, you may want to remove all sequences with putative recombination signals to avoid biasing your results. If removing recombinant sequences results in a drastically reduced dataset, you may want to mask recombinant regions instead, which is an approach that can maximize your dataset and be used for recombination-aware phylogenetics and molecular epidemiology [29].

Generally, sequences are not considered recombinant if only one of the algorithms in RDP implicates the sequence as recombinant—a three-out-of-seven methods threshold as significant evidence of recombination is the typical cutoff used in the literature. This was determined by an empirical analysis of simulated sequence datasets, where statistically significant evidence from at least three methods drastically reduced the false-positive rates for recombination detection [30]. The threshold can be set by pressing the "List all events" button in the "Data Processing Options" section of the "Options" window (Fig. 3) and toggling until the desired threshold is selected.

3.4 Refining Recombination Hypotheses

If you wish to refine the recombination hypothesis so you can properly characterize recombination patterns in your dataset (and even for generating alignments with masked recombinant fragments, you may want to manually adjust breakpoints prior to masking), then you will need to examine each individual recombination event for mistakes RDP might have made during the initial scan. Per the manual, the main issues RDP will face are:

1. Inaccurate identification of recombination breakpoint positions.
2. Incorrect identification of parental sequences as recombinants.
3. Incorrect inference that groups of identified recombinants are all descended from the same recombinant ancestor ("Over-grouping").
4. Incorrect inferences that recombinants descended from the same ancestral recombinant contain evidence of unique recombination events ("Under-grouping").

Particularly in datasets featuring frequent recombination, it is likely that RDP may have made some mistakes while interpreting recombination signals. Importantly, as stated in the manual, mistakes made early in the analysis will be more serious than the ones made at the end because RDP characterizes the strongest recombination signals first and the weakest are left for the end. If a mistake is made at any point (especially at the beginning) in the analysis, it is more likely that subsequent recombination will be mischaracterized, leading to a largely incorrect analysis. As a result, it is important to refine the recombination hypothesis by assessing any program failures from the initial scan.

RDP helpfully supplies warnings when there is low support for one of the conclusions (such as potential misidentification of parent vs. recombinant sequences). Don't panic when you see these warnings, but take note of them. They do not mean your alignment/dataset is fatally flawed—and the warnings themselves may be false alarms and the conclusion is likely accurate. The warnings are trying to draw your attention to conclusions of lower confidence—and you may choose to follow up to address the issues with additional work, and ultimately may have significant confidence in the result.

3.5 Known RDP Issue 1: Inaccurate Identification of Recombination Breakpoint Positions

Finding the correct position of recombination breakpoints is important for the identification of recombination hot/cold spots and for functional analysis (i.e., location relative to protein domains/key residues) of recombination events. Additionally, correctly identifying breakpoint locations to generate recombination-free sub-alignments is an important step for downstream phylogenetic analysis [31]. You can verify the accuracy of the identified recombination breakpoints by examining the recombination graphs produced by the different methods in the plot display in the main program window (Fig. 2). For example, you may examine a MaxChi plot for a given event by selecting it from the dropdown menu in the "Check using" section of the plot display (Fig. 4). For the MaxChi plot, you can check whether the peaks on any of the three plotted lines correspond with the borders of the detected recombinant region in pink. If the peaks do not match, it may indicate that there is uncertainty in the estimated position for the breakpoints. You may check any of the other plots for further corroboration. For interpretation of each plot, you may consult with the RDP manual.

If you are satisfied with the breakpoint positions, you can continue to examine any other program issues. However, if you'd like to adjust the position of the breakpoints, this can be done in the alignment display by clicking on the arrow in the top right corner until the "Show Relevant Sequences" option is enabled (Fig. 4). The display will change and the invariant nucleotide sites in the alignment will be shown in grey while the polymorphic sites that are shared between the putative recombinant sequences and the inferred major and minor parental sequences are colored in teal and purple, respectively. You can slide the window to the approximate position of the inferred recombination breakpoints and examine whether they are placed on the correct nucleotide sites. The breakpoint can then be moved by right-clicking on the desired position and selecting the "Place beginning/ending breakpoint here" option. Ideally, a breakpoint should be placed between two polymorphic sites, one reflecting a closer relationship to the major parent and one indicating a closer relationship to the minor parent.

In the example in Fig. 4, the beginning recombination breakpoint for event 1 (which is the well-known ancestral recombination event for the EACMV-Ug lineage) was placed at position 560 in the alignment for sequence EACMV_UG_HE814064_-Chad_2008. However, if you examine other EACMV-Ug sequences by clicking on the recombinant fragments in the schematic sequence display, you will see that the breakpoints are slightly different. In the sequence display, you will see that there is a continuous stretch of invariant sites between the teal polymorphic sites and the purple polymorphic sites (from position 544 to 575) which is where most of the beginning recombination breakpoints are placed (Fig. 4). The inconsistency in assigning the beginning breakpoint in this region for different sequences stems from the fact that the true recombination breakpoint could potentially be at any of these invariant sites but the high sequence identity between the recombinant and both parents in the region makes it difficult to pinpoint the exact recombination breakpoint. In theory, the breakpoint can be placed at any position within the invariant region but for this exercise we place it at position 575 given that after this site is where we observe that the polymorphic patterns of the recombinant match the minor parent more than the major parent. By the same approach, the ending breakpoint can be adjusted to site 1034 in the alignment (not shown).

3.6 Known RDP Issue 2: Incorrect Identification of Parental Sequences as Recombinants

Once the breakpoints are adjusted, it is important to ensure the correct sequence is identified as the recombinant. However, inferring the direction of recombination event (i.e., which sequence is the parent, and which is the recombinant) is not always straightforward. RDP5 employs a variety of tests that attempt to determine which of the three sequences involved in a recombination event is the recombinant. The results of the tests are displayed with their weighted consensus as a series of bar graphs in the "Recombination information display" panel of the main window (Fig. 2). If it is unclear which sequence is recombinant, RDP5 will display a warning that reads "Possible misidentification of recombinant" in the display, and you may want to corroborate whether the putative recombinant has been identified correctly.

One way you can evaluate whether a recombinant sequence has been correctly identified is to compare phylogenies constructed from the regions between and outside of the putative recombinant breakpoints. RDP5 will automatically produce UPGMA trees from these regions whenever a recombination event is selected (Fig. 5), and the trees can be examined by pressing the "Trees" button at the top of the "Recombination information display". In general, the position of the recombinant in the tree will change with respect to the region being analyzed, and they should cluster more closely to and descend from the parental sequence.

In our example, RDP5 has inferred that, as expected, all the EACMV-Ug sequences are descended from a common ancestor with the major parent region being closely related to the EACMV sequences and the minor parent region being closely related to the ACMV sequences (Fig. 5). However, in situations where recombination events are overprinted by subsequent recombination events, the recombinant sequences may only have trace evidence of recombination events and not appear to be monophyletic in the trees, making it more challenging to identify recombinant sequences by just inspecting the phylogenies. Another potential complication may arise from situations where parent sequences are recombinant themselves, which can make the interpretation of the placement of sequences in the tree more confusing. Pervasive recombination in the dataset could also confound interpretation even if the parental sequences are not recombinant. If it seems difficult to identify the recombinant sequence, given that RDP5 has used a variety of different approaches to select the correct one, it is advisable that you leave the results as they are. However, if you would like to change the sequence designations, you can right-click on the graphical representation of the desired recombination event in the "Schematic sequence display" (Fig. 2) and select the "Make the major/minor parent the recombinant" option.

3.7 Known RDP Issues 3 and 4: Over- and Under-Grouping of Recombination Events

It is possible that RDP4 or RDP5 may either infer that recombinants are descended from the same recombinant ancestor when they originated from separate recombination events ("over-group") or that multiple, unique recombination events generated sequences that are actually descended from the same recombinant ("under-group"). "Over-grouping" tends to occur most often since RDP will be conservative when counting the number of unique recombination signals in the dataset and will infer that recombinants with similar breakpoint locations and/or similar parent sequences have descended from a common ancestor. "Under-grouping" is less common but may occur when there is partial overprinting of older recombination events by newer ones in some sequences but not others and, as a result, RDP5 fails to group sequences properly.

To ascertain sequences demonstrating evidence of a common ancestral recombination event, you can compare BOOTSCAN or RDP plots for different potential recombinants while utilizing the same parental sequences. To achieve this in RDP5, follow the following steps:

1. Compile a list of sequences either flagged by the program as containing evidence of a similar recombination event (shown in pink in the trees) or appearing closely related to identified recombinants in phylogenetic trees constructed from various sections of the alignment.
2. Select either the BOOTSCAN or RDP plots from the "Check Using" dropdown menu on the plot display (Fig. 4).
3. Within one of the trees, position the mouse pointer over a sequence name from your list, right-click, and opt for the "Recheck plot with…as recombinant" option.

This action will compare the plots of the presently selected sequence, typically the one harboring the "best" evidence of the recombination event, with one of the sequences selected from your list. The results will be depicted by a line segment above the graph in the plot display (Fig. 6). In the segment, blue will indicate regions where recombination signals closely resemble each other, whereas dark red indicates regions where recombination signals significantly differ. If the region of the sequence covering one or

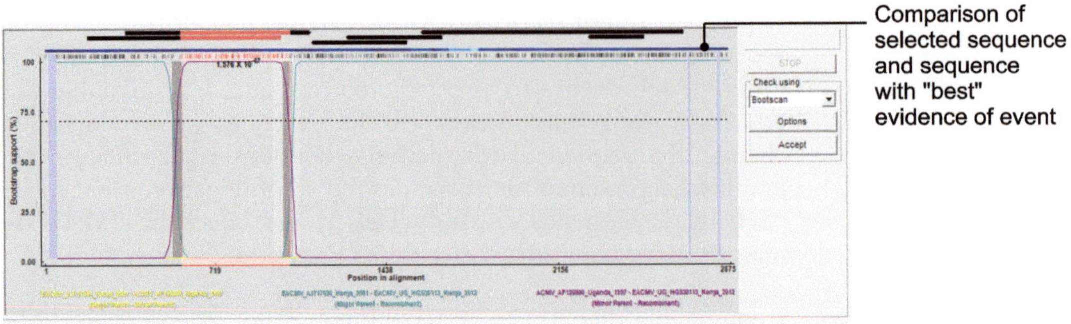

Fig. 6 Bootscan plot with comparison of selected sequence and the sequence with "best" evidence of recombination event

both recombination breakpoints aligns with a blue or green region in the segment, it suggests that the shared site patterns between the compared sequences and their presumed parents are highly similar, conceivably originating from the same event. In our example, randomly selecting another EACMV-Ug sequence from the tree and performing the comparison shows that both sequences are likely descendants of the same event since the entire segment is colored in shades of blue.

If you believe that RDP5 has either over- or under-grouped sequences under a particular recombination event, you can fix the issue through the "Trees" display (Fig. 5). On either of the trees, right-click on the sequence that has been incorrectly included or excluded as sharing the same recombination event and select the "Mark/unmark <sequence name> as having evidence of recombination event" option.

3.8 Finishing up Analyses and Saving Results

Whether you make any modifications to a putative recombination event or not, you should specify whether you are satisfied with the current characterization of the event. This is important because any modification you make to an earlier event may impact the accuracy of the characterization of subsequent events. Once you are done evaluating a particular event, you can let the program know whether you are content with the analysis by moving the mouse pointer over the desired recombination fragment in the "Schematic sequence display" (Fig. 2), pressing the right mouse button and selecting one of the "Accept/reject this event in only/all sequences" options. If the event is accepted, a red border will appear around the recombinant fragment for all sequences with evidence of the event. If you are not satisfied with the characterized event, you can either leave the event as unaccepted or reject it. If you do choose to accept/reject an event, the program will skip this event as you continue your analysis of subsequent events.

If no modifications are made to the first event, you can continue to check the next one. However, after any modification and/or acceptance/rejection of an event, you should reanalyze the dataset while taking your changes into account by pressing the "Rescan" button under the "Schematic sequence display" (Fig. 2). After the reanalysis is finished, you may continue to evaluate events as outlined previously in this work.

It is highly recommended that you save the analysis results often given that any software program will crash sometimes (particularly unstable releases like RDP5). You can save the analysis by pressing the "Save" command in the main program window (Fig. 2). This will save your results as an RDP4/5 project file (with an ".rdp4/.rdp5" file extension) that can be reloaded anytime into the program. It is good practice to regularly save your results in this format to preserve any refining done on the preliminary analysis. If you would like a table summary of the results, you can also save your results in .csv format by clicking the "Save recombination results to an excel readable .csv file" in the "Save" command dropdown menu but note that the program will not be able to reload the analysis from this .csv file.

4 Additional Features

1. Once you have refined your recombination hypothesis, there are a variety of downstream analyses that can be performed to further characterize recombination patterns found in your dataset. For example, the program allows you to create a "breakpoint distribution plot" based on detected recombination breakpoints in your dataset that can help identify recombination hot/cold spots using a breakpoint permutation test [32]. To perform the test, simply select the "Breakpoint distribution plot" option in the "Check Using" dropdown menu. Note that this feature relies on detected recombination breakpoints for every unique recombination event and will be largely based on the easiest-to-detect recombination signals. Since sometimes many recombination events may be undetected depending on program settings and variable stringency when considering evidence for recombination events (e.g., a three-out-of-seven vs. a five-out-of-seven recombination methods threshold), you should carefully consider the obtained results. This analysis is most appropriate for datasets with evidence of many unique recombination events.
2. RDP5 can also perform association tests to determine if there is any evidence suggesting that breakpoint locations are influenced by genomic features of the analyzed sequences. This includes whether breakpoints cluster within particular sites of the genome (e.g., genes, intergenic regions or secondary structures) [33] and whether recombination breakpoints are

associated with variables that may vary along the length of the sequences in the dataset such as sequence diversity and GC content. To learn more about setting up these analyses, you can consult the manual.

3. When connected to the Internet, RDP5 will automatically annotate the genomic features of the input alignment using the NCBI reference sequence database (https://www.ncbi.nlm.nih.gov/genome/viruses/) and, in this case, it will automatically test to see whether breakpoint distributions vary between individual genes and between genes and intergenic regions. These annotations also allow you to output recombination-aware, gene sub-alignments for downstream selection analyses (e.g., dN/dS analysis) that can account for variation in START/STOP codon positions, intron splicing (useful for the analysis of multiple geminivirus genera, http://ictv.global/report/geminiviridae), overlapping reading frames and frameshifts. To save the gene alignment following a completed RDP scan, right-click on the desired gene in the "ORF display" section of the main program window (Fig. 2) and select the "Save alignment file containing the coding region of <gene name>" and follow the prompts to specify the features you want to account for.
4. One of the strengths of RDP is that you do not need recombination-free reference sequences to perform the analyses [6], but that is an option in RDP5 [3]. This feature can be useful when defining recombination events between known parental sequences (e.g., ACMV and EACMV for EACMV-UG, as in our example dataset) or for experimental evolution, when the parental sequences are known.
5. In many cases, some parents of recombinants will not be identified in the analysis. The most likely explanation for this is that the contributor wasn't part of the analyzed dataset—a common situation since we do not include representatives of all species within a genus in our alignments (see curating a dataset, above—including so many distantly related sequences would be unwise, harming the overall alignment). Therefore, to track down the identity of the unknown parents of recombination events, some geminivirologists BLAST the portion of the genome associated with an unknown parent in GenBank [7, 34, 35]. However, this does not necessarily always yield very similar matches, so the major or minor contributor to a recombination event may remain unknown. When you do get a plausible BLAST hit, you can rerun RDP with an alignment including this potential parental sequence and get RDP's assessment of support for it contributing to a given recombination event.

6. A final advanced feature of RDP worth mentioning is the ability to combine the analysis of gene alignments with solved structures of the resulting protein products. As recombination events can dramatically alter protein structure [36], this is a very useful integration of additional biological data. However, few geminivirus proteins have had their structures solved [37] so this is a feature that may become more useful in the future than it is in the present for ssDNA virologists, especially as predictive folding algorithms increase in accuracy [38].

Acknowledgments

The authors acknowledge support from NSF PIRE 1545553 (to SD).

References

1. Schierup MH, Hein J (2000) Consequences of recombination on traditional phylogenetic analysis. Genetics 156:879–891
2. Arenas M, Posada D (2010) The effect of recombination on the reconstruction of ancestral sequences. Genetics 184:1133–1139
3. Martin DP, Varsani A, Roumagnac P, Botha G, Maslamoney S, Schwab T, Kelz Z, Kumar V, Murrell B (2021) RDP5: a computer program for analyzing recombination in, and removing signals of recombination from, nucleotide sequence datasets. Virus Evol 7:veaa087
4. Varsani A, Navas-Castillo J, Moriones E, Hernandez-Zepeda C, Idris A, Brown JK, Zerbini FM, Martin DP (2014) Establishment of three new genera in the family *Geminiviridae*: *Becurtovirus*, *Eragrovirus* and *Turncurtovirus*. Arch Virol 159:2193–2203
5. Lefeuvre P, Martin DP, Harkins G, Lemey P, Gray AJA, Meredith S, Lakay F, Monjane A, Lett J-M, Varsani A, Heydarnejad J (2010) The spread of tomato yellow leaf curl virus from the Middle East to the world. PLoS Pathog 6: e1001164
6. Martin DP, Murrell B, Golden M, Khoosal A, Muhire B (2015) RDP4: detection and analysis of recombination patterns in virus genomes. Virus Evol 1:vev003
7. Crespo-Bellido A, Hoyer JS, Dubey D, Jeannot RB, Duffy S (2021) Interspecies recombination has driven the macroevolution of cassava mosaic begomoviruses. J Virol 95:e0054121
8. Muhire BM, Varsani A, Martin DP (2014) SDT: a virus classification tool based on pairwise sequence alignment and identity calculation. PLoS One 9:e108277
9. Xavier CA, Godinho MT, Mar TB, Ferro CG, Sande OF, Silva JC, Ramos-Sobrinho R, Nascimento RN, Assunção I, Lima GS, Zerbini FM (2021) Evolutionary dynamics of bipartite begomoviruses revealed by complete genome analysis. Mol Ecol 30:3747–3767
10. Guadie D, Tesfaye K, Knierim D, Winter S, Abraham A (2019) Molecular analysis of maize (*Zea mays* L.)-infecting mastreviruses in Ethiopia reveals marked diversity of virus genomes and a novel species. Virus Genes 55:339–345
11. Bejerman N, Trucco V, de Breuil S, Pardina PR, Lenardon S, Giolitti F (2018) Genome characterization of an Argentinean isolate of alfalfa leaf curl virus. Arch Virol 163:799–803
12. Phillips A, Janies D, Wheeler W (2000) Multiple sequence alignment in phylogenetic analysis. Mol Phylogenet Evol 16:317–330
13. Sievers F, Wilm A, Dineen D, Gibson TJ, Karplus K, Li W, Lopez R, McWilliam H, Remmert M, Soding J, Thompson JD, Higgins DG (2011) Fast, scalable generation of high-quality protein multiple sequence alignments using Clustal Omega. Mol Syst Biol 7: 539
14. Sievers F, Higgins DG (2021) The clustal omega multiple alignment package. In: Multiple sequence alignment: methods and protocols. Humana Press, New York, pp 3–16
15. Larkin MA, Blackshields G, Brown NP, Chenna R, McGettigan PA, McWilliam H,

Valentin F, Wallace IM, Wilm A, Lopez R (2007) Clustal W and Clustal X version 2.0. Bioinformatics 23:2947–2948

16. Edgar RC (2004) MUSCLE: multiple sequence alignment with high accuracy and high throughput. Nucleic Acids Res 32:1792–1797
17. Katoh K, Standley DM (2013) MAFFT multiple sequence alignment software version 7: improvements in performance and usability. Mol Biol Evo 30:772–780
18. Simmonds P, Adriaenssens EM, Zerbini FM, Abrescia NGA, Aiewsakun P, Alfenas-Zerbini P, Bao Y, Barylski J, Drosten C, Duffy S, Duprex WP, Dutilh BE, Elena SF, Garcia ML, Junglen S, Katzourakis A, Koonin EV, Krupovic M, Kuhn JH, Lambert AJ, Lefkowitz EJ, Lobocka M, Lood C, Mahony J, Meier-Kolthoff JP, Mushegian AR, Oksanen HM, Poranen MM, Reyes-Munoz A, Robertson DL, Roux S, Rubino L, Sabanadzovic S, Siddell S, Skern T, Smith DB, Sullivan MB, Suzuki N, Turner D, Van Doorslaer K, Vandamme AM, Varsani A, Vasilakis N (2023) Four principles to establish a universal virus taxonomy. PLoS Biol 21:e3001922
19. Tamura K, Stecher G, Kumar S (2021) MEGA11: molecular evolutionary genetics analysis version 11. Mol Biol Evol 38:3022–3027
20. Larsson A (2014) AliView: a fast and lightweight alignment viewer and editor for large datasets. Bioinformatics 30:3276–3278
21. Kearse M, Moir R, Wilson A, Stones-Havas S, Cheung M, Sturrock S, Buxton S, Cooper A, Markowitz S, Duran C, Thierer T, Ashton B, Meintjes P, Drummond A (2012) Geneious basic: an integrated and extendable desktop software platform for the organization and analysis of sequence data. Bioinformatics 28: 1647–1649
22. Duchêne S, Ho SY, Holmes EC (2015) Declining transition/transversion ratios through time reveal limitations to the accuracy of nucleotide substitution models. BMC Evo Biol 15:1–10
23. Sánchez-Campos S, Domínguez-Huerta G, Díaz-Martínez L, Tomás DM, Navas-Castillo J, Moriones E, Grande-Pérez A (2018) Differential shape of geminivirus mutant spectra across cultivated and wild hosts with invariant viral consensus sequences. Front Plant Sci 9:932
24. Ben Chehida S, Filloux D, Fernandez E, Moubset O, Hoareau M, Julian C, Blondin L, Lett J-M, Roumagnac P, Lefeuvre P (2021) Nanopore sequencing is a credible alternative to recover complete genomes of geminiviruses. Microorganisms 9:903
25. Aimone CD, Lavington E, Hoyer JS, Deppong DO, Mickelson-Young L, Jacobson A, Kennedy GG, Carbone I, Hanley-Bowdoin L, Duffy S (2021) Population diversity of cassava mosaic begomoviruses increases over the course of serial vegetative propagation. J Gen Virol 102:001622
26. Varsani A, Lefeuvre P, Roumagnac P, Martin D (2018) Notes on recombination and reassortment in multipartite/segmented viruses. Curr Opin Virol 33:156–166
27. Martin DP, Murrell B, Khoosal A, Muhire B (2017) Detecting and analyzing genetic recombination using RDP4. Methods Mol Biol 1525:433–460
28. Zhou X, Liu Y, Calvert L, Munoz C, Otim-Nape GW, Robinson DJ, Harrison BD (1997) Evidence that DNA-A of a geminivirus associated with severe cassava mosaic disease in Uganda has arisen by interspecific recombination. J Gen Virol 78:2101–2111
29. Didelot X, Parkhill J (2022) A scalable analytical approach from bacterial genomes to epidemiology. Philos Trans R Soc Lond Ser B Biol Sci 377:20210246
30. Posada D, Crandall KA (2001) Evaluation of methods for detecting recombination from DNA sequences: computer simulations. Proc Natl Acad Sci 98:13757–13762
31. Cen S, Rasmussen DA (2023) Exploring the accuracy and limits of algorithms for localizing recombination breakpoints. bioRxiv:2023.2012.2008.570844
32. Heath L, Van Der Walt E, Varsani A, Martin DP (2006) Recombination patterns in aphthoviruses mirror those found in other picornaviruses. J Virol 80:11827–11832
33. Martin DP, Biagini P, Lefeuvre P, Golden M, Roumagnac P, Varsani A (2011) Recombination in eukaryotic single stranded DNA viruses. Viruses 3:1699–1738
34. Fourment M, Gibbs AJ, Gibbs MJ (2008) SWeBLAST: a sliding window web-based BLAST tool for recombinant analysis. J Virol Methods 152:98–101
35. Díaz-Pendón JA, Sánchez-Campos S, Fortes IM, Moriones E (2019) Tomato yellow leaf curl Sardinia virus, a begomovirus species evolving by mutation and recombination: a challenge for virus control. Viruses 11:45
36. Martin DP, Lefeuvre P, Varsani A, Hoareau M, Semegni JY, Dijoux B, Vincent C, Reynaud B,

Lett JM (2011) Complex recombination patterns arising during geminivirus coinfections preserve and demarcate biologically important intra-genome interaction networks. PLoS Pathog 7:e1002203

37. Bennett A, Agbandje-McKenna M (2020) Geminivirus structure and assembly. Adv Virus Res 108:1–32

38. Jumper J, Evans R, Pritzel A, Green T, Figurnov M, Ronneberger O, Tunyasuvunakool K, Bates R, Žídek A, Potapenko A (2021) Highly accurate protein structure prediction with AlphaFold. Nature 596: 583–589

Chapter 12

Detection of Tomato Leaf Curl New Delhi Virus-ES by Real-Time Quantitative PCR

Dirk Janssen and Leticia Ruiz García

Abstract

The tomato leaf curl New Delhi virus (ToLCNDV) is a bipartite, single-stranded DNA begomovirus (genus *Begomovirus*, family *Geminiviridae*) that was first identified in India in 1995 affecting solanaceous cucurbitaceous crops in India. In 2012 a new virus strain, denominated ToLCNDV-ES, was first detected in Europe affecting zucchini squash, melon, cucumber, and to a lesser degree, tomato, in Spain and other Mediterranean countries. The virus is currently listed as a quarantine pest by EPPO. ToLCNDV-ES is reported to be transmitted by *Bemisia tabaci* whiteflies. Symptoms that are produced by the virus in zucchini are curling, chlorosis and vein thickening of leaves, stunted growth, and fruit deformation and abortion However, viruses of cucurbits often cause severe symptoms and mixed infections are common. Therefore ToLCNDV needs to be confirmed through laboratory analysis, either through PCR or through ELISA. ELISA provides a good basis for virus detection and confirmation in virus surveys, while PCR-based tests overall have higher sensitivity. In this manuscript, we propose a protocol to detect and quantify the viral load of ToLCNDV in any of its horticultural hosts.

Key words Tomato leaf curl New Delhi virus, Begomovirus, qPCR, Viral load, TaqMan fluorogenic probe, Relative viral quantification

1 Introduction

The tomato leaf curl New Delhi virus (ToLCNDV) is a bipartite, single-stranded DNA begomovirus belonging to the genus *Begomovirus*, family *Geminiviridae*. Initially identified in India in 1995, it impacted solanaceous crops and subsequently caused significant damage to cucurbit crops on the Indian subcontinent [1, 2]. First reported in Europe in 2012, ToLCNDV affected zucchini squash, melon, cucumber, and to a lesser extent, tomatoes, primarily in Spain [3, 4]. Its presence was later documented in Estonia, Greece, Italy, Portugal, Tunisia, Morocco, and Algeria [5]. Recent studies on Spanish isolates of ToLCNDV indicate the existence of a new strain, designated ToLCNDV-ES, possibly evolved through recombination [6, 7]. Due to the rapid spread of ToLCNDV to different

Francisco Murilo Zerbini et al. (eds.), *Geminiviruses: Methods and Protocols*, Methods in Molecular Biology, vol. 2912,
https://doi.org/10.1007/978-1-0716-4454-6_12,

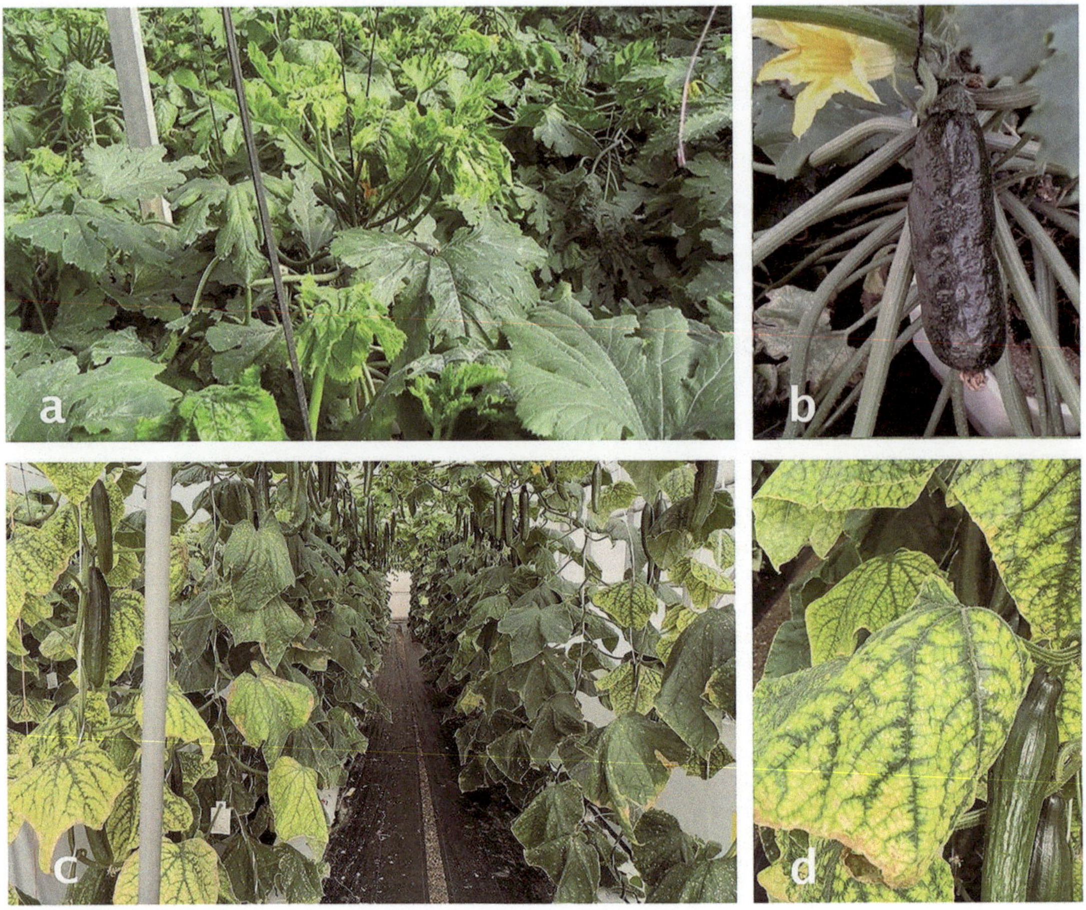

Fig. 1 (**a**) ToLCDNV infection in a zucchini crop produced in a commercial greenhouse. (**b**) Details of the symptoms expressed on zucchini fruit. (**c**) ToLCNDV infection in a cucumber crop. (**d**) Details of the symptoms expressed on the leaves from an infected cucumber plant

countries and the severity of outbreaks, particularly in Spain and Italy, the virus has been categorized as a quarantine pest by EPPO [5]. ToLCNDV-ES is known to be transmitted by the Mediterranean-Q1 *Bemisia tabaci* cryptic species in Spain and likely by the Med-Q2 species in Italy [8, 9]. Symptoms induced by ToLCNDV-ES in zucchini include leaf curling, chlorosis, vein thickening, stunted growth, and fruit deformation and abortion (Fig. 1a, b) [6]. In other crop species like cucumber, yellowing symptoms on leaves can be mistaken for those resulting from infections by other viruses (EFSA 2020) (Fig. 1c, d). Leaf curling symptoms are reminiscent of begomovirus infections; however, cucurbit-infecting viruses often exhibit severe symptoms, and mixed infections are commonly observed.

After visually inspecting and selecting samples from plants showing symptoms, the confirmation of ToLCNDV in a laboratory setting becomes necessary. This can be achieved through either

PCR or ELISA. ELISA serves as a robust method for virus detection and confirmation in surveys [10]. On the other hand, PCR-based tests generally exhibit higher sensitivity and better discrimination between TYLCV and ToLCNDV in tomatoes [11]. PCR has been shown to be considerably more sensitive (usually 100 times) for detecting plant viruses compared to ELISA [12]. However, the cost per unit and the scale of testing may constrain the application of PCR in extensive surveys. Consequently, ELISA can be employed for initial detection and confirmation of ToLCNDV in cucurbits and tomatoes, followed by discriminatory PCR for precise identification. In PCR-based detection of ToLCNDV, Sifres Cuerda et al. [13] utilized two primer pairs: To-A1F and To-A1R from DNA-A, and To-B1F and To-B1R from DNA-B [13, 14]. These primers amplified 505 and 677 bp fragments of the two viral DNAs. Panno et al. [15] conducted PCR using the A1F/A1R primer pair for the DNA-A component and the primer pair described by Ruiz et al. [4] for the DNA-B component, resulting in ~1200-bp and ~890-bp fragments of DNA-A and DNA-B, respectively [4, 16, 17]. Figàs et al. [11] employed the To-1F and To1R primers [18] in their PCR assays [11, 18]. Luigi et al. [19] developed a novel primer and probe set targeting the BC1 region of component B of the ToLCNDV genome. They established a real-time PCR protocol, validated according to the guidelines in EPPO standard PM 7/98 [20], capable of detecting ToLCNDV in both host plants and its vector, *Bemisia tabaci*.

In this chapter we describe a protocol to detect ToLCNDV-ES and quantify the viral load in any of its horticultural hosts.

2 Materials

2.1 Sample Collection and DNA Extraction

1. Ziplock plastic bags.
2. Disposable gloves.
3. Plant DNA extraction kit (*see* **Note 1**).
4. TissueLyser System (Qiagen).
5. Stainless grinding beads.
6. 1.5 mL microcentrifuge tubes.
7. 2 mL microfuge tubes.
8. Ethanol.
9. Pipettes and pipette tips.
10. Heating blocks.
11. Microcentrifuge.
12. Vortexer.
13. Disposable gloves.

14. Spectrophotometer.
15. Zymoclean Gel DNA Recovery kit (Zymo Research).
16. pUC19 plasmid vector.
17. *E. coli* XL1-BLUE competent cells.
18. Zyppy Plasmid Miniprep Kit (Zymo Research).

2.2 Real-Time PCR Assay

1. qPCR instrument.
2. Plasticware specific for qPCR instrument.
3. Primers and TaqMan probes:

   Forward primer ToLA-Up: 5′- CATTATTGCAC GAATTTCCG-3′.

   Reverse Primer ToLA-Low: 5′- ATCGTAGCC GACTGTGTCTG-3′.

   Taqman probe ToLA-Probe: 5′-FAM-CATGCACCTTAGAC CATGGACGCT-TAMRA-3′.

   Forward primer ToLB-Up: 5′- TCCGACAGCATTAATTG GAA-3′.

   Reverse Primer ToLB-Low: 5′- GAACGATGCTGCAGAGG TAA-3′.

   Taqman probe ToLB-Probe: 5′-6FAM-TGCACCTGTTCCT CAGCTGGC-TAMRA-3.

   Forward primer CUC18S-For: 5′- GGCGGATGTTGCTT TAAGGA-3′.

   Reverse Primer CUC18S-Rev (5-′-GTGGTGCCCTTCCGTCAAT-3′.

   Taqman probe CUC18S-Ana: 5′- JOE-TCCGCCAGCACCT-TATGAGAAATCAAAGTC-BHQ1-3′.
4. TaqMan Universal PCR Master Mix.
5. PCR grade water.
6. Pipettes and pipette tips.
7. Disposable gloves.

3 Methods

3.1 Sample Collection

Second or third apical leaf samples showing typical symptoms attributed to ToLCNDV (apical leaf curling and chlorotic mottling on intermediate leaves; Fig. 1) or asymptomatic, are collected from plants and temporarily stored in ziplock plastic bags.

3.2 DNA Extraction

1. DNA from plant material is extracted by using the DNeasy Plant kit protocol.
2. Fresh plant material (ca. 80 mg) is placed in 2-mL microfuge safe-lock tubes containing 400 μL lysis buffer P1 and stainless 5 mm grinding balls.
3. Plant material is then disrupted by using TissueLyser System (*see* **Note 2**).
4. After incubation at 65 °C for 10 min, 140 μL of buffer P2 is added to the lysis mixture, vortex and centrifuge at 10,000×*g* for 10 min.
5. Add 400 μL Buffer AP1 and 4 μL RNase A stock solution (100 mg/mL) (both from the DNeasy Plant kit) to a maximum of 100 mg (wet weight) or 20 mg (dried) disrupted plant tissue and vortex vigorously. Also, do not mix Buffer AP1 and RNase A before use (*see* **Note 3**).
6. Incubate the mixture for 10 min at 65 °C. Mix 2–3 times during incubation by inverting tube to lyse the cells.
7. Add 130 μL Buffer P3 to the lysate. Mix and incubate for 5 min on ice. This step precipitates detergent, proteins, and polysaccharides.
8. Centrifuge the lysate for 5 min at 20,000×*g* (14,000 rpm).
9. Pipette the lysate into the QIAshredder Mini spin column placed in a 2 mL collection tube, and centrifuge for 2 min at 20,000×*g* (14,000 rpm).
10. Transfer the flow-through fraction into a new tube without disturbing the cell-debris pellet. Typically 450 μL lysate is recovered. For some plant species less lysate is recovered. In this case, determine the volume for the next step.
11. Add the required amount of ethanol de Buffer AW1, and add 1.5 volumes of this buffer AW1 to the cleared lysate, and mix by pipetting. For example, to 450 μL lysate, add 675 μL Buffer AW1. Reduce the amount of Buffer AW1 accordingly if the volume of lysate is smaller. A precipitate may form after the addition of Buffer AW1, but this will not affect the lysate. Also, make sure to pipette Buffer AW1 directly onto the cleared lysate and to mix immediately.
12. Pipette 650 μL of the mixture, including any precipitate that may have formed, into the DNeasy Mini spin column placed in a 2 mL collection tube. Centrifuge for 1 min at ≥6000 *g*, and discard the flow-through (*see* **Note 4**).
13. Repeat **step 14** with remaining sample. Discard flow-through.
14. Add the required amount of ethanol de Buffer AW2. Place the DNeasy Mini spin column into a new 2 mL collection tube,

add 500 μL Buffer AW2 and centrifuge for 1 min at ≥6000 *g* (≥8000 rpm). Discard the flow-through and reuse the collection tube in **step 13**.

15. Add 500 μL Buffer AW2 to the DNeasy Mini spin column, and centrifuge for 2 min at 20,000×*g* (14,000 rpm) to dry the membrane. It is important to dry the membrane of the DNeasy Mini spin column, because residual ethanol may interfere with subsequent reactions. This centrifugation step ensures that no residual ethanol will be carried over during elution. Discard flow-through and collection tube.
16. Transfer the DNeasy Mini spin column to a 1.5 mL or 2 mL microcentrifuge tube, and pipette 100 μL Buffer AE directly onto the DNeasy membrane (*see* **Note 5**).
17. Centrifuge for 1 min at ≥6000×*g* (≥8000 rpm) to elute.
18. The DNA is ready for quantification and quality control. Measure DNA quality and concentration using 1 μL subsamples of the eluted DNA, using the NanoDrop ND-1000 spectrophotometer (*see* **Note 6**).
19. Store the DNA at −80 °C.

3.3 qPCR

3.3.1 Preparation of Standard Samples

ToLCNDV infectious clones of DNA-A and DNA-B can prepared as follows:

1. Rolling circle amplification (RCA) can be performed on total DNA extracted and after *Bam*HI partial digestion a 5.4 kb fragment obtained representing two full-length copies of the viral genome.
2. The DNA fragments are recovered from agarose gel using Zymoclean Gel DNA Recovery kit, cloned into a *Bam*HI-linearised pUC19 and used to transform *E. coli* XL1-BLUE competent cells. The resulting plasmids contain complete dimers for DNA-A and DNA-B, respectively and can be recovered from bacterial cultures using Zyppy Plasmid Miniprep Kit.
3. After sequencing with specific primers, the correctness of the inserts can be confirmed by comparison with sequences available in the databases (GenBank Acc. Number KM977733, KT175406 for DNA-A and KM977734, KT175407 for DNA-B).
4. The double-stranded circular molecules contain 2× DNA-A and DNA-B, and its integrity can be were analyzed by gel electrophoresis in 1% agarose gels and quantified with a NanoDrop 2000c spectrophotometer to assess purity though determination of the A260/A280 ratio, and to estimate the yield.

3.3.2 Absolute Quantification of ToLCDNV by qPCR

1. Absolute quantification of ToLCNDV DNA is carried out amplifying the target region of *AV2* (movement protein, MP) gene sequences located on DNA-A by using the ToLA-TaqMan probe, and the primers ToLA-Up and ToLA-Low (*see* **Note 7**).
2. In addition, qPCR is performed targeting a gene sequence within *BC1* (movement protein, MP) located on DNA-B ToLCNDV-DNA-B, using the following primers and ToLB-TaqMan probe, and primers ToLB-Up and ToLB-Low.
3. qPCR can be performed in any compatible qPCR equipment, using 25 μL of a reaction mix that contained 12.5 μL TaqMan Universal PCR Master Mix, 10.75 μL of nuclease free water, 50 nM (0.05 μM) of each forward and reverse primer, 50 nM (0.05 μM) TaqMan probe and 1 μL of total DNA (10 ng) (0.01 μg) for each genomic component of ToLCNDV.
4. Cycling conditions consisted of incubation at 95 °C for 10 min, and 40 cycles of 95 °C for 15 s and 60 °C for 1 min. In each run, the qPCR software may plot the fluorescence intensity against the number of cycles and provided the quantification cycle (Cq) value.
5. ToLCNDV dimeric clones of DNA-A and DNA-B is to be used as standards for quantitative analyses. Conversion of double stranded DNA (dsDNA) to nanograms are performed considering the average molecular weight of a base pair of deoxynucleotide (650 Da) and the recombinant DNA base pair number. Avogadro's constant (6.023×10^{23} molecules/mol) are used to estimate the dsDNA copy number. To generate external standard curves for absolute quantification, tenfold serial dilutions containing 10^9–10^0 molecules of circular dsDNA per μL of each viral genomic component, are to be prepared and analyzed by qPCR with the two designed probes: ToLA-Probe (*AV2* gene) and ToLB-Probe (*BC1* gene) (points 1 and 2). Total DNAs extracts without viral DNA from healthy host plants can be run in parallel to ensure the absence of any ToLCNDV amplification.
6. Standard curves for each TaqMan probe can be constructed plotting Cq values per three replicates per standard dilution versus the DNA copy number logarithm. The amplification efficiency is calculated from the slope of the corresponding curve using the formula $(10^{(-1/\text{slope of the standard curve})} - 1) \times 100$ (% values). Quantification of each DNA is obtained by interpolation of Cq data with the corresponding standard curve. Data from dsDNA quantification are multiplied by two since each dsDNA clone molecule contains two dsDNAs genome copies.
7. In order to evaluate the qPCR assay repeatability and reproducibility, the tenfold serial dilutions of each standard sample,

containing 10^9–10^0 molecules of circular dsDNA per μL, can be analyzed in triplicate and in three independent qPCR runs. Furthermore, tenfold serial dilutions of DNA extracts from infected plants of zucchini squash were used to prepare dilution curves for both viral genomic components in each case. The efficiency variation and accuracy were compared between both types of templates, standards and infected ToLCNDV DNA extracts. The Cq mean values and its standard deviation (SD), correlation coefficients and the calculated amplification efficiencies, across the entire linear dynamic range assayed, are calculated for every condition.

8. The standard curves, containing 10^9–10^0 copies for ToLCNDV DNA-A and DNA-B, cover a wide dynamic range of eight log units of concentration. This procedure enables detection of as few as 10^2 *AV2* gene copies, although the quantification of such a low number may not be reliable as it may fall off the linear range of the standard curve. Consequently, the limit of detection (LOD) may be fixed at higher copy numbers (e.g., 10^3 copies for DNA-A and 10^2 copies for DNA-B) (Fig. 2).
9. For each run include the suitable control samples and NTC (no template control).
10. Prepare the real-time PCR reaction in a final volume of 25 μL by using: (a) 50 nM each forward and reverse primer; (b) 50 nM TaqMan probe; (d) 12.5 μL TaqMan Universal Master Mix and 1 μL total DNA (10 ng) for each genomic

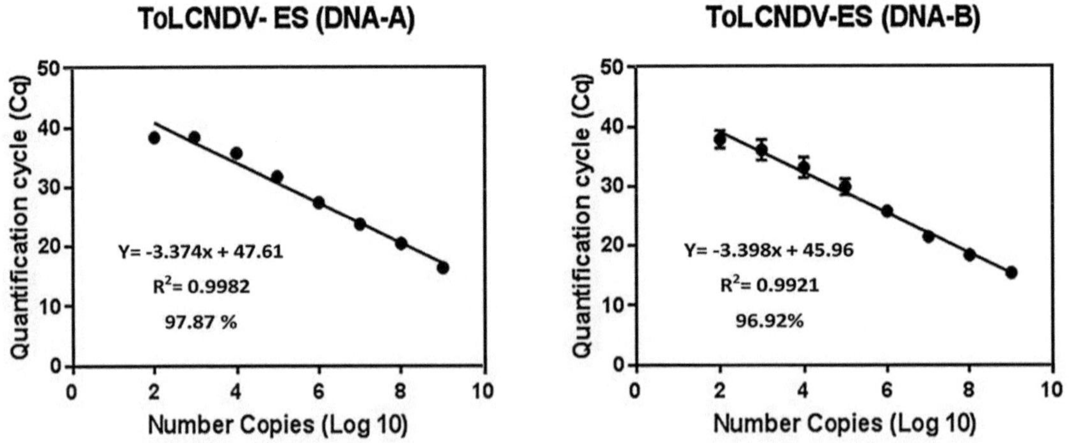

Fig. 2 An example of amplification efficiency and dynamic range of amplification of the target (AV2 and BC1 genes) specific DNA templates. Mean Cq values were obtained from serial log 10 dilutions of dimeric clones of ToLCNDV-ES DNA-A and DNA-B as standards. The figure shows the regression functions, the coefficients of correlation and the efficiencies values obtained. Bars represent SD. (Reprinted from Simón et al. [21])

component of ToLCNDV. Cycling conditions consisted on: incubation 95 °C for 10 min and 40 cycles of 95 °C 10 s, 60 °C 1 min.

11. In each run, the real-time PCR software, provide the quantification cycle (Cq) value. Each sample were analyzed in triplicate and the mean and SD were calculated. The Cq mean was extrapolated on the standard curve. ToLCNDV copy number was extrapolated from the formula $10^{(Cq-b(\text{slope of the standard curve}))}$ where b is the intercept.

3.3.3 Relative Quantification by Duplex qPCR

A duplex assay detects the variation of ToLCNDV DNA and host (cucumber or zucchini) DNA during the infection process (*see* **Note 8**).

1. Total DNA should be extracted from a sample of an apical leaf collected using the DNeasy Plant kit protocol as described in Subheading 3.2.
2. The primers and probe for the ToLCNDV TaqMan assay are the same as described in Subheading 3.3.2. DNA levels in samples are normalized using CUC18S-For and CUC18S-Rev primers and CUC18S-Ana Taqman probe for amplification of the internal controls are based on a fragment within the 18S ribosomal region of the cucurbit mitochondrial genome [22].
3. Three technical replications are performed per sample.
4. For each run the suitable control samples and NTC (no-template control) must be included.
5. Prepare the real-time PCR reaction mix in a final volume of 25 μL by using: 50 nM each forward and reverse primer; 50 nM TaqMan probe; and 12.5 μL TaqMan Universal Master Mix.
6. Add 1 μL total DNA (10 ng) and run the tests as follows: 1 min at 95 °C, 40 cycles of 15 s at 95 °C and 1 min at 60 °C.
7. The relative accumulation level of ToLCNDV in the plants is calculated using the formula $2^{-\Delta\Delta Ct}$, where $\Delta\Delta Ct$ is the difference between the ΔCt of each sample (mean of the three technical repetitions) and the ΔCt of the internal control (mean of the three technical repetitions) (Fig. 3).

4 Notes

1. This kit takes advantage of the selective binding properties of silica-based membranes. The lysed samples are buffered to promote optimum binding of the viral DNA to the membrane, and the sample is loaded onto the column. The DNA binds to the membrane, and the contaminants are washed away in two

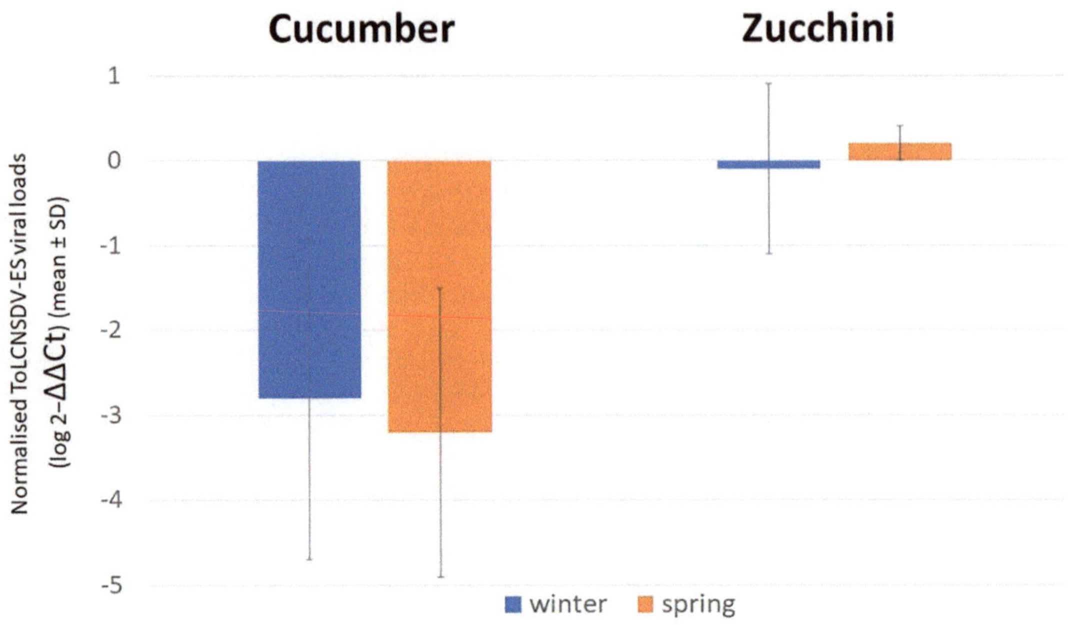

Fig. 3 Duplex qPCR assay of ToLCDNV DNA-A in cucumber and zucchini leaves collected from naturally infected crops during the winter and spring season. Each value is the average delta Ct value (between Ct ToLCNDV DNA-A and Ct host-S18) +/– S.D. (standard deviation) of leaves from ten plants

steps using two different washing buffers. High-quality DNA is eluted and ready for direct use or safe storage. The purified DNA is free of protein, nucleases, and other contaminants and inhibitors.

2. First, freeze the tubes on dry ice for 30 s. Tubes are then placed into the adaptor sets, which are fixed into the clamps of the TissueLyser. Disruption is performed in two 1- to 2-min high-speed (20–30 Hz) shaking steps. To prevent variation in sample homogenization, it is advised to remove the adaptor sets removed from the TissueLyser and disassemble after the first disruption step. Then proceed with a second disruption step, on which the adaptor sets should be reassembled so that the tube order is reversed. Rotating the racks of tubes in this way ensures that all samples are thoroughly and equally disrupted.
3. No tissue clumps should be visible. Vortex or pipette further to remove any clumps. Clumps of tissue will not lyse properly and will therefore result in a lower yield of DNA. In rare cases, where clumps cannot be removed by pipetting and vortexing, a disposable micropestle may be used.
4. All columns must be closed during the spin process to avoid cross-contamination. After centrifugation, if the solution has not entirely passed through the membrane, repeat the centrifugation step at higher speed until all the solution has passed through.

5. Incubate for 5 min at room temperature.
6. Concentration is given by the OD measure at 260 nm. An OD 260/280 ratio of approximately 1.8 indicates a good quality of the purified DNA [23].
7. The design of specific oligonucleotides and internal fluorogenic probe is fundamental for the accurate quantification of the virus. Taqman probes presenting the same oligonucleotide sequence but labeled with different fluorophores at their 5′ extremities can generate distinct fluorescent signals in the analysis of a sample, resulting in differences on the quantification values. The qPCR assay can be performed as a one-step reaction, and ideally, primer design should be focused in a conserved region of the viral genome.
8. This qPCR can be validated in a mixture containing viral DNA and plant DNA (e.g., cucumber or zucchini), in serial dilutions with healthy tissue.

Acknowledgments

This study was funded by projects from IFAPA and FEDER/ERDF AVA 2023.019 and AVA 2023.025.

References

1. Padidam M, Beachy RN, Fauquet CM (1995) Tomato leaf curl geminivirus from India has a bipartite genome and coat protein is not essential for infectivity. J Gen Virol 76:25–35
2. Zaidi SS, Martin DP, Amin I et al (2017) Tomato leaf curl New Delhi virus: a widespread bipartite begomovirus in the territory of monopartite begomoviruses. Mol Plant Pathol 18:901–911
3. Juárez M, Tovar R, Fiallo-Olivé E, Aranda MA et al (2014) First detection of tomato leaf curl New Delhi virus infecting zucchini in Spain. Plant Dis 98:857
4. Ruiz ML, Simón A, Velasco L et al (2015) First report of tomato leaf curl New Delhi virus infecting tomato in Spain. Plant Dis 98:894
5. EPPO (2021) EPPO global database tomato leaf curl New Delhi virus (ToLCNDV). Available online: https://gd.eppo.int/taxon/TOLCND. Accessed on 20 Dec 2021
6. Ruiz L, Simon A, Velasco L et al (2017) Biological characterization of tomato leaf curl New Delhi virus from Spain. Plant Pathol 66: 376–382
7. Fortes IM, Sanchez-Campos S, Fiallo-Olive E et al (2016) A novel strain of tomato leaf curl New Delhi virus has spread to the mediterranean basin. Viruses 8:307
8. Janssen D, Simon A, Crespo O et al (2017) Genetic population structure of Bemisia tabaci in Spain associated with tomato leaf curl New Delhi virus. Plant Protect Sci 53:25–31
9. Bertin S, Luigi M, Parrella G et al (2018) Survey of the distribution of *Bemisia tabaci* (Hemiptera: Aleyrodidae) in Lazio region (Central Italy): a threat for the northward expansion of tomato leaf curl New Delhi virus (*Begomovirus*: *Geminiviridae*) infection. Phytoparasitica 46:171–182
10. Juárez M, Rabadan MP, Martinez LD et al (2019) Natural hosts and genetic diversity of the emerging tomato leaf curl New Delhi virus in Spain. Front Microbiol 10:140
11. Figàs MR, Alfaro-Fernández A, Font MI et al (2017) Inoculation of cucumber, melon and zucchini varieties with tomato leaf curl New Delhi virus and evaluation of infection using different detection methods. Ann Appl Biol 170:405–414
12. Alfaro-Fernández A, Sánchez Navarro J, Landeira M et al (2016) Evaluation of PCR and non-radioactive molecular hybridization

techniques for the routine diagnosis of tomato leaf curl New Delhi virus, tomato yellow leaf curl virus and tomato yellow leaf curl Sardinia virus. J Plant Pathol 98:245–254

13. Sifres Cuerda AG, Sáez-Sánchez C, Ferriol-Molina M et al (2018) First report of tomato leaf curl New Delhi virus infecting zucchini in Morocco. Plant Dis 102:1045–1045
14. Sáez C, Martínez C, Ferriol M et al (2016) Resistance to tomato leaf curl New Delhi virus in Cucurbita spp. Ann Appl Biol 169: 91–105
15. Panno S, Caruso AG, Troiano E et al (2019) Emergence of tomato leaf curl New Delhi virus in Italy: estimation of incidence and genetic diversity. Plant Pathol 68:601–608
16. Panno S, Iacono G, Davino M et al (2016) First report of tomato leaf curl New Delhi virus affecting zucchini squash in an important horticultural area of southern Italy. New Dis Rep 33. https://doi.org/10.5197/j.2044-0588.2016.033.006
17. Mizutani T, Daryono BS, Ikegami M et al (2011) First report of tomato leaf curl New Delhi virus infecting cucumber in Central Java, Indonesia. Plant Dis 95:1485
18. López C, Ferriol M, Picó MB (2015) Mechanical transmission of tomato leaf curl New Delhi virus to cucurbit germplasm: selection of tolerance sources in *Cucumis melo*. Euphytica 204: 679–691
19. Luigi M, Manglli A, Bertin S et al (2020) Development and validation of a specific real-time PCR protocol for the detection of tomato leaf curl New Delhi virus. Eur J Plant Pathol 157:969–974
20. EPPO (2019) PM 7/98 specific requirements for laboratories preparing accreditation for a plant pest diagnostic activity. EPPO Bull 51: 468–498
21. Simón A, Ruiz L, Velasco L, Janssen D (2018) Absolute quantification of tomato leaf curl New Delhi virus Spain strain, ToLCNDV-ES: virus accumulation in a host-specific manner. Plant Dis 102:165–171
22. Gil-Salas FM, Colyer A, Boonham N et al (2009) Resistance screening against cucumber vein yellowing virus using a real-time (Taqman) RT-PCR assay in cucumber (*Cucumis sativus*). Crop Prot 28:109–112
23. Thermo Scientific (2009) T042-technical bulletin nanodrop spectrophotometers. http://www.nhm.ac.uk/content/dam/nhmwww/our-science/dpts-facilities-staff/Coreresearchlabs/nanodrop.pdf

Chapter 13

Detection of Cassava Mosaic Geminiviruses Using Loop-Mediated Isothermal Amplification (LAMP)

Gonçalo Silva and Neil Boonham

Abstract

A real-time loop-mediated isothermal amplification (LAMP) is described to diagnose cassava mosaic disease (CMD). The disease continues to cause great damage in Sub-Saharan African countries threatening food security. Early detection of the pathogen is paramount to control the spread of the disease and promote the safe exchange of clean planting material. Real-time LAMP in combination with a crude but rapid method of DNA extraction can be used to detect the two most widely distributed species of cassava mosaic geminiviruses in Sub-Saharan Africa, African cassava mosaic virus (ACMV) and East African cassava mosaic virus (EACMV), in less than 30 min at a single operation temperature (65 °C) without the need for any expensive instrumentation. Further, this protocol avoids the laborious extraction of high-quality DNA and making it suitable to be used in poorly resourced laboratories and in field settings.

Key words Begomovirus, ACMV, EACMV, LAMP, On-site detection, Virus diagnostics

1 Introduction

Cassava mosaic disease (CMD) is a viral disease that causes substantial yield losses in Sub-Saharan Africa and more recently in Southeast Asia, endangering food security in these regions [1, 2]. CMD is caused by 11 known cassava mosaic geminivirus species all belonging to the genus *Begomovirus* in the family *Geminiviridae* [3]. In Sub-Saharan Africa the two most widely distributed species of cassava mosaic geminivirus are African cassava mosaic virus (ACMV) and East African cassava mosaic virus (EACMV) [4]. Coinfection of two or more virus species is a common feature in the etiology of the diseases that usually leads to increased symptom severity. Cassava mosaic geminiviruses are known to be transmitted either by infected stem cuttings or by members of the cryptic whitefly species complex *Bemisia tabaci* (Gennadius) (Hemiptera: Aleyrodidae) [5].

Francisco Murilo Zerbini et al. (eds.), *Geminiviruses: Methods and Protocols*, Methods in Molecular Biology, vol. 2912, https://doi.org/10.1007/978-1-0716-4454-6_13,

Early detection of CMD is critical to achieve effective control, both from a biosecurity and an endemic pest perspective [6, 7]. The use of virus-free planting materials remains one of the most effective methods to control the spread of the disease. The development and implementation of specific, sensitive, and rapid diagnostic methods is paramount in seed systems to achieve this goal.

Several serological and PCR-based methods have been developed and applied for the diagnosis of CMD [4, 5]. Different factors must be taken into consideration when selecting the most appropriate detection method, including sensitivity, specificity, cost, and the time required to obtain results. PCR-based assays are frequently favored due to their high sensitivity and specificity [4], however they require trained personnel and sophisticated equipment that might be difficult to implement in poorly equipped laboratories or in field settings. Furthermore, these methods usually need the extraction of high-quality DNA from the sample material, which is time-consuming and frequently involves hazardous chemicals.

Isothermal amplification methods, like the Loop-mediated isothermal AMPlification (LAMP) [8] overcome the disadvantages of the PCR-based methods, offering rapid detection systems with specificity and sensitivity similar to PCR assays [9]. LAMP is a rapid amplification method that uses two pairs of primers and a *Bst* DNA polymerase with strand displacing activity to generate amplification products containing stem-loop structures. Amplification can be accelerated by the addition of loop primers [10] which bind to the looped amplicons. Whilst loop primers are not essential for the amplification mechanism to proceed, assays with two loop primers typically amplify target DNA in a shorter period. The Bst DNA polymerase used in LAMP assays is more robust and less affected by proteins, polysaccharides or polyphenolic compounds present in plant material that can inhibit PCR assays. As a result, there is no need to use high-quality DNA and simple crude tissue lysis methods can be used to generate extracts for LAMP assays [11–14]. LAMP products can be visualized by color change reactions (Fig. 1) [15] although weak positive results can be difficult to interpret. LAMP amplification results can also be visualized through agarose gel electrophoresis, lateral flow devices (LFDs) [16] or in real-time using a fluorescent intercalating dye of probe. Real-time detection is preferred as the close tube reaction greatly reduces risk of post-amplification contamination. Portable fluorescent devices like the Genie II (Fig. 2) have been developed for real-time isothermal amplification. These devices are particularly suitable for use in a diagnostic lab or in remote locations due to its small size and portability, and its ability to run on battery power for several hours.

In this chapter, we describe an alkaline polyethylene glycol protocol for preparation of fast, crude extracts that can be used with LAMP for the detection of ACMV and EACMV.

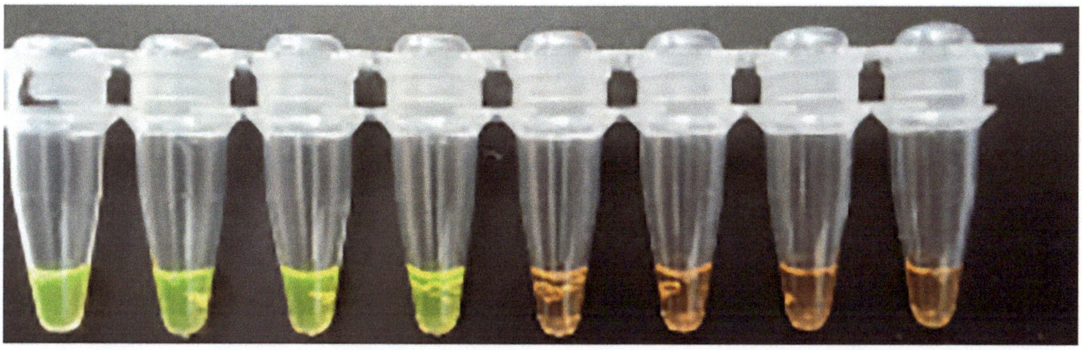

Fig. 1 Example of LAMP products visualized by color change reactions. Inclusion of SYBR Green in the reaction creates a color change at the end of LAMP reactions. The green and orange solutions in the tubes represent positive and negative reactions, respectively

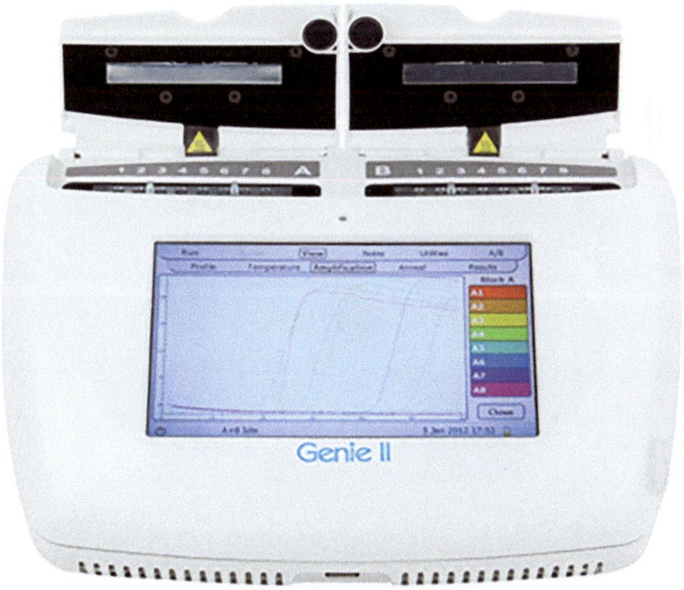

Fig. 2 Image of a Genie II portable fluorescent devices (Optisense Ltd.)

2 Materials

2.1 Crude Extract Preparation

1. Cassava leaf samples (*see* **Note 1**).
2. Alkaline PEG buffer: add 20 mM KOH (or NaOH), pH 13.3–13.5 to 6% Polyethylene glycol (PEG) 200.
3. Sterile nuclease-free water.
4. Screw cap tubes.
5. Stainless steel ball bearings (8–10 mm diameter).

6. Ice bucket and ice.
7. Vortex.

2.2 Real-Time LAMP

1. LAMP mastermix (e.g., GspSSD2.0 Isothermal Mastermix, OptiGene) (*see* **Note 2**).
2. ACMV and EACMV LAMP primers (Table 1).
3. Microcentrifuge.
4. Fluorometer/real-time PCR instrument (e.g., Genie II, Optigene) (*see* **Note 3**).
5. A set of pipettes and corresponding sterile/filter tips.
6. Sterile 1.5 mL microfuge tubes and a microfuge rack.
7. Genie Strips tubes (Optigene) (*see* **Note 4**).

Table 1
LAMP primer sequences and volume of each primer needed to prepare the primer mix

Primer	Sequence 5′–3′	Volume in microliters (μL) (concentration of starting solution)	Reference
ACMV_F3	GCTCGTAATTATGTCGAAGCG	0.5 (10 μM)	[12]
ACMV_B3	TAGGTATGTCTGGGCTTCTGTA	0.5 (10 μM)	
ACMV_FIP_dg	CTGTATGGGCTGTCGAAG TTCAGACCAGGAGATATCATCA TTTMCA	0.5 (100 μM)	
ACMV_BIP_dg	GAACCKTGCTACTGCCCCCACTTTCTG TACATGGGYCTGTT	0.5 (100 μM)	
ACMV_FL_dg	ACGAACCTTGGAKYCTGG	0.25 (100 μM)	
ACMV_BL	TCCACGTCACAAATCGAAAACG	0.25 (100 μM)	
EACMV_F3dg	CTGTTACATYTKGAGCAGGAATA	0.5 (10 μM)	
EACMV_B3dg	GGTGACGCGGACAGTRGG	0.5 (10 μM)	
EACMV_FIPdg	TCTCCTGGTCGCTTCGACATAAGTACTG TTGGKGCKGAGT	0.5 (100 μM)	
EACMV_BIPdg	CCCKTATCCAAGG TGCGGACAACAACACGGTTCKTGTATG	0.5 (100 μM)	
EACMV_FLdg	TTACACCGTAGMACMCCTAT	0.25 (100 μM)	
EACMV_BLdg	AGGCTGAACTTCGACASYC	0.25 (100 μM)	

ACMV African cassava mosaic virus, *EACMV* East African cassava mosaic virus, *B & F* backward and forward, *FIP & BIP* forward and backward inner primer, *FL & BL* forward and backward loops, *dg* indicates presence of degeneracies in the primer sequence, *μM* micro molar

3 Methods

3.1 Alkaline PEG DNA Extraction

1. Add 1 mL Alkaline PEG buffer and a stainless-steel ball-bearing to a screw cap tube.
2. Place a small piece (1–2 cm^2) of leaf material to be tested into the tube.
3. Replace cap and shake bottle vigorously for 1–2 min, or until the sample is a mid-green color (*see* **Note 5**).
4. Dilute the PEG extract by a factor of one in 10 by transferring 10 μL PEG extract into a tube containing 90 μL nuclease-free water and shake or vortex to mix. The DNA sample is now ready to be used for LAMP amplification (*see* **Note 6**).

3.2 Preparation of Primer Mix

1. Prepare the primer mix according to Table 1. Prepare one primer mix for each target virus.

3.3 Real-Time LAMP Amplification

1. For each target virus, set up the LAMP reaction mixture (total reaction volume 25 μL) as follows: 15 μL of LAMP master mix, 2.5 μL of primer mixture (*see* Table 1) and 5.5 μL of nuclease-free water (*see* **Note 7**).
2. Pipette 23 μL of LAMP master mix into the Genie tube-strips.
3. Keep strip tubes on ice until ready to use. Reactions can be stored on ice for several hours prior to use.
4. Add 2 μL of diluted plant extract to each tube and close the lids firmly (*see* **Note 8**). Use a fresh tip for each sample.
5. Spin the 8-well strip briefly.
6. Place the 8-well strip into the Genie II machine.
7. Run the LAMP for 30 min at 65 °C to allow real-time data capture followed a melting process from 98 °C to 80 °C with a ramp rate of −0.05 °C/s (*see* **Note 9**).
8. The results can be observed as amplification plots along with the annealing profile of the amplified DNA (*see* **Note 10**).

4 Notes

1. It is important to collect both symptomatic and asymptomatic cassava leaf samples as some cassava varieties might be infected with viruses but not showing disease symptoms.
2. Several commercial isothermal master mixes are available to purchase. The New England Biolabs mastermix, WarmStart LAMP kit, is a good alternative to the Optigene mastermix used in this study. These master mixes contain the necessary reagents including DNA polymerase and fluorescence dye to perform reactions in real-time.

3. Real-time LAMP can be run in any fluorescent reading device including real-time PCR instruments. In this protocol the Genie II (Optisense Ltd.) instrument was used.
4. The Genie Strips tubes are specifically designed to fit the Genie II machine used in this protocol. If using another fluorometer/ real-time PCR instrument other 0.2 mL tubes or 8-well strips can be used.
5. If the extract is too clear it might not contain enough DNA in solution due to poor cell disruption. Avoid dark green extracts as these might contain higher levels of plant contaminants that can interfere with LAMP reaction that could result in false-negative results.
6. Ideally crude extracts would be prepared just prior to amplification. When handling several samples it is recommended to put extracts on ice until use in LAMP reactions.
7. As a guide, multiply the volume of each component by the numbers of samples to be tested +3. One extra sample will be the negative control (where DNA is replaced with molecular biology grade water), one the positive control and one to accommodate pipetting errors. To minimize pipetting errors and reduce the risk of losing small volumes of liquid, add the components in a particular order, starting with larger volumes first.
8. The tubes are designed to be closed once and have a locking mechanism preventing the tubes from being reopened after amplification.
9. Do not open the tubes after the completion of the amplification reaction, as this carries the risk of contamination with amplification product.
10. The amplification plot (Fig. 3) shows, on the *y*-axis the fluorescence values and on the *x*-axis the time in minutes. The threshold reflects a significant increase of fluorescence over the baseline signal. It is set to distinguish relevant amplification signal from the background. Any reaction with an amplification curve that goes above the threshold is considered a positive reaction. Any straight line, that stays below the threshold is considered a negative reaction. The negative control or no-template control (NTC) should appear as a straight line. The threshold line can be automatically defined by the software or manually adjusted by the user. The time of amplification can also be an indication of the amount of target we have in the samples. The more diluted the sample is, or the less amount of target in the sample, more time is needed to detect it.

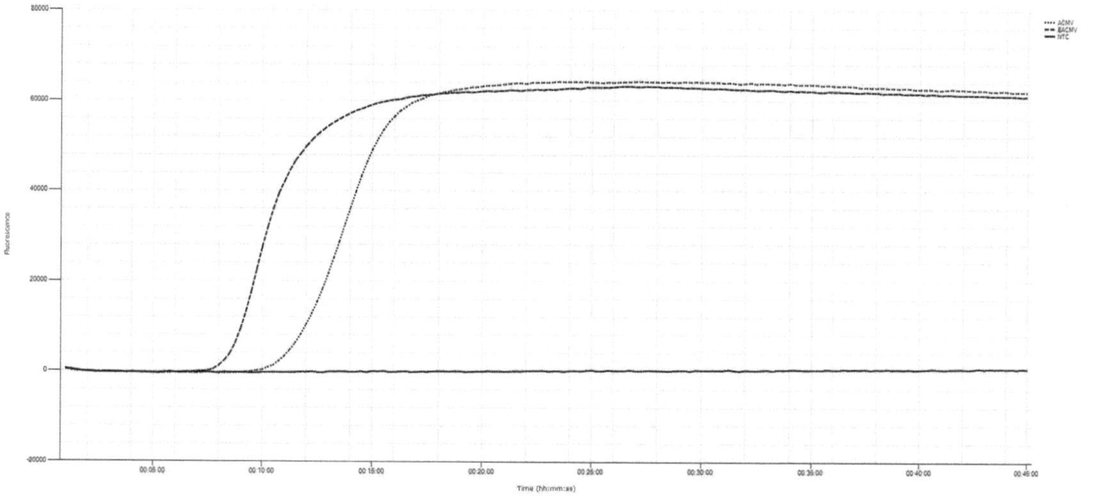

Fig. 3 Real-time loop-mediated isothermal amplification for detection of ACMV and EACMV. *NTC* no-template control

Acknowledgments

This work was supported by the Biotechnology and Biological Sciences Research Council under the "CONNECTED—COmmunity Network for africaN vECTor borne plant viruses" project (project reference BB/R005397/1) and the Bill and Melinda Gates Foundation under the "Renewal: Enabling Research Tools for Cassava and Yam Virologists and Breeders" project (Investment ID INV-007697/OPP1149777).

References

1. Carvajal-Yepes M, Cardwell K, Nelson A et al (2019) A global surveillance system for crop diseases. Science 364:1237–1239
2. Kreuze J, Cuellar W, Lava Kumar P, Boddupalli P, Omondi AB (2023) New technologies provide innovative opportunities to enhance understanding of major virus diseases threatening global food security. Phytopathology 113:1622–1629
3. Rey C, Vanderschuren H (2017) Cassava mosaic and brown streak diseases: current perspectives and beyond. Annu Rev Virol 4:429–452
4. Abarshi MM, Mohammed IU, Jeremiah SC et al (2012) Multiplex RT-PCR assays for the simultaneous detection of both RNA and DNA viruses infecting cassava and the common occurrence of mixed infections by two cassava brown streak viruses in East Africa. J Virol Methods 179:176–184
5. Legg JP, Kumar PL, Makeshkumar T et al (2015) Cassava virus diseases: biology, epidemiology, and management. Adv Virus Res 91: 85–142
6. Mumford RA, Macarthur R, Boonham N (2016) The role and challenges of new diagnostic technology in plant biosecurity. Food Secur 8:103–109
7. Silva G, Tomlinson J, Onkokesung N et al (2021) Plant pest surveillance: From satellites to molecules. Emerg Top Life Sci 5:275–287
8. Notomi T, Okayama H, Masubuchi H et al (2000) Loop-mediated isothermal amplification of DNA. Nucleic Acids Res 28:e63
9. Boonham N, Kreuze J, Winter S et al (2014) Methods in virus diagnostics: from ELISA to next generation sequencing. Virus Res 186: 20–31
10. Nagamine K, Hase T, Notomi T (2002) Accelerated reaction by loop-mediated isothermal

amplification using loop primers. Mol Cell Probes 16:223–229

11. Tomlinson JA, Boonham N, Hughes KJD et al (2005) On-site DNA extraction and real-time PCR for detection of Phytophthora ramorum in the field. Appl Environ Microbiol 71:6702–6710
12. Okereke N, Tomlinson J, Adams I et al (2017) Protocol for cost effective detection of cassava mosaic virus. Nig Agr J 48:96–102
13. Nkere CK, Oyekanmi JO, Silva G et al (2018) Chromogenic detection of yam mosaic virus by closed-tube reverse transcription loop-mediated isothermal amplification (CT-RT-LAMP). Arch Virol 163:1057–1061
14. Festus RO, Seal SE, Prempeh R et al (2022) Improved reverse transcription loop-mediated isothermal amplification (RT-LAMP) for the rapid and sensitive detection of yam mosaic virus. Viruses:1592. https://doi.org/10.3390/v15071592
15. Tomlinson JA, Boonham N, Dickinson M (2010a) Development and evaluation of a one-hour DNA extraction and loop-mediated isothermal amplification assay for rapid detection of phytoplasmas. Plant Pathol 59:465–471
16. Tomlinson JA, Dickinson MJ, Boonham N (2010b) Rapid detection of *Phytophthora ramorum* and *P. kernoviae* by two-minute DNA extraction followed by isothermal amplification and amplicon detection by generic lateral flow device. Phytopathology 100:143–149

Chapter 14

Tissue Printing Hybridization Using Digoxigenin-Labeled DNA Probes for the Detection of Geminiviruses and Associated DNA Satellites

Elvira Fiallo-Olivé and Jesús Navas-Castillo

Abstract

Nucleic acid hybridization is a fundamental technique in plant virus research, enabling precise detection of plant pathogens. Tissue printing hybridization exhibits high sensitivity and specificity in detecting viral genomes, providing particularly valuable for screening a large number of samples without the need for DNA purification. This method virtually eliminates contamination and false positives. This chapter presents a detailed and effective protocol for nucleic acid hybridization of geminiviruses using digoxigenin-labeled probes. Specifically, the tissue printing hybridization technique is outlined for a particular geminivirus and its associated deltasatellite. However, the methodology is adaptable to a diverse range of geminiviruses and host plants, rendering it versatile and applicable across various geminivirus research contexts.

Key words Nucleic acid hybridization, Tissue printing, Geminiviruses, Begomoviruses, Digoxigenin-labeled probes, Plant virus diagnosis

1 Introduction

Geminiviruses pose a significant threat to global agriculture, causing severe economic losses by infecting a wide range of plant species [1]. Within the family *Geminiviridae*, the genus *Begomovirus* is an especially successful group of emerging viruses. These viruses are transmitted by whiteflies and infect a wide range of dicotyledonous plants, causing a variety of symptoms in their hosts. They are a limiting factor in the production of many crops, both in greenhouses and open fields [2, 3]. In some cases, DNA satellites (alphasatellites, betasatellites, and deltasatellites) are associated with begomoviruses, influencing the pathogenesis and success of the helper viruses [3–8].

Accurate and timely detection of geminiviruses is crucial for effective disease management and for developing strategies to prevent their spread [9]. Traditional diagnostic methods face

Francisco Murilo Zerbini et al. (eds.), *Geminiviruses: Methods and Protocols*, Methods in Molecular Biology, vol. 2912,
https://doi.org/10.1007/978-1-0716-4454-6_14,

challenges due to the complex biology of geminiviruses, which are often associated with satellites, making their detection a multifaceted task. Tissue printing hybridization using digoxigenin (DIG)-labeled DNA probes offers a solution to these challenges. This method leverages the principles of nucleic acid hybridization, which has evolved into a highly specific and sensitive molecular biology technique, enabling the analysis of large numbers of samples with minimal risk of false positives. By using nylon membranes, this protocol captures plant sap directly from cross-sectional cuts of plant material, eliminating the need for time-consuming DNA purification steps. This not only simplifies the process but also reduces the risk of cross-contamination, ensuring reliable results.

This chapter presents a comprehensive protocol for tissue printing hybridization using DIG-labeled DNA probes, a powerful method designed for the specific and sensitive detection of geminiviruses, a group of single-stranded DNA plant viruses known for causing diverse and economically significant infections. Specifically, the protocol allows for the detection of the emergent begomovirus tomato leaf curl New Delhi virus (ToLCNDV) [10–12], and sweet potato leaf curl deltasatellite 1 (SPLCD1) [13]. However, it can be adapted for detecting any geminivirus and associated DNA satellites, underscoring the importance of this technique in geminivirus research.

2 Materials

Prepare all solutions using ultrapure water and analytical grade reagents. Prepare and store all reagents at room temperature unless indicated otherwise.

2.1 Reactive and Solutions

1. BIOTAQ DNA polymerase (Bioline) and reagents for PCR.
2. Full-length clones of ToLCNDV DNA-A and SPLCD1 inserted into the pBSK+ plasmid.
3. Pairs of oligonucleotides for specific amplification of ToLCNDV and SPLCD1.
4. Expand High Fidelity Enzyme mix; HF Buffer, 10× conc. with $MgCl_2$; and PCR DIG probe synthesis mix, 10× conc. (nucleotide mix containing 2 mM each dATP, dCTP, dGTP, 1.3 mM dTTP, 0.7 mM DIG-11-dUTP, alkali-labile; pH 7.0) (included in the PCR DIG Probe Synthesis Kit, Roche Diagnostics).
5. Standard prehybridization solution: 5× SSC, 0.1% N-lauroylsarcosine, 0.02% SDS, 1% blocking reagent (Roche Diagnostics).
6. Anti-Digoxigenin conjugated with alkaline phosphatase (Roche Diagnostics).

7. CDP-Star, a chemiluminescent alkaline phosphatase substrate (Roche Diagnostics).
8. Hybridization solution: 25 μL of the digoxigenin-labeled probe diluted in 25 mL of standard prehybridization solution.
9. Solution I: 0.1 M maleic acid, 0.15 M NaCl, adjust pH to 7.5 with 6 N NaOH.
10. Solution II: 1% blocking reagent in Solution I.
11. Solution III: 0.1 M Tris–HCl, pH 9.5, 0.1 M NaCl.
12. Washing buffer: 0.3% Tween 20 in Solution I.

2.2 Required Material and Equipment

1. Nylon membranes, positively charged.
2. Razor blades.
3. UV crosslinker.
4. Hybridization oven and tubes.
5. Orbital shaker.
6. Bench centrifuge.
7. Transparency films (high-resistance clear polyester film).
8. Autoradiography film (for example, KODAK X-OMAT AR).

3 Methods

3.1 Digoxigenin Labeling: DNA Probe Synthesis

1. A PCR is carried out for the specific detection of tomato leaf curl New Delhi virus (ToLCNDV). Primers MA1788 (5′-CG TGTCGTTTCGATCTGGTGTC-3′) and MA1789 (5′-GTT TGTGGATCTAAACTTGGTGAG-3′) were designed to target the intergenic region of the DNA-A component of the ToLCNDV isolate Spain-MU-8.1-Squash-2012 (GenBank Accession Number KF749224) [14, 15]. PCR amplification is performed in a 50 μL reaction volume containing approximately 100 ng of a full-length clone of ToLCNDV DNA-A, 1 μL each of primers MA1788 and MA1789 (100 ng μL^{-1}), 1× BIOTAQ DNA polymerase buffer (Bioline), 1.5 μL of 50 mM $MgCl_2$, 2 μL of 2.5 mM dNTP mix and 5 U BIOTAQ DNA polymerase. The PCR includes an initial denaturation at 95 °C for 3 min, followed by 35 cycles of denaturation at 95 °C for 1 min, annealing at 54 °C for 1 min, and extension at 72 °C for 30 s, with a final extension at 72 °C for 5 min.
2. A PCR is carried out for the specific detection of sweet potato leaf curl deltasatellite 1 (SPLCD1). Primers MA465 (5′-CCT TAGCTTCGCACGTAGCT-3′) and MA466 (5′-CTGCTTA GCGTAGCGGTTTGG -3′) were designed to amplify the complete deltasatellite (GenBank Accession Number FJ914390) [5]. PCR amplification is performed in a 50 μL

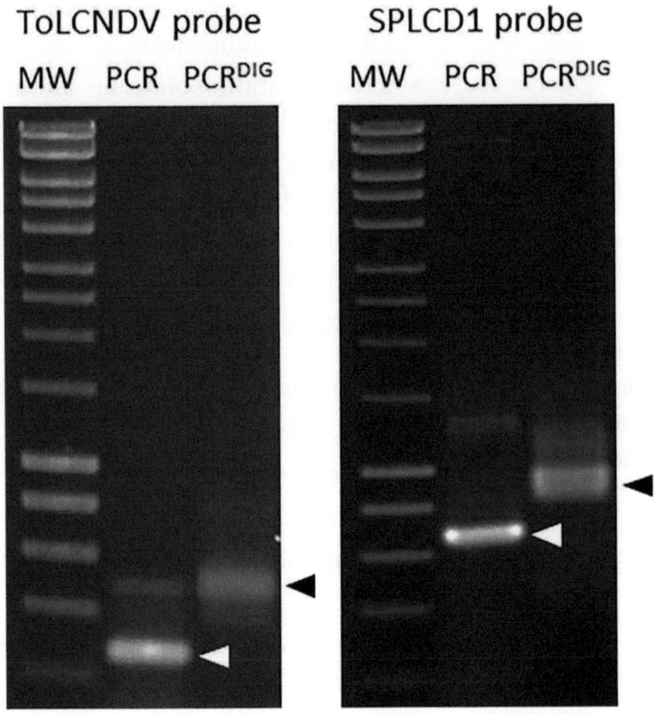

Fig. 1 Generation of DIG-labeled probes specific to ToLCNDV and SPLCD1. Aliquots of unlabeled (PCR, white arrowheads) and DIG-labeled (PCR^{DIG}, black arrowheads) PCR products were visualized on 0.8% agarose gels. MW, 1 kb DNA ladder

reaction volume containing approximately 100 ng of a dimeric clone of SPLCD1, 1 μL each of primers MA465 and MA466 (100 ng μL^{-1}), 1× BIOTAQ DNA polymerase buffer (Bioline), 1.5 μL of 50 mM $MgCl_2$, 2 μL of 2.5 mM dNTP mix, and 5 U BIOTAQ DNA polymerase (Bioline). The PCR protocol includes an initial denaturation at 95 °C for 3 min, followed by 35 cycles of denaturation at 95 °C for 30 s, annealing at 58 °C for 30 s, and extension at 72 °C for 30 s, with a final extension at 72 °C for 5 min.

3. Visualize the amplified DNA fragments on a 0.8% agarose gel.
4. To prepare the probes, repeat the PCRs using 1 μL of the previous PCR products as templates, employing the PCR DIG Probe Synthesis Kit.
5. Visualize the digoxigenin-labeled PCR fragments on a 0.8% agarose gel. The electrophoretic mobility of the digoxigenin-labeled PCR products (probes) will be slower than that of the unlabeled PCR products (Fig. 1). *See* **Note 1**.

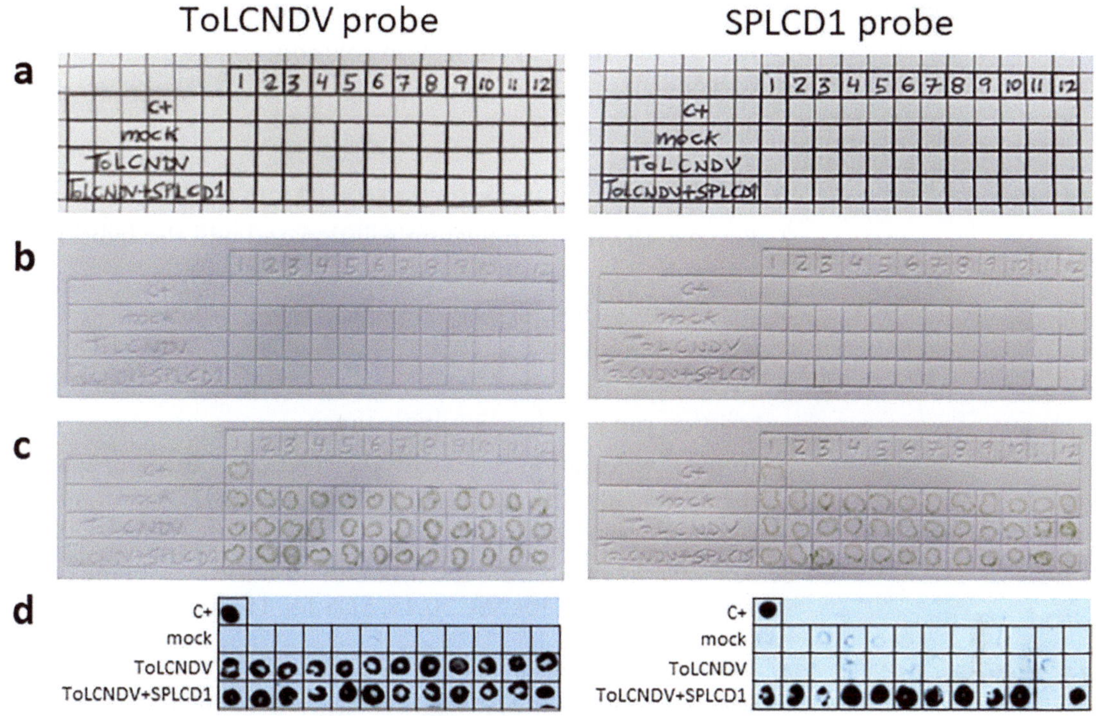

Fig. 2 Plant tissue imprinting and detection of virus (ToLCNDV probe) and deltasatellite (SPLCD1 probe) DNA on nylon membranes. (**a**) Marking a 5 × 5 mm grid on the nylon membrane using preprinted protective paper. (**b**) Appearance of the grid on the nylon membrane after tracing. (**c**) Imprinting of plant tissue (petiole cross-sections) onto the grid-marked membrane. (**d**) Chemiluminescent detection of hybridized virus and deltasatellite DNA using DIG-labeled probes, CDP-Star substrate and autoradiographic film exposure

3.2 Application of Plant Tissue Imprints

Mark a 5 × 5 mm grid on the nylon membrane, which is protected on both sides by paper preprinted with the grid. Place the membrane on a flat surface and, using a pen and a ruler, carefully trace the grid from the paper onto the nylon membrane (Fig. 2a, b).

1. Prepare a separate membrane for each virus or deltasatellite being analyzed. *See* **Notes 2** and **3**.
2. For each plant to be tested, make a cross-sectional cut in the petiole using a new razor blade. Press the cut surface onto one of the squares marked on the membrane until the plant sap is absorbed (Fig. 2c).
3. Repeat this process for each plant, using a new blade between samples.
4. Include both healthy and infected controls.
5. Allow the membrane to dry, then fix the nucleic acids with UV light using a UV crosslinker (120,000 microjoules/cm^2).
6. Store the membrane in a dry place at room temperature. *See* **Notes 4** and **5**.

3.3 Prehybridization

1. Place the membrane in the hybridization tube.
2. Add 20 mL of prehybridization solution.
3. Prehybridize for 2 hours at 65 °C with rotation in a hybridization oven.

3.4 Hybridization

1. Heat the hybridization solution for 10 min at 100 °C.
2. Remove the prehybridization solution and add the hybridization solution.
3. Incubate overnight at 65 °C with rotation in the hybridization oven.
4. Collect the hybridization solution and store it at −20 °C. This solution can be reused multiple times.
5. In the hybridization tube (with the rotation in the oven), wash the membrane with 50 mL of 2× SSC, 0.1% SDS for 10 min at room temperature.
6. Remove the liquid from the tube and wash the membrane twice with 50 mL of 0.1× SSC, 0.1% SDS for 15 min at 65 °C.

3.5 Detection

1. Remove the solution, avoiding the membrane from drying out, and transfer it to a tray slightly larger than its dimensions to ensure even exposure to the treatment solutions. From this point, the process is carried out at room temperature with gentle agitation. *See* **Note 6**.
2. Wash the membrane with washing buffer for 5 min.
3. Wash the membrane with Solution I for 1 min.
4. Wash the membrane with Solution II for 30 min.
5. Wash the membrane with Solution II plus antibody (anti-digoxigenin conjugated with alkaline phosphatase 1:20,000; centrifuge the antibody for 2 min at 4 °C, 5000 rpm before dilution, and carefully take the antibody from the supernatant).
6. Wash the membrane with washing buffer for 15 min.
7. Repeat **step 6**.
8. Wash the membrane with Solution I for 1 min.
9. Wash the membrane with Solution III, 5 min.
10. Dilute the chemiluminescent alkaline phosphatase substrate (CDP-Star) in Solution III at a 1:100 ratio in an Eppendorf tube covered with aluminum foil, and keep it on ice.
11. Transfer the membrane to a transparency film, evenly distribute the substrate over it using a micropipette, and cover it with a second transparency film.
12. Incubate for 5 min in darkness.

13. Remove the excess substrate by gently pressing a tissue paper against the transparency film and carefully pushing the liquid outwards. *See* **Note 7**.
14. Place an autoradiographic film on the membrane in darkness.
15. Perform a standard photographic development after the desired exposure time (Fig. 2d). Typically, two exposures are carried out: one lasting 1–3 h and a second overnight exposure, although in some cases a 5-min exposure may be sufficient. *See* **Notes 8** and **9**.

4 Notes

1. An easy way to double-check that digoxigenin has been incorporated into the DNA is to compare the electrophoretic mobility of digoxigenin-labeled DNA with that of labeled DNA in agarose gels. If digoxigenin has been successfully incorporated, the electrophoretic mobility of the labeled DNA will be slower than that of the unlabeled DNA.
2. Grids measuring 5 × 5 mm are routinely drawn on the nylon membranes, and one or two imprints are made depending on the size of the petiole section (e.g., one imprint for cucurbit samples and two for tomato samples).
3. Larger grids (greater than 5 × 5 mm) can be used if necessary.
4. If the tissue-imprinted membrane is not hybridized immediately after UV fixation, it can be stored for an extended period. It is important to keep the membrane between two smooth surfaces (for example, between the pages of a closed book, with preprinted protective papers).
5. If fresh plant material is not available for tissue printing, but plant DNA extracts are accessible, the same hybridization procedure can be performed applying 1 μL of each sample to the membrane (dot blot). However, the risk of false positives is increased in this case.
6. During detection (**steps 1–9**), it is crucial to adjust the solution volumes to the size of the membrane (600 $\mu L/cm^2$) to prevent it from drying out.
7. An excess of substrate in **step 13** of the detection can cause the membrane to appear completely black.
8. When tissue imprinting is performed with certain plant species, false positives can occur, for example with pepper plants. This issue can sometimes be resolved by using an RNA probe.
9. Used membranes can be re-hybridized with the same or a different probe. To do this, rinse the membrane in water, then incubate it for 20 min at 37 °C in a solution of 0.2 M

NaOH and 0.1% SDS, twice. Finally, transfer the membranes to 2xSSC at room temperature. The membranes can be reused immediately or allowed to dry for later use.

Acknowledgments

This work was supported by a grant from the Ministerio de Ciencia e Innovación (MICINN, Spain) (PID2021-128445OA-I00/AEI/10.13039/501100011033), cofinanced by the European Regional Development Fund, awarded to E.F.O.

References

1. Navas-Castillo J, Fiallo-Olivé E (2021) Geminiviruses (*Geminiviridae*). In: Zuckerman M, Bamford DH (eds) Encyclopedia of virology, 4th edn. Academic Press, Cambridge, MA
2. Navas-Castillo J, Fiallo-Olivé E, Sánchez-Campos S (2011) Emerging virus diseases transmitted by whiteflies. Annu Rev Phytopathol 49:219–248
3. Fiallo-Olivé E, Navas-Castillo J (2023) Begomoviruses: what is the secret(s) of their success? Trends Plant Sci 28:715–727
4. Zhou X (2013) Advances in understanding begomovirus satellites. Annu Rev Phytopathol 51:357–381
5. Hassan I, Orílio AF, Fiallo-Olivé E et al (2016) Infectivity, effects on helper viruses and whitefly transmission of the deltasatellites associated with sweepoviruses (genus *Begomovirus*, family *Geminiviridae*). Sci Rep 6:30204
6. Fiallo-Olivé E, Tovar R, Navas-Castillo J (2016) Deciphering the biology of deltasatellites from the New World: maintenance by New World begomoviruses and whitefly transmission. New Phytol 212:680–692
7. Nogueira AM, Nascimento MB, Barbosa TMC et al (2021) The association between New World alphasatellites and bipartite begomoviruses: effects on infection and vector transmission. Pathogens 10:1244
8. Ferro CG, Zerbini FM, Navas-Castillo J et al (2021) Revealing the complexity of sweepovirus-deltasatellite-plant host interactions: expanded natural and experimental helper virus range and effect dependence on virus-host combination. Microorganisms 9:1018
9. Gaur RK, Sharma P, Czosnek H (eds) (2022) Geminivirus: detection, diagnosis and management. Academic Press, Cambridge, MA
10. Zaidi SSEA, Martin DP, Amin I et al (2017) Tomato leaf curl New Delhi virus: a widespread bipartite begomovirus in the territory of monopartite begomoviruses. Mol Plant Pathol 18:901–911
11. Panno S, Caruso AG, Troiano E et al (2019) Emergence of tomato leaf curl New Delhi virus in Italy: estimation of incidence and genetic diversity. Plant Pathol 68:601–608
12. Moriones E, Praveen S, Chakraborty S (2017) Tomato leaf curl New Delhi virus: an emerging virus complex threatening vegetable and fiber crops. Viruses 9:264
13. Lozano G, Trenado HP, Fiallo-Olivé E et al (2016) Characterization of non-coding DNA satellites associated with sweepoviruses (genus *Begomovirus*, *Geminiviridae*) – definition of a distinct class of begomovirus-associated satellites. Front Microbiol 7:162
14. Fortes IM, Sánchez-Campos S, Fiallo-Olivé E et al (2016) A novel strain of tomato leaf curl New Delhi virus has spread to the Mediterranean Basin. Viruses 8:307
15. Juárez MA, Tovar R, Fiallo-Olivé E et al (2014) First detection of *tomato leaf curl New Delhi virus* infecting zucchini in Spain. Plant Dis 98:857

Chapter 15

High-throughput Sequencing (HTS)-Based Diagnosis of Geminiviruses

Ayane F. F. Quadros and Francisco Murilo Zerbini

Abstract

The development of high-throughput sequencing (HTS) technologies has revolutionized plant virology. One of the many application of HTS is the detection and diagnostics of plant viruses. The main advantage of HTS compared to other diagnostics methods is its unbiased nature, meaning that it is capable of detecting any virus present in the sample. Thus, it is particularly suitable for the discovery of new viruses. This chapter provides a step-by-step guide on how geminivirus diagnosis is performed using short-read HTS.

Key words Virome, Next-generation sequencing, Illumina, Bioinformatics, Virus detection, Diagnostics

1 Introduction

Detection and diagnosis of geminiviruses is traditionally carried out using PCR-based methods (serological methods such as ELISA were used in the early days but have been largely supplanted by molecular methods) [1]. The nature of the geminivirus genome (small, circular DNA, with both single-stranded and double-stranded forms accumulating in infected plants) greatly facilitates the use of PCR for detection and diagnosis. Degenerate ("universal") primers have been available for PCR-based detection of begomoviruses [2, 3] and are used in laboratories worldwide. Species-specific primers can also be used when the objective is to detect the presence of a specific virus. The sensitivity, convenience, versatility, and simplicity of PCR-based diagnostics are currently unmatched by other methods, and it is likely that PCR-based methods will continue to be the standard for geminivirus diagnostics in the foreseeable future, especially in developing countries.

The development of high-throughput sequencing (HTS) technologies has revolutionized biology in general, and plant virology is no exception [4]. One of the many application of HTS is the

Francisco Murilo Zerbini et al. (eds.), *Geminiviruses: Methods and Protocols*, Methods in Molecular Biology, vol. 2912,
https://doi.org/10.1007/978-1-0716-4454-6_15,

detection and diagnostics of pathogens, including plant viruses [5]. Compared to PCR-based methods, the use of HTS has a number of unequivocal advantages as far as detection and diagnosis is concerned. The main advantage is that HTS is a completely unbiased method, capable of detecting any virus/pathogens present in the sample [5, 6]. Thus, it is particularly suitable for the discovery of new viruses [6, 7].

The two most obvious limitations in the use of HTS for geminivirus diagnosis are the cost and the complexity of the analysis [8]. As much as costs have been decreasing in developed countries (nowadays being comparable to the cost of quantitative, real-time PCR), they remain high in developing countries, where geminiviruses are more common and thus the need for quick and reliable diagnosis is more pressing. But more than cost, the main limitation to the widespread use of HTS for geminivirus diagnosis is lack of expertise in bioinformatics analysis of HTS data.

One recent development is the use of long-read HTS (such as Oxford Nanopore Technologies, ONT). In theory, these technologies can sequence the full-length geminivirus genome in a single read, greatly simplifying (or even eliminating) bioinformatics analysis [9]. ONT in particular has the additional advantage of portability, being suitable for field diagnostics (with no electricity or an Internet connection) [8, 9]. But its costs are still high, and its error rate is much higher than that of short-read HTS [10]. Nevertheless, their use will certainly become more widespread in the future.

The objective of this chapter is to provide a step-by-step guide on how geminivirus diagnosis is performed using short-read HTS, and not to describe how sequencing itself is performed (nowadays sequencing is almost always performed at facilities or commercial companies). It is hoped that this protocol will allow researchers who are not familiar with bioinformatics to use HTS for geminivirus diagnosis.

2 Materials

2.1 Raw Data

The analyses that will be presented below begin when the raw data from a sequencing run is received. The raw files are generated by the sequencing facilities/companies and, after preliminary quality checks, are sent to the user.

2.2 Software for Sequence Quality Analysis

The software FastqC is freely available at https://www.bioinformatics.babraham.ac.uk/projects/fastqc/. To use the command line version, go to https://github.com/s-andrews/FastQC (*see* **Note 1**).

2.3 Software for Preprocessing Sequencing Data

Several programs are available for preprocessing (removal of adapters and low-quality sequences), including TrimGalore, Trimmomatic, and Cutadapt. We will use Trimmomatic due to its functionalities, but users are free to choose the software they are most familiar with. Trimmomatic performs a range of useful trimming tasks for both Illumina paired end and single end data. The selection of trimming steps and parameters is provided via the command line. The program is freely available at https://github.com/timflutre/trimmomatic (*see* **Note 2**).

2.4 Software for Sequence Assembly

It is recommended to use different sequence assemblers, as each may produce slightly different final results. There are several programs available for assembling short sequences, including SPAdes, MEGAHIT, MaSuRCA, Supernova, Unicycler, ABySS, Velvet, and SOAPdenovo2. We will use SPAdes and Velvet, but users are encouraged to try other programs that may be more convenient for their needs.

SPAdes constructs contigs using De Bruijn graphs and *k*-mer distance calculations, offering various options depending on the type of data being assembled. Most SPAdes pipelines support a hybrid mode, allowing the integration of long reads as supplementary data. For more information or to download the Linux or macOS versions, go to https://github.com/ablab/spades (*see* **Note 3**).

Velvet is a software tool used for DNA assembly from short reads by working with De Bruijn graphs. It can generate long contigs, with an N50 of over 150 kb, from paired-end short reads. To use Velvet, you need to run two commands: velveth and velvetg. The velveth command creates a hash table of *k*-mers, while velvetg assembles the genome. The *k*-mer length, also known as hash length, refers to the length in base pairs of the sequences from the reads that are hashed. You can download the latest version of Velvet from https://github.com/dzerbino/velvet (*see* **Note 4**).

2.5 Software for Analysis of Contigs by Similarity Searches

To identify sequences related to geminiviruses in assembled contigs by similarity search programs, we commonly use local alignment methods to compare these sequences against a database. The most widely used tool for this purpose is BLAST (Basic Local Alignment Search Tool). BLAST is specifically designed to find significant matches between a query sequence and sequences in a database. BLAST is accessed through its online version at NCBI (https://blast.ncbi.nlm.nih.gov/Blast.cgi). There is also a command line suite known as BLAST+ (*see* **Note 5**).

3 Methods

3.1 Downloading the Raw Data

Raw data can be downloaded directly from the links provided by the sequencing facility/company. In this chapter, we will work with raw data from paired-end short reads in FASTQ format.

3.2 Quality Analysis of the Raw Data

1. Run FastQC from the terminal or command prompt:

   % fastqc <reads_R1>.fastq.

   % fastqc <reads_R2>.fastq.

2. After quality analysis, two sets of files will be generated:

   <reads_R1_fastqc>.html and <reads_R1_fastqc>.zip;

   <reads_R2_fastqc>.html and <reads_R2_fastqc>.zip.

3. To visually analyze the data, open the .html files in a web browser. The report includes a results section for each FastQC module. For each module, the report provides graphs or lists data, and assigns a status flag: 'Pass', 'Warning' or 'Fail' (*see* **Note 6**). These graphs help assess the quality and characteristics of sequencing reads by providing a visual overview of the data.
4. When interpreting the flags 'Warning' or 'Fail', be cautious about considering them as strictly unacceptable. It is important to understand what these results mean in the context of your specific sample.
5. Based on these results, the user must decide how to preprocess the raw data.

3.3 Preprocessing the Raw Data

1. Run Trimmomatic from the terminal or command prompt:

   % trimmomatic PE-threads <number_of_threads> <input_file_1> <input_file_2> <output_paired_1> <output_unpaired_1> <output_paired_2> <output_unpaired_2> ILLUMINACLIP:TruSeq3-PE-2.fa:2:30:10 SLIDINGWINDOW:5:30 LEADING:20 TRAILING:20 MINLEN:100 AVGQUAL:30 (*see* **Note 7**).

2. For paired-end sequencing data, two input files and four output files are specified in the Trimmomatic command. The four output files are as follows:
   - Two files for "paired" reads, where both reads survived the trimming process.
   - Two files for "unpaired" reads, where one read survived the trimming process, but its partner did not.
3. Re-run the evaluation step with FastQC to verify that the poor quality sequences have been removed:

% fastqc <output_paired_1>.fastq.

% fastqc <output_paired_2>.fastq.

4. To perform visual analysis of the data, open the .html files in a web browser.
5. If needed, adjust the parameters and repeat the analysis.
6. The reads are now ready for the assembly step.

3.4 Running the Sequence Assembly

3.4.1 Using Spades

1. Run Spades from the terminal or command prompt. To use only the 'paired' sequences type the following command:

   % spades.py -o <output_directory> -1 <forward_reads.fastq> -2 <reverse_reads.fastq> --threads <number_of_threads> -k 27,39,77,87,97,107,117,123 (*see* **Note 8**).

2. To use both the 'paired' and 'unpaired' sequences type the following command:

   % spades.py -o <output_directory> -1 <forward_reads.fastq> -2 <reverse_reads.fastq> -s <unpaired_reads.fastq> --threads <number_of_threads> -k 27,39,77,87,97,107,117,123.

3. Examine the output. There should be five (or more) new files in the output directory, including *scaffolds.fasta* (resulting scaffolds), *contigs.fasta* (resulting contigs), *params.txt* (information about SPAdes parameters in this run), and other files for statistics about these.

3.4.2 Using Velvet

1. Run Velvet from the terminal or command prompt:

   % velveth <output_directory> 21 -fastq -shortPaired <forward_reads.fastq> <reverse_reads.fastq> (*see* **Note 9**).

2. After running velveth, the next step is to run velvetg on the <output_directory> and files generated from velveth. Run the command:

   % velvetg <output_directory> -min_contig_lgth <length> (*see* **Note 9**).

3. Check the directory after velvetg. The output FASTA file *contigs.fasta* is the final Velvet output that contains the assembled contigs.

3.5 Analysis of Contigs by Similarity Searches

Contigs are subjected to a BLAST search against the RefSeq viral genome sequence database from NCBI.

1. Download the reference viral sequences in the NCBI RefSeq Viral genome sequence database using the wget command (*see* **Note 10**).

   - For nucleotide sequences, type:

     % wget https://ftp.ncbi.nlm.nih.gov/refseq/release/viral/viral.1.1.genomic.fna.gz.

- For amino acid sequences, type:

  % wget https://ftp.ncbi.nlm.nih.gov/refseq/release/viral/viral.1.protein.faa.gz.

2. Search for geminivirus sequences in the contigs obtained by the assembly, then index the reference sequences that were just downloaded.

   - For nucleotide, type:

     % makeblastdb -in viral.1.1.genomic.fna -dbtype nucl (*see* **Note 11**).

   - For amino acids, type:

     % makeblastd -in viral.1.protein.faa -dbtype prot.

3. Proceed with the comparison process. Use blast*n* to compare nucleotide sequences of the contigs with nucleotide sequences of viruses. Use blast*x* to compare the contigs with the amino acid sequences of the viral proteins.

   - For nucleotide sequences, type:

     % blastn -query contigs_sequences.fasta -db viral.1.1.genomic.fna -out contigs_results_blast_results.tab -evalue 1e-5 -outfmt 6 -max_target_seqs 1 -num_threads <number_of_threads> (*see* **Notes 11** and **12**).

   - For amino acid sequences, type:

     % blastx -query contigs_sequences.fasta -db viral.1.protein.faa -out contigs_results_blast_results.tab -evalue 1e-5 -outfmt 6 -max_target_seqs 1 -num_threads <number_of_threads>.

4. After completing the analysis, review the *contigs_results_blast_results.tab* file to identify geminivirus sequences by evaluating the coverage and identity results.

4 Notes

1. FastQC is a widely used tool that provides an overview of basic quality control metrics for raw HTS data. The tool includes several different analyses, known as modules, that can be applied to a sequence dataset. The user manual can be found at the links provided above, and (as always) it is highly recommended reading.
2. The code for Trimmomatic is available under the GPL license. Since version 0.27, Trimmomatic can be run using Java with the -jar option. For detailed instructions, refer to the complete user manual (http://www.usadellab.org/cms/uploads/supplementary/Trimmomatic/TrimmomaticManual_V0.32.pdf).

3. Download SPAdes binaries for Linux or MacOS from this link: https://github.com/ablab/spades/releases/tag/v4.0.0. Alternatively, you can compile SPAdes from source, which requires g++ version 9.0 or higher, cmake version 3.16 or higher, and the libraries zlib and libbz2. Note that SPAdes requires Python 3.8 or later.
4. Velvet is primarily compatible with Linux and macOS, but it can also be used in Windows via WSL (Windows Subsystem for Linux) or virtual machines. It is widely used in bioinformatics and has been optimized for Unix-based platforms. Velvet should work on any standard 64-bit Linux environment with gcc. It is recommended to have a good amount of physical memory (starting with 12 GB, although more is better). For the complete user manual, visit https://github.com/dzerbino/velvet/blob/master/Manual.pdf.
5. Download and install BLAST+ at https://ftp.ncbi.nlm.nih.gov/blast/executables/blast+/LATEST/. You can find the necessary databases to download (see the database section below) or create your own. For detailed instructions, refer to the BLAST+ user manual.
6. These are the parameters available in the output html report provided by FastQC:
   - Basic Statistics: Provides essential details about the input FastQ file, including its name, quality score encoding type, total number of reads, read length, and GC content.
   - Per Base Sequence Quality: Displays the quality scores across each base position; ideally, initial bases should have scores around 32, increasing to 38–40 for high quality; some variability in the last bases is expected, but overall a score >20 is considered good.
   - Per Sequence Quality Scores: Shows the average quality score on the *x*-axis and the number of sequences with that score on the *y*-axis.
   - Per Base Sequence Content: Represents the proportion of each base at each position across the reads.
   - Per Sequence GC Content: Plots the number of reads against their GC content percentage.
   - Per Base N Content: Indicates the percentage of bases at each position with no base call (i.e., 'N').
   - Overrepresented Sequences: Lists sequences that appear more frequently than expected.
   - Adapter Content: Displays a cumulative plot showing the fraction of reads with identified adapter sequences at various base positions, specific to the library type used.
   - Kmer Content: Measures the frequency of each *k*-mer (default length = 7) across the reads.

7. Meaning of the parameters:
   - ILLUMINACLIP: Cuts adapter and other illumina-specific sequences from the reads (https://github.com/timflutre/trimmomatic/tree/master/adapters).
   - SLIDINGWINDOW: Performs a sliding window trimming approach; it starts scanning at the 5′-end and clips the read once the average quality within the window falls below a threshold.
   - LEADING: Cuts bases off the start of a read, if below a threshold quality.
   - TRAILING: Cuts bases off the end of a read, if below a threshold quality.
   - MINLEN: Drops the read if it is below a specified length.
   - AVGQUAL: Drops the read if the average quality is below the specified level.
8. Meaning of the parameters:
   - -o: Directory to store all the resulting files.
   - -1 and -2: Files with forward and reverse paired end reads, respectively, in FASTQ or FASTA.
   - -k: List of *k*-mer sizes.
9. Meaning of the parameters:
   - -file_format: File format options (FASTQ, FASTA, BAM or SAM).
   - -read_type: Read type options.
   - -min_contig_lgth: Minimum contig length exported to *contigs.fasta* file.
10. You can download reference sequences directly from the BLAST online portal at: https://www.ncbi.nlm.nih.gov/labs/virus/vssi/#/.
11. Meaning of the parameters:
    - -in: Input file/database name.
    - -dbtype: Database type (nucl for nucleotide and prot for protein).
    - -query: Query file name.
    - -db: BLAST database name.
    - -out: Output file name.
    - -evalue: *e* value of the alignment.
    - -outfmt: Output format (alignment view options), the available options are:

      0 = Pairwise.

      1 = Query-anchored showing identities.

2 = Query-anchored no identities.

3 = Flat query-anchored, show identities.

4 = Flat query-anchored, no identities.

5 = XML Blast output.

6 = Tabular.

7 = Tabular with comment line.

8 = Text ASN.1.

9 = Binary ASN.1.

10 = Comma-separated values.

11 = BLAST archive format (ASN.1).

- -max_target_seqs: The maximum number of best hits per query.
- -num_threads: Number of processors.

12. The output format 6 (tabular) typically includes the following columns:
    - query_id: Query identifier.
    - subject_id: Target sequence identifier (from the database).
    - percent_identity: Percentage of identity between the query and the target.
    - alignment_length: Alignment length.
    - mismatches: Number of differences between the target and the query.
    - gap_opens: Number of gap openings in the alignment.
    - evalue: *e* value of the alignment.
    - bit_score: Alignment score.

References

1. Haible D, Kober S, Jeske H (2006) Rolling circle amplification revolutionizes diagnosis and genomics of geminiviruses. J Virol Met 135:9–16
2. Rojas MR, Gilbertson RL, Russell DR, Maxwell DP (1993) Use of degenerate primers in the polymerase chain reaction to detect whitefly-transmitted geminiviruses. Plant Dis 77:340–347
3. Brown JK, Idris AM, Torres-Jerez I, Banks GK, Wyatt SD (2001) The core region of the coat protein gene is highly useful for establishing the provisional identification and classification of begomoviruses. Arch Virol 146:1581–1598
4. Wu Q, Ding SW, Zhang Y, Zhu S (2015) Identification of viruses and viroids by next-generation sequencing and homology-dependent and homology-independent algorithms. Annu Rev Phytopathol 53:425–444
5. Maree HJ, Fox A, Al Rwahnih M, Boonham N, Candresse T (2018) Application of HTS for routine plant virus diagnostics: state of the art and challenges. Front Plant Sci 9:1082
6. Villamor DEV, Ho T, Al Rwahnih M, Martin RR, Tzanetakis IE (2019) High throughput sequencing for plant virus detection and discovery. Phytopathology 109:716–725
7. Blawid R, Silva JMF, Nagata T (2017) Discovering and sequencing new plant viral genomes by next-generation sequencing: description of a practical pipeline. Ann Appl Biol 170:301–314

8. Boykin LM, Sseruwagi P, Alicai T, Ateka E, Mohammed IU et al (2019) Tree lab: portable genomics for early detection of plant viruses and pests in Sub-Saharan Africa. Genes 10:632
9. Ben Chehida S, Filloux D, Fernandez E, Moubset O, Hoareau M et al (2021) Nanopore sequencing is a credible alternative to recover complete genomes of geminiviruses. Microorganisms 9:903
10. Pecman A, Adams I, Gutiérrez-Aguirre I, Fox A, Boonham N et al (2022) Systematic comparison of Nanopore and Illumina sequencing for the detection of plant viruses and viroids using total RNA sequencing approach. Front Microbiol 13:883921

Chapter 16

CRISPR-Cas-Based Diagnosis of Geminiviruses

Tripti Singhal and Ashish Srivastava

Abstract

Successful disease management relies on rapid and accurate identification of the causal agent. Begomoviruses (family *Geminiviridae*) cause severe economic losses and pose a serious threat to sustainable agriculture. Here, we describe a clustered regularly interspaced short palindromic repeats (CRISPR)-based nucleic acid detection method utilizing the CRISPR/Cas12a and CRISPR/Cas13a system for begomoviruses used in our laboratory. CRISPR-based diagnostic tools are very precise and sensitive and visual readout-compatible reporters do not need expensive laboratory equipment such as qRT-PCR. The assay detects the targeted begomoviruses in infected plants with high sensitivity and specificity, and can provide highly sensitive and specific detection visual readouts using a simple, low-cost blue light lamp, ideal for on-site use.

Key words Begomovirus, CRISPR/Cas12a, Point-of-care testing, RT-RAA, RT-RPA, RT-LAMP

Abbreviations

Cas protein	CRISPR-associated protein
CRISPR	Clustered, regularly interspaced, short palindromic repeats
DETECTR	DNA endonuclease targeted CRISPR trans reporter
gRNA	guide RNA
HOLMES	1-h low-cost multifunctional highly efficient system
PAM	Protospacer adjacent motif
RT-LAMP	Reverse transcription-loop-mediated isothermal amplification
RT-RAA	Reverse transcription-recombinase-aided amplification
RT-RPA	Reverse transcription-recombinase polymerase amplification
TAE buffer	Tris-acetate-EDTA buffer

1 Introduction

In the past two decades, as transportation has increased and economically important crops have expanded to new regions, the

Francisco Murilo Zerbini et al. (eds.), *Geminiviruses: Methods and Protocols*, Methods in Molecular Biology, vol. 2912,
https://doi.org/10.1007/978-1-0716-4454-6_16,

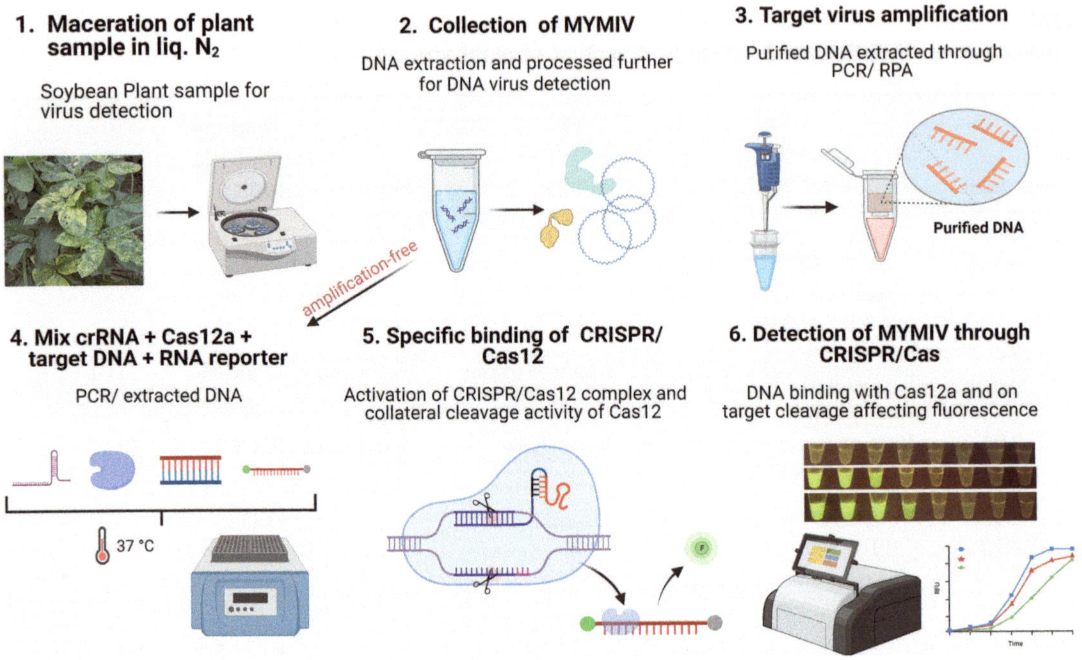

Fig. 1 Graphical representation of CRISPR/Cas12a technique (**1-2**) isolation of virus, (**3**) amplification of target sequence through RTPCR, (**4-5**) collateral cleavage through Cas12a, signal-readout, and (**6**) fluorometric detection of cleaved ssDNASingle stranded DNA (ssDNA) probes

3. 1× reaction buffer (50 mM NaCl, 10 mM Tris–HCl, 10 mM $MgCl_2$, 100 μg/mL Recombinant Albumin, pH 7.9).
4. PCR/RCA/Lamp-amplified DNA fragment.
5. Substrate DNA.
6. ssDNA fluorescent probe (5′-/56-FAM/TTATT/3IABKFQ/-3′) or DNase alert.
7. In vitro transcription kit (*see* **Note 4**).
8. Ultrapure deionized water (18 MΩ-cm at 25 °C).
9. 384-well black polypropylene microplate.

3 Methods

3.1 Synthesis of sgRNA

1. The LbCas12a (Cpf1) crRNA is a single, 40–44 base, guide RNA, comprising a 20-nt constant region (loop domain) and a 20- to 24-nt target-specific region (protospacer domain). Download the genome components of your target virus from GenBank and align using Sequence Demarcation Tool (SDT) [19] for scoring and identifying conserved regions.
2. Design PCR primers to amplify a 300–1200 bp fragment from the conserved regions identified in the previous step.

3. Download the conserved regions and open in SnapGene Viewer (https://www.snapgene.com/).
4. Search for a unique protospacer-adjacent motif (PAM) region TTTV ($V = A,C,G$).
5. A 20- to 24-nt RNA complementary to the target DNA and downstream to PAM must be identified and either subjected to a BLASTn search or mapped against the plant genome in CLC Genomics Workbench; sgRNA with off-targets must be removed, and only those on-target should be considered for synthesis.
6. Synthesize two sgRNAs per target for PCR amplified target detection, and 15–30 sgRNA per virus for amplification-free detection (*see* **Note 5**).
7. Perform in vitro transcriptions with a T7 sense primer and an in vitro transcription kit.
8. Treat the synthesized sgRNA with DNase I (*see* **Note 6**).
9. Dilute the sgRNA to 100 nM for stock and use 30 nM in the final reaction.

3.2 Target Amplification

1. Collect begomovirus-infected leaf samples (grown under controlled condition) and extract total DNA (*see* Chapter 1).
2. Perform PCR using DNA-A-specific degenerate primers [20] with the following cycling parameters: 94 °C for 5 min; 30 cycles of denaturing at 94 °C for 45 s, annealing at 55 °C for 45 s and extension at 72 °C for 45 s; final extension of 10 min at 72 °C. *See* **Note 7**.
3. Elute amplicons and record their concentration.
4. Group sgRNA based on the target amplicon for detection.

3.3 Begomovirus Detection

1. Mix 3 μL of 300 nM sgRNA, 1 μL of Cas12a (Cpf1) enzyme, 3 μL of 10× reaction buffer, and 20 μL of nuclease-free water and incubated for 10 min at room temperature (total reaction volume of 27 μL).
2. Add 5 μL probe DNA (500 nM) to the reaction mix and incubate for 1 min.
3. Add up to 3 μL of 30 nM substrate DNA and incubate for 10–30 min at 37 °C; observe in blue light (450–470 nm).
4. Real-time reading of fluorescence can be taken in Cytation 3 microplate reader (BioTek) or Quantus Fluorometer (Promega). *See* **Note 8**.

conserved genome sequences as well as rolling circle amplification (RCA) using Phi29 DNA polymerase with random-nucleotide primers [4]. PCR-based methods suffer from primer-template affinity issues, causing viral template loss [5] while RCA is less prone to primer complementarity bias and results in hyper-branched, high molecular weight, concatenated products requiring linearization via restriction enzymes or mechanical shearing before sequencing [6]. However, the use of these restriction enzymes necessitates prior knowledge of conserved restriction sites, leading to the loss of viral sequences without or with multiple restriction sites. An alternative, polymerase cloning (ploning), uses endonucleases and DNA repair enzymes for linearization, followed by shotgun sequencing and genome assembly [7].

Recent long-read sequencing advancements allow direct full-length RCA product sequencing, necessitating complex DNA sequence product resolution algorithms. Adaptation of library preparation protocols and development of novel bioinformatics methods make long-read technologies such as Single Molecule Real-Time (SMRT) sequencing (Pacific Biosciences and Oxford Nanopore) suitable to overcome similar DNA sequence assembly challenges, as shown in comparative Illumina and SMRT sequencing studies of bacterial genomes and comprehensive SMRT sequencing analyses for viral and bacterial genome identification and sequencing [8, 9].

Provided below is the laboratory protocol for CIDER-Seq (Circular DNA Enrichment sequencing); for sequence-independent circular DNA virus enrichment and assembly-free SMRT long-read sequencing [10, 11]. CIDER-Seq, employing a ploning-based enrichment protocol, requires only an estimate of virus genome size and, optionally, a reference sequence. A novel algorithm, DeConcat, parses concatenated DNA strands from RCA, enabling complete virus genome sequencing without reference-based or de novo assembly. Finally, we also provide an update to the CIDER-Seq pipeline that works with Oxford Nanopore sequencing in addition to the PacBio sequencing. In the updated pipeline the existing output limitations of Pacbio sequencing [12], that might be critical for in-depth analysis of virus populations, have been overcome by using Oxford Nanopore sequencing technology.

2 Materials

Use ultrapure water (double-distilled and deionized) for preparing all solutions. Prepare and store all reagents at room temperature, unless indicated otherwise. Strictly follow all biosafety and waste disposal regulations.

2.1 Plant Material

This method can be adapted for any sample type infected with circular DNA virus. In this protocol, we used cassava cultivar 60,444, available at the International Institute of Tropical Agriculture (IITA, Nigeria) in vitro cassava germplasm collections. Cassava cv. 60,444 plants were agroinoculated with African cassava mosaic virus (ACMV; family *Geminiviridae*) infectious clone using the previously described protocol [13, 14], to obtain virus-infected plant material.

2.2 Reagents

1. 2-Mercaptoethanol.
2. Cetyltrimethylammonium bromide (CTAB).
3. Deoxynucleotide triphosphates, 10 mM.
4. Disodium ethylenediamine (EDTA).
5. DNA-binding magnetic beads.
6. *E. coli* DNA Polymerase 1.
7. Ethanol, >99.8%.
8. Ethanol, 80%, prepared in DNase-free distilled water.
9. Exo-Resistant Random Primer, 100 mM.
10. Fast AP Thermosensitive Alkaline Phosphatase.
11. Geneclean kit (Optional).
12. Inorganic Pyrophosphatase, U/μL.
13. NEBuffer 2, 10×.
14. NEB Exonuclease V.
15. Phi29 Buffer, 10×.
16. Phi29 DNA Polymerase, 10 U/μL.
17. Polyvinylpyrrolidone (PVP).
18. Qubit DNA Broad Range measurement kit.
19. S1 Nuclease Buffer, 5×.
20. S1 Nuclease, 100 U/μL.
21. SMRTBell™ Barcoded Adapter Complete Prep Kit-96.
22. Sodium Acetate, 3 M, prepared in DNase-free distilled water.
23. T4 DNA Polymerase.
24. Tris-hydrochloride (Tris–HCl).
25. Ultrapure DNase/RNase-free distilled water.
26. NEBNext FFPE DNA Repair module.
27. NEBNext Ultra II End Repair/dA-Tailing module.
28. Nanopore ligation sequencing kit.

2.3 Equipment and Consumables

1. This method requires a dedicated desktop or computational server utilizing a UNIX-based system (MacOS X or a 64-bit Linux OS), with a preference for multi-threaded processors to ensure rapid performance.
2. PacBio RS2/Sequel/Sequel2 instrument.
3. Fridge (4 °C) and freezer (−20 °C and −80 °C).
4. Thermalcycler.
5. Qubit Fluorometer.
6. NanoDrop system.
7. Magnetic microfuge tube rack.
8. Refrigerated centrifuge.
9. Micropipette.
10. Mortar and pestle.
11. pH meter.
12. Pipette aid.
13. Precision balance.
14. Spatula, scalpel, and forceps.
15. Vortexer.
16. Safety mask/goggles (UV protection).
17. Microfuge tubes (1.5 and 2 mL).
18. Microfuge LoBind tubes (1.5 mL).
19. Sterile polypropilene Falcon tubes, 15 and 50 mL.
20. Nanopore Flow Cell (R10.4.1).
21. Nanopore instrument.

2.4 Software

1. Bio-MUST-Core (https://metacpan.org/release/Bio-MUST-Core).
2. Biopython (https://biopython.org/).
3. BLAST (ftp://ftp.ncbi.nlm.nih.gov/blast/executables/blast+/LATEST/).
4. CIDER-Seq Data Analysis Package 2 (https://github.com/devang-mehta/ciderseq2).
5. Click (https://click.palletsprojects.com/en/5.x/).
6. Git (https://git-scm.com/).
7. Matplotlib (https://matplotlib.org/).
8. MUSCLE (http://www.drive5.com/muscle/).
9. NumPy (http://www.numpy.org/).
10. Python 3 (https://www.python.org/download/releases/3.0/).
11. Guppy (https://www.nanoporetech.com).

12. Porechop (https://github.com/rrwick/Porechop).
13. MinKNOW software (https://www.nanoporetech.com).

3 Methods

3.1 Total DNA Extraction from Infected Tissues

Here we provide the CIDER-Seq protocol for amplifying ACMV from virus-infected leaves of cassava. This method can be adapted for any sample type infected with circular DNA virus, after extracting high-quality DNA from the infected samples.

3.1.1 Sample Collection

Collect ~500 mg of young leaves from infected cassava plants in an aluminum foil or falcon tube. Flash freeze the harvested leaf samples by immediately transferring them to liquid nitrogen. The samples are processed as soon as they arrive at the laboratory, or they can be stored at −80 °C for long-term storage.

3.1.2 Total Nucleic Acid Isolation

This protocol is adapted from the standard CTAB protocol used for nucleic acid isolation from plant leaf tissues [15].

1. Grind 50–100 mg of leaf tissue in liquid nitrogen with a pre-chilled pestle and mortar. Add more liquid nitrogen if needed, until a fine powder is obtained.
2. Transfer the ground leaf tissue to a 2 mL microfuge tube and add 1 mL of CTAB extraction buffer.
3. Shake vigorously using a vortex until you get a homogeneous suspension and centrifuge the tubes for 5 min at 13,000×*g* at RT.
4. Collect 750 μL of the supernatant and transfer it to a new 2 mL microfuge tube.
5. Incubate the new tube at 65 °C for 45 min. Mix the samples by shaking the tubes every 10–15 min.
6. Add an equal volume (750 μL) of chloroform, mix vigorously, and centrifuge the tubes at 13,000×*g* for 10 min.
7. Transfer the supernatant to a new 1.5 mL microfuge tube and add one volume of pre-chilled Isopropanol. Mix gently by inverting the tubes and incubate the tubes at −20 °C for at least 60 min.
8. Centrifuge the tubes at 13,000×*g* for 15 min at 4 °C, discard the supernatant and preserve the pallet by inverting the tube.
9. Wash the pellet with 500 μL of 70% pre-chilled ethanol and centrifuge a 13,000×*g* for 10 min.
10. Discard the supernatant and air dry the pellets.
11. Resuspend the pellet in 50 μL of nuclease-free water.

12. Check the extent of DNA degradation using agarose gel electrophoresis or a Bioanalyzer.

3.2 Size Selection on Silica Beads

This step uses GeneClean kit (MP Biomedicals, cat. no. 111001200) to perform silica-based purification and partial size selection (200 bp–20 kb) on total DNA. This step is optional (*see* **Note 1**).

1. Take 5 μg DNA and makeup 20 μL volume with H_2O.
2. Add 60 μL (3 volumes) of NaI solution. This keeps the final concentration of NaI above 4 M.
3. Resuspend glassmilk by vortexing for 1 min.
4. Add 10 μL glassmilk to the DNA-NaI solution and vortex gently or stir with a pipet tip to mix.
5. Incubate at room temperature for 5 min, mixing every 1–2 min to ensure that glassmilk stays in suspension.
6. Centrifuge at 14,000×*g* for 5 s and discard the supernatant. This will pellet the glassmilk with the bound DNA.
7. Add 500 μL prepared NEW Wash and resuspend (*see* **Note 2**).
8. Carefully resuspend the pellet by pipetting up and down while stirring the pellet with the pipet tip.
9. Centrifuge at 14,000×*g* for 5 s and discard supernatant.
10. Repeat the wash procedure (as detailed in **steps 7–9**).
11. Dry the pellet to remove residual ethanol.
12. After the supernatant from the final wash has been removed, centrifuge the tube again at 14,000×*g* for a few seconds and remove the last bit of liquid with a small-bore pipet tip to avoid diluting the eluate with the prepared NEW Wash.
13. Add 10 μL water or TE and carefully resuspend the pellet by gently pipetting up and down with a wide-bore pipet tip or by tapping the side of the tube with a finger to mix and elute DNA.
14. Centrifuge at 14,000×*g* for 30 s to pellet.
15. Carefully remove the supernatant containing the eluted DNA and place it in a new tube. Approximately 80% of the bound DNA will elute in this first step. Save the tube containing the pellet until recovery of DNA has been verified.

3.3 Linear DNA Removal

Linear DNA can be removed using NEB Exonuclease V or Lucigen PlasmidSafe Exonuclease (E3101K), below is the protocol for NEB ExoV. This step is optional (*see* **Note 3**).

1. Set up the reaction containing 100–200 ng DNA, 5 μL NEBuffer 4 (10×), 5 μL ATP (10 mM), and 8 μL Exonuclease V (10 U/μL).

2. Add nuclease-free water until 50 μL.
3. Incubate at 37 °C for 6 days.
4. To stop reaction, add EDTA to 11 mM.
5. Heat inactivate by incubating at 70 °C for 30 min.
6. To clean up treated samples, go to steps of Subheading 3.4 (ethanol cleanup).

3.4 Ethanol Cleanup

1. To 1 volume of reaction add 0.1 volume of 3 M sodium acetate.
2. Add 1 μL of 20 mg/mL molecular biology-grade glycogen.
3. Mix thoroughly by pipetting.
4. Add 2.0–2.5 vol. (50 μL) of ice-cold 100% ethanol.
5. Incubate for 10–30 min at −20 °C.
6. Spin at 13,000×*g* for 30–60 min at 4 °C.
7. Remove the ethanol, and add 200 μL of freshly prepared 80% ethanol.
8. Spin at 13,000×*g* for 2 min at RT.
9. Air-dry the pallet and resuspend in nuclease-free water.

3.5 Rolling Circle Amplification

1. Set up the reaction containing 1 pg–100 ng DNA, 2 μL Phi29 buffer (10×), 5 μL dNTPs (10 mM), 5 μL Exo-resistant random primers (100 mM), 1 μL Phi29 DNA polymerase (10 U/μL), and 0.2 μL inorganic pyrophosphatase (0.1 U/μL).
2. Add nuclease-free water until 20 μL.
3. Incubate at 30 °C for 18 h.
4. Heat inactivate the reaction by incubation at 65 °C for 2 min.
5. Perform the ethanol clean up as described in Subheading 3.4.

3.6 Phi29 Debranching

1. Set up the reaction containing 15.5 μL DNA from Subheading 3.5, 2 μL Phi29 buffer (10×), 2 μL dNTPs (10 mM) and 0.5 μL Phi29 DNA polymerase (10 U/μL).
2. Incubate at 30 °C for 2 h.
3. Stop the reaction by heating at 65 °C for 2 min.
4. To clean up treated samples, follow steps of Subheading 3.4 (ethanol cleanup).

3.7 S1 Nuclease Treatment

1. Set up the reaction containing 15.5 μL DNA from Subheading 3.6, 4 μL S1 buffer (5×), 0.5 μL S1 Nuclease (100 U/μL).
2. Incubate at 37 °C for 30 min.
3. To clean up treated samples, follow steps of Subheading 3.4 (ethanol cleanup).

3.8 DNA Repair

1. Set up the reaction containing 20 μL DNA from Subheading 3.7, 5 μL NEBuffer 2 (10×), 1 μL dNTPs (10 mM), 1 μL DNA polymerase 1 (10 U/μL), and 1 μL T4 DNA polymerase (5 U/μL) (*see* **Note 4**).
2. Add nuclease-free water until 50 μL.
3. Incubate at RT for 30 min.
4. Add 5 U (5 μL) of Fast AP (alkaline phosphatase).
5. Incubate at 37 °C for 10 min.
6. Stop the reaction by incubating at 75 °C for 5 min.

3.9 Magnetic Bead Purification

1. Add 1.5 vol. of magnetic beads (KAPA Pure or AMPure) to each sample (85 μL beads to 55 μL sample).
2. Mix, and incubate at RT for 15 min.
3. Place the tubes on a magnetic rack and allow beads to pellet.
4. Discard the supernatant.
5. Add 1 vol. (140 μL) freshly prepared 80% ethanol to each tube.
6. After 30 s, remove the ethanol.
7. Repeat the ethanol wash.
8. Dry the tubes for 5 min.
9. Remove the tubes from the magnet and resuspend in 20–50 μL of nuclease-free water.
10. Incubate at RT for 10 min.
11. Place the tubes on the magnet.
12. Recover the supernatant once the magnets pellet.
13. Measure DNA concentration on a Qubit (dsDNA BR dye).

3.10 Library Preparation and Sequencing

3.10.1 SMRT Library Preparation and PacBio Sequencing

1. Prepare sequencing libraries using the SMRTBell Barcoded Adapter Complete Prep Kit-96 following the manufacturer's instructions.
2. Use ~200 ng of enriched DNA from Subheading 3.9 per sample as input (*see* **Note 5**).
3. Size-select libraries using the desired cutoffs (*see* **Note 6**).
4. Prepare sequencing complexes using the latest available MagBead kit and use the PacBio MagBead loading protocol (Pacific Biosciences: Template Preparation and Sequencing Guide) to load samples on the PacBio RS II, Sequel, or Sequel II instrument (*see* **Note 7**).

3.10.2 Nanopore Library Preparation and Sequencing

1. Prepare the library by ligation of sequencing adapters to be repaired and end-prepped complete dsDNAs.

2. Take DNA sample (~1000 ng) and mix with the components of NEBNext FFPE DNA Repair and NEBNext Ultra II End Repair/dA-Tailing modules.
3. Incubate at 20 °C for 15 min and 65 °C for 5 min.
4. Perform AMPure XP Beads DNA cleaning and adapter ligation with Nanopore ligation sequencing kit v14 according to the manufacturer's instructions.
5. Prepared library (~200 ng) can be loaded into the Nanopore flow-cell (R10.4.1) for sequencing with MinKNOW software according to the manufacturer's instructions.

3.11 Sequencing Data Analysis

3.11.1 Demultiplexing of PacBio Sequencing Data and CCS Analysis

1. Process the raw sequencing data using the SMRT Link software to demultiplex sample barcodes and perform CCS analysis (refer to the Pacific Biosciences: SMRT Link User Guide).
2. Set the CCS analysis parameters for high stringency, 0.999 quality, and minimum read length at 1 kp, to obtain high-quality sequencing reads for further analysis.
3. Store the processed reads, post-demultiplexing and CCS analysis, as fastq files for downstream analyses.

3.11.2 Nanopore Data Basecalling

1. Perform basecalling on the raw Nanopore sequencing data using neural network Guppy basecaller software.
2. Perform adapter trimming on the basecalled data using Porechop tool.

3.12 Setting up CIDER-Seq Parameters

1. Download the latest version of the CIDER-Seq software package from github (https://github.com/devang-mehta/ciderseq2). Ensure that all required software has been installed (*see* **Note 8**).
2. Use the terminal on Linux or MacOS and navigate to the 'ciderseq2' folder. Ensure that all required software has been installed.
3. Open the 'examples' folder and edit the ciderseq_config.json file using any text editor. Edit the parameter values based on the guidelines in Table 1. Default parameters should suffice for most applications; however, modify the file locations to suit your local setup. For virus metagenomics, only the "deconcat" parameters require editing. The other parameters are critical for generating annotated virus genomes from one or more reference genomes. Save the file.

3.13 Extracting the Virus Genomes

1. After completing the configuration file with accurate parameter values (*see* Subheading 3.12), return to the primary ciderseq2 directory.

Table 1
CIDER-Seq parameters filled in for East African cassava mosaic virus (EACMV) data analysis as a working example

Module	Parameter	Default	Comments
settings	outputdir	logs	Provide the path to the directory for saving process logs
separate	outputdir	separate	Directory containing separate.py outputs
	blastinit	[blank]	Python code link for BLAST env. Leave blank unless necessary
	blastexe	blastn	Set path to BLAST executable. Use default if BLAST executables are not found in PATH
	blastndb	./examples/blastdb/EACMV_RefSeq.fasta	Location of BLAST database of reference sequences. Presented here is a database of EACMV. Change according to the needs of experiment
	evalue	1	Change to calibrate BLAST results, only if required
align	outputdir	align	Name of the output directory
	muscleinit	[blank]	Link to Python code for running MUSCLE. Leave blank unless necessary
	muscleexe	/opt/bin/muscle/muscle3.8.31_i86linux64	Path to MUSCLE executable. Edit to point to your local MUSCLE installation
	targets	{"EACMV_DNA_A": ./examples/blastdb/EACMV_DNA_A.fa "EACMV_DNA_B": ./examples/blastdb/EACMV_DNA_B.fa}	List of target virus genomes and locations of their reference genome .fasta files. Number of targets in the list can be increased or decreased. Here we use EACMV DNA-A and EACMV DNA-B. Change according to the needs of experiment
deconcat	outputdir	deconcat	Name of the output directory
	muscleinit	[blank]	Link to Python code for running MUSCLE. Leave blank unless necessary
	muscleexe	/opt/bin/muscle/muscle3.8.31_i86linux64	Path to MUSCLE executable. Edit to point to your local MUSCLE installation
	Fragmentsize	30	The fragment size used by the DeConcat algorithm. Leave unchanged unless strictly required. Deafult value 30 works best for the geminivirus genomes with size ~3 kb
	statistics	1	Replace with 0 to turn off the generation of DeConcat stats files

(continued)

Table 1
(continued)

Module	Parameter	Default	Comments
annotate	outputdir		Name of output directory
	blastinit	[blank]	Link to Python code for running the BLAST environment. Leave blank unless necessary
	blastexe	blastn	Path to BLAST executable. Use default unless BLAST executables are not in $PATH
	tblastndb	./examples/blastdb/ ACMV_Proteins.fasta	Location of reference protein sequences used to annotate virus genomes
	evalue	0.01	
phase	outputdir	phased	
	Outputformat	["genbank", "fasta"]	Format of results. The default produces both .fasta and .genbank files as outputs
	phasegenomes	"EACMV_DNA_A": {"proteins": {"AC1": {"strand": -1}, "AC2": {"strand": -1}, "AC3": {"strand": -1}, "AC4": {"strand": -1}, "AC5": {"strand": -1}, "AV1": {"strand": 1}, "AV2": {"strand": 1}}, "phaseto": "AV2", "offset":10}, "EACMV_DNA_B": {"proteins": {"BC1": {"strand": 1}, "BV1": {"strand": -1}}, "phaseto": "BC1", "offset": 10}	The 'annotate' step lists proteins for each target genome based on the protein .fasta file. 'Strand' indicates the ORF direction on the reference genome. The 'phaseto' setting determines the gene order in the annotated genomes

2. Launch the software by typing the following instructions into the command line interface, and alter the pathways to the configuration file and input file as necessary:

```
python3 cs-tools.py split [OPTIONS] [CONFIG-FILE] [INPUTSEQUENCE]
python3 cs-tools.py join [OPTIONS] [CONFIG-FILE] [INPUTSEQUENCE]
```

For example:

```
python3 cs-tools.py split examples/ciderseq_config.json examples/example 1.fastq
```

3. Upon initiation of the primary command, the program will ask a series of questions to ascertain the operational parameters:

```
Format (fasta, fastq, tab, gb) [fastq]:
```

```
Numjobs [1]:
Cluster []:
Mode (full, deconcat)[full]:
```

Default settings employed when no response is given are presented in brackets. The 'Format' option inquires about the format of the sequences in the input file. The default is the fastq format. The Numjobs option will divide the task into multiple subprocesses to harness multiple CPUs in a system. The Cluster option exists for use with HPC clusters, in which typically a separate job management command must be supplied. By default, no job management command is supplied. For annotated virus genomes, use the 'full' option for the 'Mode' parameter. The time needed to complete the CIDER-Seq analysis will vary according to the size of the input file and the number of available processors. Utilize the 'ps' command to verify the process status and proceed only after the process has ended.

4. Once the split command is run and completed, execute an additional join command:

```
python3 cs-tools.py join --mode full --clean examples/
ciderseq_config.json examples /example 1.fastq
```

The --clean option removes intermediate files created in the split process.

5. Generate a set of graphs displaying key outcomes and process statistics by running the following command:

```
python3 cs-tools.py plot examples/ciderseq_config.json
examples/ example 1.fastq
```

6. Running the CIDER-Seq data analysis package in the virus sequencing mode will result in the creation of multiple output files. For annotated virus sequencing applications, a successful run of the program will produce a set of virus genomes as a multisequence .fasta file and a multisequence .genbank file containing annotated virus sequences. These files are stored in the /Fasta and /Genbank directories, respectively, in the output folder specified in the config.json file. Optionally, using the plot command a set of DeConcat statistic graphs can also be generated. For unannotated virus sequencing, virus genomes are produced as a multisequence .fasta file stored in the /Fasta directory.
7. Running the CIDER-Seq data analysis package in the virus sequencing mode will result in several output files. If the experiment involves annotated virus sequencing, the program will

produce a set of virus genomes as a multi-sequence FASTA file, and a multi-sequence GenBank file containing annotated virus data. These files will be stored in the /Fasta and /Genbank directories, respectively, within the output folder specified in the config.json file. Graphs depicting DeConcat statistics can be obtained using the plot command. For unannotated virus sequencing, virus genomes are produced as a multi-sequence FASTA file, which is stored in the /Fasta directory.

4 Notes

1. Before this step, please check if size selection is the requirement of the experiment. If no size selection is required, move directly to the RCA.
2. Make sure ethanol and water have been added to the NEW Wash Concentrate before using.
3. Before this step, please check if linear DNA removal is the requirement of the experiment. If not, then move directly to the RCA.
4. Set up the DNA repair reaction in Low-Bind 1.5 mL microfuge tubes if possible.
5. Using less than 200 ng of enriched DNA sample for sequencing may result in low read counts.
6. We recommend normalizing libraries to equal concentrations before sequencing. Sequencing providers may be able to assist with size-selection parameters and equipment.
7. Generally, SMRT library preparation and PacBio sequencing (steps in Subheading 3.10) are completed by a sequencing provider.
8. Prerequisite software required to run CIDER-Seq package include BLAST, Python 3 and MUSCLE.

Acknowledgments

The authors acknowledge financial support from the Belgian FNRS (Fonds National de la Recherche Scientifique) grant numbers 1. B456.20, F.4515.17, and J.0187.21.

References

1. Simmonds P, Adams MJ, Benkő M et al (2017) Consensus statement: Virus taxonomy in the age of metagenomics. Nat Rev Microbiol 15: 161–168
2. Mavromatis K, Ivanova N, Barry K et al (2007) Use of simulated data sets to evaluate the fidelity of metagenomic processing methods. Nat Methods 4:495–500

3. Jurasz H, Pawłowski T, Perlejewski K (2021) Contamination issue in viral metagenomics: Problems, solutions, and clinical perspectives. Front Microbiol 12:745076
4. Dean FB, Nelson JR, Giesler TL, Lasken RS (2001) Rapid amplification of plasmid and phage DNA using Phi 29 DNA polymerase and multiply-primed rolling circle amplification. Genome Res 11:1095–1099
5. Callanan J, Stockdale SR, Shkoporov A, Draper LA, Ross RP, Hill C (2021) Biases in viral metagenomics-based detection, cataloguing and quantification of bacteriophage genomes in human faeces, a review. Microorganisms 9:524
6. Inoue-Nagata AK, Albuquerque LC, Rocha WB, Nagata T (2004) A simple method for cloning the complete begomovirus genome using the bacteriophage phi29 DNA polymerase. J Virol Methods 116:209–211
7. Zhang K, Martiny AC, Reppas NB et al (2006) Sequencing genomes from single cells by polymerase cloning. Nat Biotechnol 24:680–686
8. Ardui S, Ameur A, Vermeesch JR, Hestand MS (2018) Single molecule real-time (SMRT) sequencing comes of age: applications and utilities for medical diagnostics. Nucleic Acids Res 46:2159–2168
9. Teng JLL, Yeung ML, Chan E et al (2017) PacBio but not Illumina technology can achieve fast, accurate and complete closure of the high GC, complex *Burkholderia pseudomallei* two-chromosome genome. Front Microbiol 8:1448
10. Mehta D, Hirsch-Hoffmann M, Were M et al (2019) A new full-length circular DNA sequencing method for viral-sized genomes reveals that RNAi transgenic plants provoke a shift in geminivirus populations in the field. Nucleic Acids Res 47:e9
11. Mehta D, Cornet L, Hirsch-Hoffmann M, Zaidi SS, Vanderschuren H (2020) Full-length sequencing of circular DNA viruses and extrachromosomal circular DNA using CIDER-seq. Nat Protoc 15:1673–1689
12. Rhoads A, Au KF (2015) PacBio sequencing and its applications. Genom Proteom Bioinf 13:278–289
13. Vanderschuren H, Alder A, Zhang P, Gruissem W (2009) Dose-dependent RNAi-mediated geminivirus resistance in the tropical root crop cassava. Plant Mol Biol 70:265–272
14. Zaidi SS, Vasudevan K, Lentz EM, Vanderschuren H (2020) Virus-induced gene silencing (VIGS) in cassava using geminivirus agroclones. Methods Mol Biol 2172:51–64
15. Doyle JJ, Doyle JL (1987) A rapid DNA isolation procedure for small quantities of fresh leaf tissue. Phytochem Bull 19:11–15

Chapter 18

Subcellular Localization of Geminivirus Proteins by Laser Scanning Confocal Microscopy

Christiane Eliza Motta Duarte, João Paulo Batista Machado, Bianca Gouveia-Mageste, Fredy Davi Albuquerque Silva, and Elizabeth Pacheco Batista Fontes

Abstract

In eukaryotic cells, the subcellular localization of proteins is inherently linked to their function. Since viruses rely on the host cellular machinery to complete their life cycle, viral proteins are expected to employ the host transport machinery to reach various compartments. Several factors, including the multifunctional nature of viral proteins, the stage of virus infection, and interactions with both viral and host proteins, influence the final destination of viral proteins. For instance, NSP (nuclear shuttle protein) from bipartite begomoviruses and CP (coat protein) from monopartite begomoviruses typically exhibit nuclear localization, yet their subcellular distribution can vary depending on coexpression partners and stage of infection. Virtually all viral proteins display dynamic subcellular distribution patterns that change under their specific functions at different stages of the virus life cycle. Thus, identifying the subcellular distribution of viral proteins is essential for comprehending their multiple roles during infection. This chapter outlines a protocol for efficiently determining the subcellular localization of viral proteins during infection or when expressed with protein partners. The protocol essentially consists of three steps: (i) cloning the viral protein and protein partners fused to fluorescent tags, (ii) transiently expressing the tagged proteins in *N. benthamiana* leaves, and (iii) determining the subcellular localization of the tagged proteins using confocal microscopy.

Key words Transient expression, Agroinoculation, Geminiviral proteins, CabLCV, Confocal microscopy, Subcellular localization

1 Introduction

Eukaryotic cells feature intracellular membranes that encompass distinct compartments known as organelles [1]. These organelles are essential components within all eukaryotic cells. Some primary organelles in these cells include the nucleus, endoplasmic reticulum (ER), Golgi apparatus, mitochondria, lysosomes, endosomes, and peroxisomes. Additionally, plant cells contain plastids, like chloroplasts. Each organelle houses a specific set of proteins responsible

Francisco Murilo Zerbini et al. (eds.), *Geminiviruses: Methods and Protocols*, Methods in Molecular Biology, vol. 2912, https://doi.org/10.1007/978-1-0716-4454-6_18,

for carrying out its specialized functions [2]. Therefore, determining the precise location of proteins within these subcellular structures is crucial for uncovering their functions.

In addition to compartmentalizing specialized functions, eukaryotic cells utilize their specific organelles and membranes, including the plasma membrane, to introduce additional layers for protein function regulation [2]. Growing evidence shows that stimuli-induced transcription factors can be synthesized under normal conditions but remain inactive by sequestration in distinct cellular compartments [3, 4]. One typical example of this phenomenon is observed with the ER stress transcription factors ATF6 (in mammalian cells) and bZIP28/17 (in Arabidopsis and their orthologs in other plant species) [5–7]. Under normal conditions, these transcription factors are tethered to the ER membrane. However, they are released from the ER membrane and translocate to the Golgi apparatus in response to ER stress. In the Golgi apparatus, these membrane-associated transcription factors are proteolytically processed, released from the Golgi membrane, and translocated to the nucleus to execute their transcriptional activator function. This intricate process adds a sophisticated layer of regulation to gene expression, ensuring that responses to cellular stress are finely tuned and controlled.

Like other viruses, geminiviruses rely extensively on the host cell's machinery to carry out essential functions for completing the virus life cycle [8]. Consequently, the precise localization of viral proteins within the host cell's organelles is a critical event that dictates their function and regulation. For example, as geminiviruses replicate in the nucleus of plant cells, viral proteins responsible for replication, transcription of viral genes, and translocation of newly synthesized viral DNA to the cytosol must migrate to the nucleus to perform their functions [9]. Similarly, viral proteins involved in facilitating the cell-to-cell movement of viral DNA need to be directed to the plasmodesmata, while those responsible for suppressing host defenses must be targeted to various organelles, including the cytoplasm and plasma membrane [10]. This orchestration of protein localization is essential for the virus to effectively manipulate the host cell's processes and successfully complete its life cycle.

As multifunctional proteins, viral proteins often change their subcellular distribution, which can depend on factors such as the stage of virus infection, host partners, inherent proviral function, or their role in suppressing host defenses [11, 12]. For example, consider the nuclear shuttle protein (NSP) encoded by the DNA-B of bipartite begomoviruses. When transiently expressed in leaves or protoplasts, NSP is localized in the nucleus (Figs. 1 and 2) [13]. However, during infection or when co-expressed with the viral movement protein (MP) or the host NSP-interacting GTPase (NIG), it is redirected to the cell periphery or cytosol (Figs. 1 and

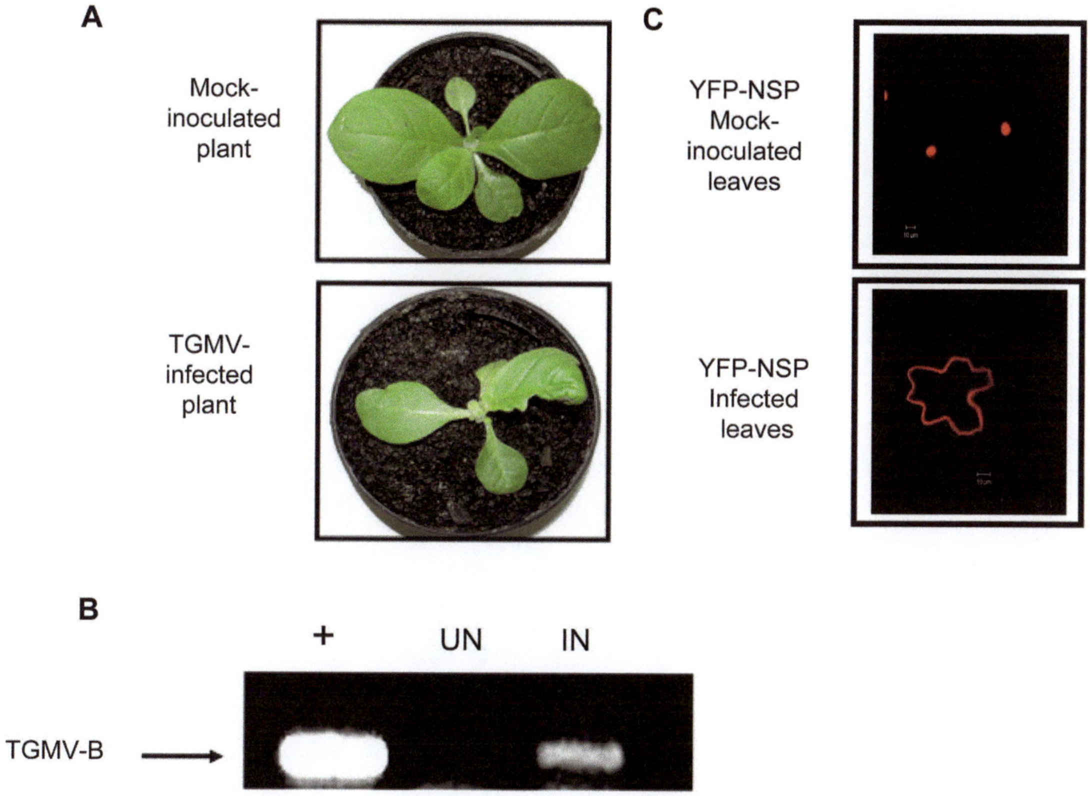

Fig. 1 NSP is nuclear localized but redirected to the cell periphery during infection. (**a**) Infection of *Nicotiana tabacum* leaves with tomato golden mosaic virus (TGMV) infectious clones. Tandemly repeated TGMV DNA-A and DNA-B were inoculated into *N. tabacum* leaves by biolistics. The top plants were bombarded with tungsten particles without viral DNA. The bottom shows infected plants at 7 days post-inoculation (dpi) displaying typical symptoms of TGMV infection. (**b**) Viral DNA accumulation in TGMV-inoculated leaves. Viral DNA was detected by PCR using total DNA from inoculated leaves and DNA-B specific primers. IN, TGMV-inoculated plants; UN, mock-inoculated plants; +, control plasmid DNA as a template. (**c**) Subcellular localization of NSP in mock-inoculated and infected plants. Both uninfected (top) and infected (bottom) tobacco leaves were agroinfiltrated with YFP-NSP, and the subcellular localization of the YFP-tagged protein was monitored by confocal microscopy. In mock-inoculated plants, NSP fused to YFP is nuclear localized, and in infected plants, it is redistributed to the cytosol

2) [13, 14]. Similarly, NSP from cabbage leaf curl virus (CabLCV) relocates to endosomes when co-expressed and interacted with the host protein NSP-interacting Syntaxin 6 domain-containing protein (NISP) (Figs. 3 and 4) [15]. This redistribution provides an intracellular route for translocating the NSP-vDNA complex toward the plasmodesmata.

The coat protein (CP or V1) from monopartite begomoviruses replaces the nuclear-shuttling function of NSP from bipartite begomoviruses [13]. Like NSP, V1 (CP) initially exhibits nuclear localization but can change its subcellular distribution depending on coexpression partners. The nucleocytoplasmic movement of CP

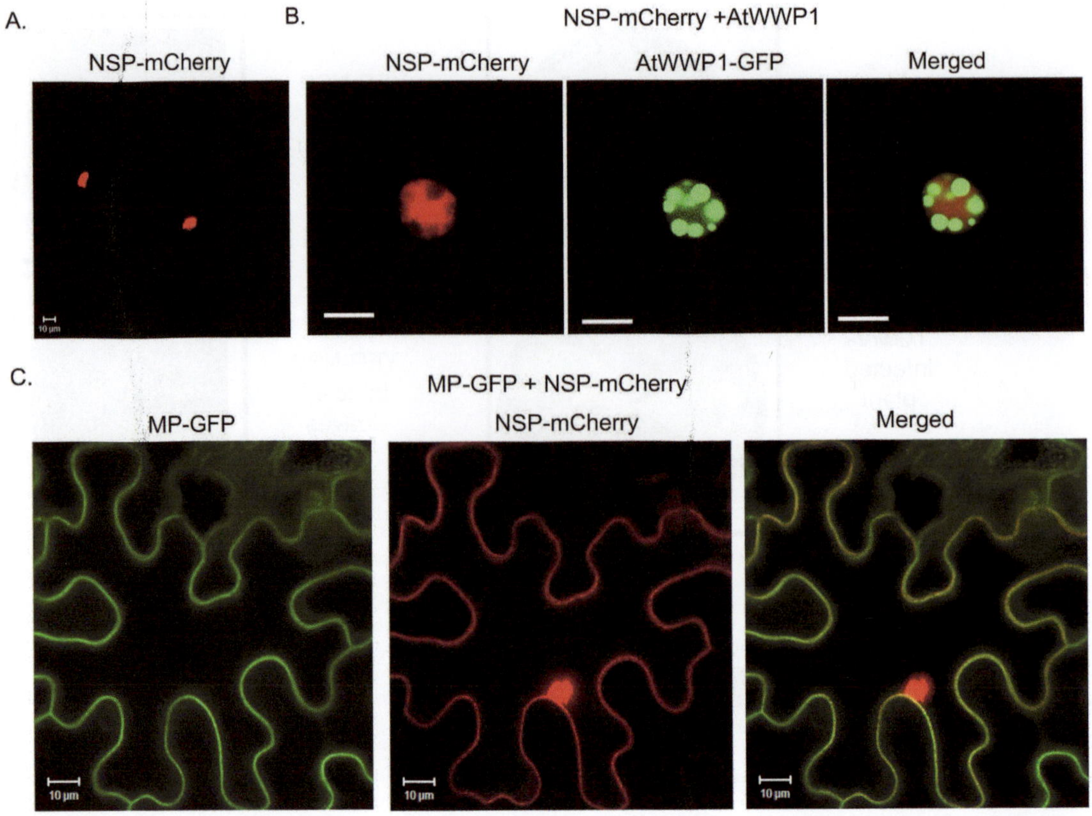

Fig. 2 CabLCV-encoded MP redirects the nuclear NSP to the cytosol. (**a**) Nuclear localization of NSP from cabbage leaf curl virus (CabLCV). *Nicotiana benthamiana* leaves were agroinfiltrated with NSP fused to mCherry under the control of the 35S promoter, and the subcellular localization of NSP-mCherry was monitored by confocal microscopy. Scale bar, 10 μm. (**b**) The nuclear body-forming protein AtWWP1 does not redirect NSP from the nucleoplasm to the membraneless nuclear bodies. *N. benthamiana* leaves were agroinfiltrated with NSP-mCherry and AtWWP1-GFP, and the subcellular localization of the fluorescently tagged proteins was monitored by confocal microscopy. NSP localizes in the nucleoplasm, and AtWWP1 forms punctuate nuclear foci and has been used as a nucleus-associated molecular marker. Scale bars, 20 μm. (**c**) Coexpression of NSP and MP promotes the translocation of NSP from the nucleus to the cytosol. *N. benthamiana* leaves were agroinfiltrated with NSP-mCherry and MP-GFP, and the subcellular localization of the fluorescently tagged proteins was monitored by confocal microscopy. MP localizes in the cytoplasm and translocates NSP to the cytosol. Scale bars, 10 μm

requires the host cell's nuclear transport machinery, involving interactions with importin (for nuclear entry) and exportin (for exit) [13]. Furthermore, the nuclear export of CP is facilitated by interactions with the viral protein V2, and this process is contingent on specific V1-V2 interactions, which are crucial for viral spread and systemic infection [16]. Additionally, V2 is associated with a small ORF in monopartite begomoviruses, C5, which assists its nuclear export and subsequent relocation to the plasmodesmata [17]. Notably, the subcellular distribution of virtually all viral proteins is dynamic and varies with different stages of infection and

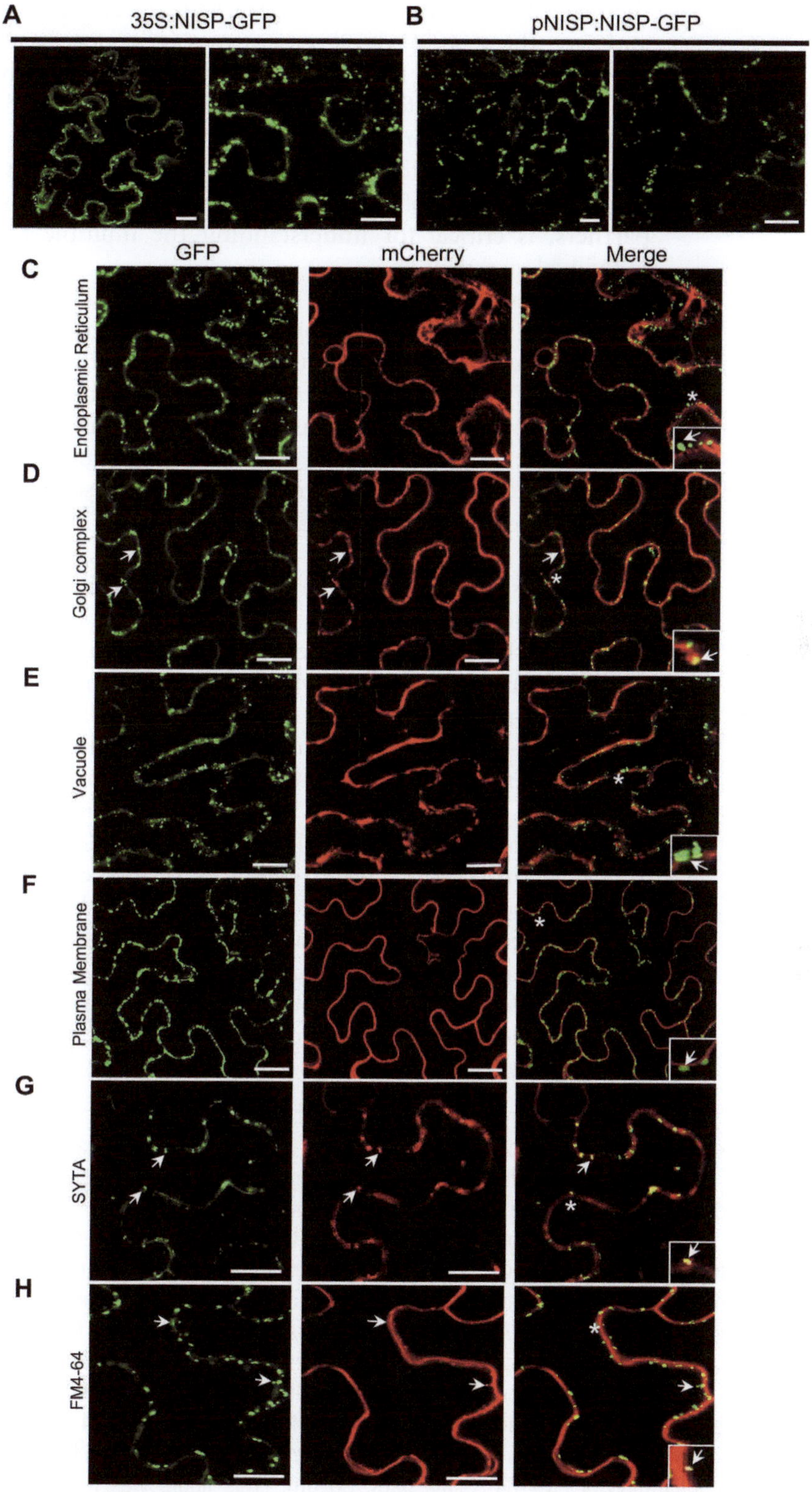

Fig. 3 Organelle-associated molecular markers to define the subcellular localization of an endosomal viral protein partner, NSP-interacting syntaxin 6 domain-containing protein (NISP). (**a**) NISP-GFP distribution in intracellular vesicles. *N. benthamiana* leaves were infiltrated with *A. tumefaciens* carrying a DNA construct

their specific functions. Physiological state, infection by pathogens, and even the stage of development may influence the localization pattern of a protein. Depending on the research objectives, it may be necessary to perform localization experiments under specific conditions, such as virus-infected cells, for example [18]. Therefore, identifying viral protein subcellular localization, both in the presence and absence of viral protein- and host protein-interacting partners, is critical for understanding the multiple functions of individual viral proteins.

This chapter describes a protocol for detecting subcellular localization of viral proteins by confocal microscopy. For transient expression of GFP, YFP- or mCherry-fused protein, we use agroinfiltration of *Nicotiana benthamiana* leaves because it is an experimental host for geminiviruses. For viral protein subcellular localization and dynamics of subcellular distribution, we employ NSP from CabLCV fused to different fluorescent tags in the absence and presence of interacting partners. Figure 1 shows a subcellular localization assay conducted in healthy and tomato golden mosaic virus (TGMV)-infected leaves, illustrating the viral infection-induced subcellular redistribution of the begomovirus NSP from the nucleus to the cell periphery. Figure 2 demonstrates the NSP subcellular nucleocytoplasmic redistribution induced by coexpression of the viral MP. For subcellular localization experiments, protein fusions must be expressed with at least one molecular marker. For the nuclear colocalization assays, we used the nuclear body-forming WWP1, an excellent nucleus-associated molecular marker in plant cells (Fig. 2) [19]. Other cell biology molecular markers are ideal references for protein localization in specific subcellular compartments (Fig. 3). Furthermore, in colocalization experiments, the fusion proteins must be extensively evaluated individually before coexpression. It is worth remembering that colocalization and protein-protein interaction are not the same phenomenon. Two proteins with the same subcellular

Fig. 3 (continued) expressing NISP-GFP under the control of the 35S promoter. Confocal images were taken 36 h post-infiltration. Scale bars, 10 μm (left image) and 20 μm (right image). (**b**) Confocal images of NISP-GFP transiently expressed under the control of the endogenous promoter. Scale bars, 10 μm (left image) and 20 μm (right image). (**c**–**g**) Coexpression of NISP-GFP and an ER-associated ER-mCherry molecular marker (**c**), a Golgi-associated G-mCherry molecular marker (**d**), a tonoplast-associated vac-mCherry molecular marker (**e**), the plasma membrane-associated FLS2-mCherry (**f**), or the endosome-associated SYTA-mCherry (**g**) in *N. benthamiana* leaves. *N. benthamiana* leaf cells expressing the indicated fusion proteins were examined by confocal microscopy 2 days after infiltration. The asterisks indicate the localization of the amplified insets, and the arrows indicate the merged pattern of GFP-associated vesicles in (**c**–**h**). Scale bars, 20 μm. In (**g**), scale bars, 30 μm. (**h**) Colabeling of vesicles with NISP-GFP and FM4-64 in epidermal cells of *N. benthamiana*. Images were taken 2 days post-infiltration of *Agrobacterium* carrying a NISP-GFP expression vector and 1 h after infiltration of FM4-64. Scale bars, 30 μm. (This figure was reproduced from Plant Physiology, 2021, 187: 158–173, https:/doi.org/10.1093/plphys/kiab252, license number 5625931314027)

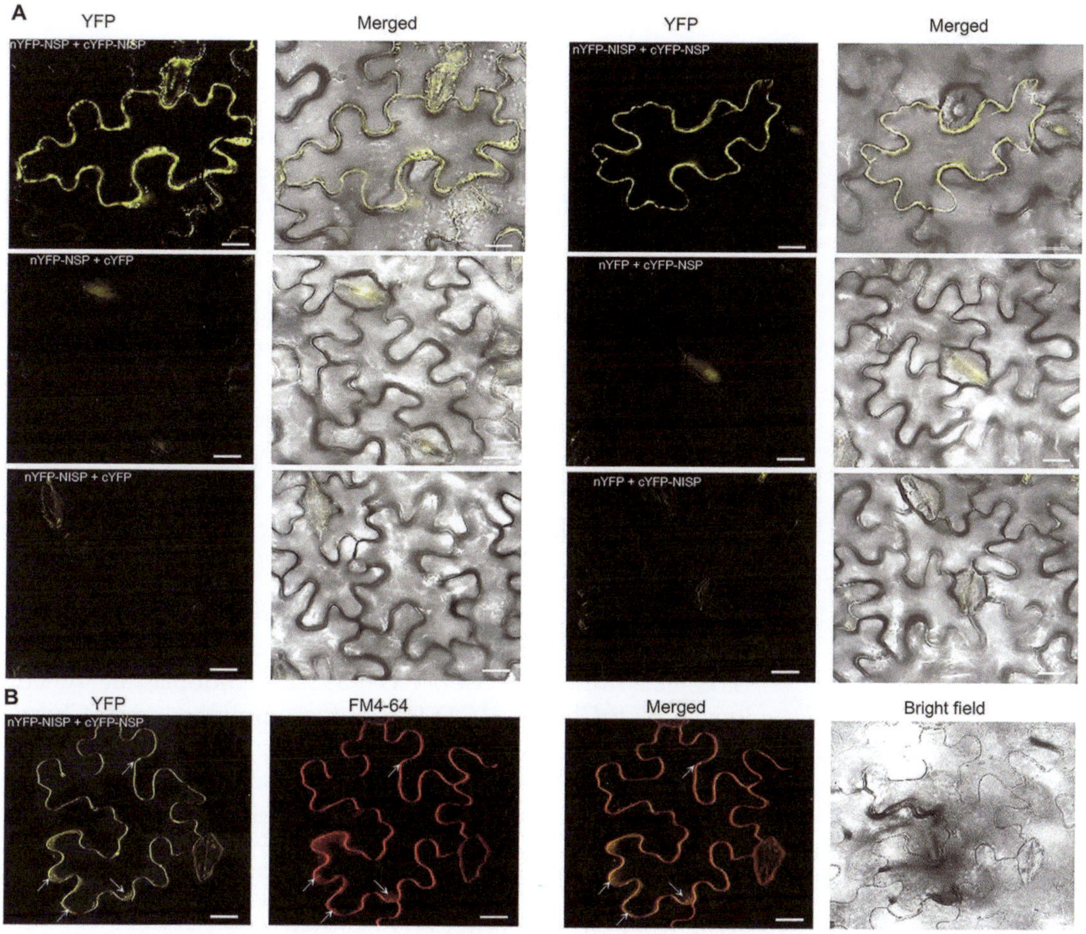

Fig. 4 NISP redirects NSP to the endosomes via direct interaction with the viral protein. (**a**) NISP interacts with NSP in vesicle-like compartments as demonstrated by BiFC. *N. benthamiana* leaves were infiltrated with *A. tumefaciens* carrying DNA constructs expressing NISP and NSP fused to the C-terminus (cYFP) or N-terminus (nYFP) of YFP, or in combination with the empty vectors. The fluorescence was observed by confocal microscopy 3 days after infiltration. Scale bars, 10 μm. (**b**) NISP-NSP complex-containing vesicles are stained by FM4-64, a marker for vesicle components of the plant endocytic pathway. *N. benthamiana* cells expressing nYFP-NISP and cYFP-NSP were observed 2 days post-agroinfiltration and 30 min after infiltration of FM4-64 by confocal microscopy. Arrows indicate vesicle-associated reconstituted fluorescent signals that were co-stained by FM4-64. Scale bars, 10 μm. (This figure was reproduced from Plant Physiology, 2021, 187: 158–173, https:/doi.org/10.1093/plphys/kiab252, license number 5625931314027)

location may not interact with each other. Evaluating interactions between proteins requires appropriate tools such as bimolecular fluorescence complementation (BiFC) and co-immunoprecipitation (Co-IP) assays. A colocalization assay of CabLCV NSP and host NISP is shown in Fig. 3. In Fig. 4, a BiFC assay demonstrates that these two proteins do indeed interact with each other in vesicle-like compartments.

2 Materials

2.1 Cloning Vectors and Organelle-Associated Markers

1. Gene-specific primers with appropriate extensions for recombination-based cloning (https://assets.thermofisher.com/TFS-Assets/LSG/brochures/710_01784_Gateway_bro.pdf) of genes *NSP* and *MP* from cabbage leaf curl virus (CabLCV) by PCR (*see* **Note 1**).
2. Coding regions of the NSP-interacting proteins NIG and NISP and the subcellular molecular markers AtWWP1, synaptotagmin A (SYTA), and leucine-rich repeat serine/threonine protein kinase (FLS2) (*see* **Note 2**).
3. pDONR207 Gateway entry vector; alternatively, a sequence encoding the proteins of interest can be produced synthetically and inserted into donor plasmids.
4. Plant-compatible vectors 35S-YFP-casseteA-Nos-pCAMBIA1300, pK7FWG2 and pH7m34GW (*see* **Notes 3–6**).
5. BiFC vectors SPYNE and SPYCE [20] (*see* **Note 3**).
6. Organelle-associated markers: ER-mCherry (Arabidopsis Biological Resource code CD-959, for endoplasmic reticulum), G-mCherry (CD-967, for Golgi), vac-mCherry (CD-975, for tonoplast), FLS2-mCherry (for plasma membrane), SYTA-mCherry (for endosome), FM4-64 (N-(3-Triethylammoniumpropyl)-4-(6-(4-(Diethylamino) Phenyl) Hexatrienyl) Pyridinium Dibromide) dye (for vesicles in epidermis cells) (*see* **Note 7**).
7. *Escherichia coli* cells (e.g., DH5α strain).
8. LB (Luria-Bertani) medium (*see* **Note 8**).
9. Stock solutions of antibiotics according to the selection of the plasmids (*see* **Note 9**).

2.2 Agrobacterium tumefaciens *Transformation*

1. *Agrobacterium tumefaciens* strain GV3101 (*see* **Note 10**).
2. Antibiotic solutions.
3. GYT medium (*see* **Note 11**).
4. LB medium.

2.3 Agroinfiltration of Nicotiana benthamiana *Leaves*

1. 1 M magnesium chloride ($MgCl_2$ 100×).
2. 1 M 2-(N-Morpholino) ethanesulfonic acid (MES100×).
3. 200 mM 3′,5′-dimethoxy-4′-hydroxyacetophenone (acetosyringone 1000×) (*see* **Note 12**).
4. Agroinfiltration buffer (*see* **Note 13**).
5. *N. benthamiana* plants grown in separated pots, 4- to 6-weeks old.

2.4 Transient Expression Verification (Protein Expression or mRNA Accumulation)

2.4.1 Protein Expression

1. 1 M phosphate buffer, pH 8.0 (phosphate buffer 10×).
2. 100 mM phenylmethylsulfonyl fluoride (PMSF 100×) (*see* **Note 14**).
3. 200 mM benzamidine (100×).
4. Lysis buffer: 100 mM phosphate buffer, pH 8.0, 150 mM sodium chloride (NaCl), 5 mM ethylenediaminetetraacetic acid (EDTA), 5 mM ethylene glycol tetraacetic acid (EGTA), 0.1% (v/v) triton X-100, 1 mM phenylmethylsulfonyl fluoride (PMSF), and 2 mM benzamidine (*see* **Note 15**).
5. Tris–HCl (pH 6.8) stock.
6. Sample buffer (6×): 12% (w/v) sodium dodecyl sulfate (SDS), 0.06% (w/v) bromophenol blue, 47% (v/v) glycerol, 60 mM Tris–HCl (pH 6.8), and 5% (v/v) β-mercaptoethanol (dithiothreitol (DTT) can be used at a final concentration of 350 mM to replace β-mercaptoethanol).
7. Precast SDS-polyacrylamide gels.
8. Pre-stained protein ladder.
9. SDS-PAGE running buffer: 0.025 M Tris–HCl base, 0.192 M glycine (electrophoresis grade), 0.1% (w/v) sodium dodecyl sulfate (SDS).
10. Nitrocellulose or polyvinylidene difluoride (PVDF) membranes.
11. Western blot transfer buffer: 0.025 M Tris base, 0.192 M glycine, 20% (v/v) methanol.
12. TBS (10×): 0.2 M Tris–HCl, pH 7.6, 1.5 M NaCl.
13. TBST: TBS containing 0.1% (v/v) Tween-20.
14. Blocking solution: 5% (w/v) milk in TBS.
15. Primary antibodies: Antibodies against fluorescent tags (e.g., anti-GFP, anti-YFP, anti-mCherry) (*see* **Note 16**).
16. Secondary antibodies: Antibodies against primary antibodies, conjugated to tags, such as the enzymes horseradish peroxidase (HRP) and alkaline phosphatase (AP) (*see* **Note 16**).
17. Substrates for detection of conjugated antibodies (e.g., signal west pico chemiluminescent substrate for HRP-linked antibodies and nitro blue tetrazolium (NBT)/5-bromo-4-chloro-3-indolyl phosphate (BCIP) for AP-conjugated antibodies).

2.4.2 For mRNA Accumulation

1. TRIzol reagent.
2. Chloroform (molecular biology grade).
3. Isopropanol (molecular biology grade).
4. RNAse-free water.
5. RNase-free DNase.

6. M-MLV reverse transcriptase.
7. Oligo(dT).
8. SYBR Green PCR Master Mix.
9. Specific primers for target genes.

2.5 General Equipment

1. Spectrophotometer.
2. Cuvettes.
3. Refrigerated microcentrifuge with rotor for 1.5-mL tubes.
4. Refrigerated centrifuge with rotor for 50-mL tubes.
5. Laminar flow hood.
6. Incubator at 28 °C and 37 °C.
7. Incubator/shaker at 28 °C and 37 °C.
8. Plant growth chambers.
9. Laser scanning confocal microscope (*see* **Note 17**).
10. Glass microscope slides and cover slips.
11. Electroporation system (e.g., Bio-Rad Gene Pulser).
12. Electroporation cuvettes with gap widths of 0.1 or 0.2 cm.
13. pH meter.
14. 1.5 mL polypropylene microfuge tubes.
15. 100 × 15 mm sterile disposable Petri plates.
16. Glass spreader.
17. Porcelain mortar with pestle.
18. Electrophoresis and transfer apparatus (e.g., Mini-PROTEAN Tetra Handcast Systems and Trans-Blot Turbo Transfer System).
19. Real-time PCR thermocycler.
20. Sterile 1 mL insulin syringe.

3 Methods

3.1 Cloning Viral Proteins Fused to Fluorescent Tags

1. Transfer viral ORFs, as well as host protein-coding sequences of interest, from donor plasmids NSP-NS-pDONR207, MP-NS-pDONR207, AtWWP1-NS-pDONR207, NISP-NS-pDONR207, NIG-NS-pDONR207, SYTA-NS-pDONR207, FLS2-NS-pDONR207 to binary vectors that allow their fusion with fluorescent tags. Cloning can be done by cleavage and ligation or performing an LR recombination reaction between an attL-containing entry clone and an attR-containing destination vector to generate an expression clone (Gateway). The binary vectors must be compatible with the Gateway system.

For constitutive expression of viral and host proteins fused to YFP (N-terminus) and GFP (C-terminus), transfer the coding region of the genes of interest to the 35S-YFP-casseteA-Nos-pCAMBIA1300 and pK7FWG2 vector, respectively, through LR recombination reaction. The fusion to mCherry (C-Terminus) is obtained in the binary vector pH7m34GW through recombinational cloning with three entry clones: pDONR-P4-P1R containing the CaMV 35S promoter with a duplicated enhancer (2 × 35S), pDONR207 containing the coding sequence of the proteins of interest, and pDONR-P2R-P3 containing the mCherry coding sequence, resulting in the clone with the gene of interest containing mCherry fluorescent tag. Likewise, the NISP fusion with GFP (C-terminus) under the control of its endogenous promoter is obtained in the binary vector pH7m34GW by multiple recombinational cloning with the following donor vectors: pDONR-P4-P1R containing the sequence of the NISP endogenous promoter, pDONR207 containing the coding sequence of NISP, and pDONR-P2R-P3 containing the GFP coding sequence. To obtain the constructs required for the BiFC assay, transfer, through recombination, the NISP and NSP coding sequences into the SPYNE and SPYCE binary vectors, which contain the N-terminal (nYFP) and C-terminal (cYFP) portions of YFP fused in frame at the C-terminal position of the proteins.

2. After constructing the recombinant expressions plasmids, transform *Escherichia coli* cells (e.g., DH5α strain) following your preferred protocol.
3. Spread *E. coli* cells on LB agar plates supplemented with appropriate antibiotics and incubate at 37 °C overnight. The pK7FWG2 and pH7m34GW vectors contain the spectinomycin resistance gene. The 35S-YFP-casseteA-Nos-pCAMBIA1300, SPYNE, and SPYCE vectors contain the kanamycin resistance gene. Therefore, the clones YFP-NSP, NSP-nYFP, NISP-nYFP, NSP-cYFP, and NISP-cYFP are selected in LB medium containing kanamycin 100 mg/L, and the clones MP-GFP, AtWWP1-GFP, NISP-GFP, NSP-mCherry, SYTA-mCherry, FLS2-mCherry, and pNISP:NISP-GFP are selected in LB medium containing spectinomycin 100 mg/L.
4. Use PCR to confirm the insertion of plasmid DNA constructs in colonies with specific primers.
5. Select individual colonies and incubate in 5 mL of LB liquid medium with the appropriate antibiotics at 37 °C under a rotation of 200 rpm on a horizontal shaker.
6. Purify the plasmid DNA using a miniprep kit according to the manufacturer's instructions.
7. Confirm the correct insertion of the plasmids by sequencing.

3.2 Agrobacterium Transformation

3.2.1 Preparation of Competent Cells

1. Properly clean the laminar flow hood to avoid contamination.
2. Inoculate a colony of *A. tumefaciens* GV3101 in a tube containing 50 mL of LB medium and 50 mg/L of gentamicin. Incubate the culture overnight at 28 °C on a rotary shaker until it reaches an OD_{600} of 0.4–0.6.
3. Centrifuge the cells at 3000×*g* for 10 min at 4 °C. Discard the supernatant and resuspend the cell pellet in 50 mL of ice-cold pure water. Repeat this procedure 4–5 times.
4. Centrifuge the cells at 3000×*g* for 10 min at 4 °C. Carefully discard the supernatant (*see* **Note 18**) and resuspend the pellet in 2 mL of ice-cold GYT medium (*see* **Note 19**).
5. Aliquot 40 μL of the cell suspension into a sterile 0.5 mL microfuge tube, place in a liquid nitrogen bath, transfer to an ultrafreezer (−80 °C) and use as needed.

3.2.2 Electroporation

1. Properly clean the laminar flow hood to avoid contamination.
2. Remove the required number of *Agrobacterium* cell aliquots from the −80 °C freezer and defrost the cells on ice. Add 0.5–1 μL of plasmid DNA (1–10 ng/mL) to 40 μL of recipient cells (*see* **Note 20**).
3. Transfer, using a pipette, the DNA/cell mixture to an electroporation cuvette. Make sure that all the transferred volume is at the bottom of the cuvette.
4. Perform electroporation by applying a single electrical pulse of 25 μF capacitance, 2.4 kV, and 200 Ω resistance (*see* **Note 21**).
5. After applying the pulse, add 1 mL of LB medium to the electroporation cuvette in a laminar flow hood.
6. Transfer the cells to a 1.5 mL microfuge tube and incubate at 28 °C for 2 h.
7. Centrifuge the cells briefly, resuspend in 100 μL of LB medium, and spread on LB agar medium containing the appropriate antibiotics. Thus, *A. tumefaciens* GV3101 carrying expression vectors containing the constructs of interest, described previously (Subheading 3.1), are selected in LB medium containing gentamycin 50 mg/L (for selection of *Agrobacterium* GV 3101 cells) and kanamycin 100 mg/L (for constructs in 35S-YFP-casseteA-Nos-pCAMBIA, SPYNE, and SPYCE vectors) or spectinomycin 100 mg/L (for constructs in pK7FWG2 and pH7m34GW vectors).
8. Incubate the plates at 28 °C for 48–72 h.

3.3 Agroinfiltration in N. benthamiana Leaves

1. Inoculate *Agrobacterium* cultures previously transformed with the plasmids of interest into 5 mL of LB medium plus appropriate antibiotics. Cultures should remain at 28 °C under shaking at 200 rpm, overnight (*see* **Note 22**).
2. Centrifuge the *Agrobacterium* cultures containing the vectors of interest at 3000×*g* for 5 min at room temperature and discard the supernatant.
3. Resuspend the pellet in 3 mL of agroinfiltration buffer without acetosyringone.
4. Centrifuge the cells at 3000×*g* for 5 min at room temperature and discard the supernatant. Repeat **steps 3** and **4** twice.
5. Resuspend the cells in 2 mL of agroinfiltration buffer containing acetosyringone (*see* **Note 23**).
6. Keep cultures at room temperature in the dark for a minimum of 2 h and a maximum of 4 h to activate virulence gene expression.
7. Take an absorbance reading (OD_{600}) of each agrobacterial culture using 100 μL of the cell suspension diluted in 900 μL of water.
8. Dilute each agrobacterial suspension to appropriate OD_{600} in agroinfiltration buffer supplemented with acetosyringone. To evaluate subcellular localization of proteins using the N-terminal or C-terminal fusion fluorescent tags, use an OD_{600} of 0.1–0.3 (*see* **Note 24**). For BiFC assays use an OD_{600} of 1.0. If it is necessary to co-express two or more proteins by agroinfiltration (e.g., with Hc-Pro or P19 or a BiFC partner), simply mix equal parts of cell suspensions transformed with each of the different constructs.
9. Infiltrate each suspension into two *N. benthamiana* leaves (*see* **Note 25**). For infiltration, use an insulin needle to make a smooth groove on the abaxial surface of the leaf (be careful not to puncture the leaf). With the help of an insulin syringe, infiltrate the material through this small groove (*see* **Notes 26** and **27**).
10. Keep the plants in a growth chamber at 25 °C under long-day conditions (16 h light/8 h dark).
11. Analyze the material under confocal microscopy or collect it to verify protein expression/mRNA accumulation (*see* **Note 28**) 48–72 h after infiltration (*see* **Note 29**).

3.4 Determination of Protein Expression and mRNA Accumulation

3.4.1 Protein Expression

1. Grind 200–300 mg of leaf tissue in a mortar and pestle in liquid nitrogen.
2. When the material is completely pulverized, add 750 μL lysis buffer. Be sure the sample does not defrost before coming into touch with the lysis buffer.

3. Transfer the extract from the mortar to 1.5 mL microfuge tube. Leave on ice under stirring for 20 min.
4. Centrifuge at 16,000×*g* for 10 min at 4 °C. Remember to cool the centrifuge before starting the extraction!
5. Transfer the supernatant to a new microfuge tube.
6. Separate an aliquot of the extract to perform SDS-PAGE (sodium dodecyl sulfate-polyacrylamide gel electrophoresis) for subsequent detection of fusion proteins with anti-GFP, anti-YFP, or anti-mCherry antibodies. Add sample buffer (Laemmli buffer; 6×) to a final 1× concentration. Boil the samples (100 °C) for 5 min. The remainder of the extract can be stored at −80 °C indefinitely.
7. Proceed with the separation of proteins by SDS-PAGE, carried out using standard protocols. Stops electrophoresis when the dye front reaches the end of the gel.
8. Transfer the separated proteins to a blotting PVDF membrane according to standard protocols.
9. After Western blot transfer and disassembly of the apparatus, place the membrane in a suitable container and add 50–100 mL of TBST. Rinse to remove excess transfer buffer and discard.
10. Incubate the membranes for 2–3 h at room temperature or overnight at 4 °C in a blocking solution with continuous shaking.
11. Discard the blocking buffer and incubate the membranes for 2 h at room temperature with the primary antibodies in TBST. Alternatively, the incubation with the antibody can be done overnight at 4 °C with continuous shaking.
12. Remove the primary antibody (which can be reused several times) and wash the membrane three times with TBST for 5 min each under constant agitation. If the antibody against the fluorescent tag is conjugated to a label (e.g., horseradish peroxidase and alkaline phosphatase), skip to **step 15** (*see* **Note 16**).
13. Incubate the membrane for 1–2 h at room temperature with the secondary antibody with continuous shaking.
14. Remove the secondary antibody (which can be reused several times) and wash the membrane three times with TBST for 10 min each under constant agitation.
15. Detect the reactivity of the conjugated antibody using appropriate substrates, considering the label used and the chosen method (*see* **Note 30**).

3.4.2 mRNA Accumulation

Alternative or additionally, transcript levels can be assessed by real-time RT-PCR.

1. Extract total RNA from frozen leaves. We use the standard protocol with TRIzol (Thermo-Fisher Scientific) and chloroform for extraction, according to the manufacturer's instructions (*see* **Notes 31** and **32**).
2. Treat the RNA with RNase-free DNase and purify it. For total RNA isolation, we use RNeasy Mini kit columns (Qiagen).
3. Synthesize first-strand cDNA from total RNA using oligo-dT_{18} and reverse transcriptase. We use the M-MLV reverse transcriptase according to the manufacturer's instructions.
4. Perform real-time RT-PCR reactions using specific oligonucleotides for the genes of the respective proteins analyzed in the subcellular localization assays, as well as an endogenous gene that can be actin, for example. Our real-time RT-PCR reactions are performed on an ABI7500 instrument (Thermo-Fisher Scientific) using a SYBR green PCR master mix.
5. Absolute gene expression is quantified using the $2^{-\Delta\Delta Ct}$ method and values normalized to the endogenous control [21].

3.5 Confocal Microscopy

1. Obtain small cuts of the leaf (~1 cm^2) with a scalpel, paying attention to the region previously delimited with a marker pen, which highlights the region where the agroinfiltration was carried out (*see* **Note 33**).
2. As the confocal microscope is usually inverted, mount the leaf sections with the abaxial side facing up. Add a drop of water (enough to cover the leaf) and cover with a glass cover slip (*see* **Note 34**).
3. It is not necessary to seal the cover slip. Position the slide with the cover slip facing down on the stage. Use the X-Y controls to move the specimen slide in both the X (right and left) and Y (back and forth) axes.
4. Before capturing images, it is necessary to turn on the lasers and select the appropriate filters and mirrors. Depending on the constructions and fluorophores to be used, it will be necessary to use different lasers for excitation. The user must know the excitation and emission maxima for the fluorophores being used. In most confocal devices, the operator also may alter the lasers' output power and the detectors' sensitivity (*see* **Notes 35** and **36**).
5. Choose a filter setup for the specific fluorophores you are utilizing. Here we will use the Zeiss LSM 510 Meta as an example of manual adjustments. In "Channel mode," select Single-track (if only one fluorophore) or Multi-track (if more than one). *See* **Note 37**.

6. By selecting "Scan" from the Acquire menu, you may change the scan control. By selecting "Mode," you may additionally choose the following parameters: frame size (256, 512, or 1024), scan speed (optimal), scan direction (8-bit, line or frame), and scan average (2, 4, 8, and 16). The images shown here (Figs. 1, 2, 3, and 4) were acquired with 8 scans in average line mode and a 512 × 512 pixels resolution.
7. Set the pinhole by clicking "Channels" (*see* **Note 38**).
8. Scan and acquire the images. If necessary, optimize the images (*see* **Note 39**).
9. Save captured images and adjust brightness and contrast if necessary. Utilize the Zeiss LSM 510 software and Adobe Photoshop to process images (*see* **Note 40**).

4 Notes

1. Any other geminivirus can be used as a template to amplify coding regions of viral proteins for cloning into expression vectors.
2. These should be isolated by RT-PCR using total leaf cDNA from *Arabidopsis*.
3. It is crucial that fusion proteins are cloned into vectors with tags at both the N-terminal and C-terminal positions. Vectors encoding different N-terminal (YFP) or C-terminal (GFP) and (mCherry) fluorescent tags are available commercially. The N-terminal tagging with a fluorescent tag such as GFP can affect protein localization, while C-terminal tagging generally better preserves native protein localization. However, in some cases, proteins located in the endoplasmic reticulum and cell wall can be negatively affected by C-terminal fusions. Therefore, it is advisable to consider switching tag positions.
4. To perform C-terminal fusions, the coding region of the genes of interest should be cloned without a stop codon.
5. The 35S-YFP-casseteA-Nos-pCAMBIA1300 vector contains YFP fused in frame to the N-terminal position of the proteins of interest, and is used to obtain YFP fluorescent tags. The pK7FWG2 vector is used for the C-terminal fusion of the GFP fluorescent tag. The pH7m34GW vector contains the C-terminal fusions of mCherry under the control of the CaMV 2 × 35S promoter and the NISP fusion with GFP under the control of its endogenous promoter. This vector is designed for use in the MultiSite Gateway three-fragment LR recombination reaction with the three entry clones. Three-fragment LR recombination facilitates the rapid construction of an expression clone containing your choice of promoter, a

gene of interest, and fluorescent tags. Other sequences of interest may be substituted or incorporated, providing greater flexibility for your vector construction.

6. It is essential to evaluate combinations with a constitutive promoter (such as 35S from cauliflower mosaic virus), which is highly active in most plant cells of transgenic plants, and the endogenous promoter, since overexpressed proteins may be mislocalized or form promiscuous associations within cellular compartments. Furthermore, expression levels produced by vectors with duplicated promoters (such as double 35S) may be significantly greater than those produced by vectors with only one promoter. However, the protein fusion may end up being mislocalized as a result.
7. For FM 4-64 preparation, dissolve 100 μg of dye in 100 μL of ultrapure water to prepare a stock solution of 1000 μg/mL. Recover with aluminum foil to minimize light exposure and store at −20 °C. Immediately before use, dilute the stock solution in water to prepare a staining solution of 10 μg/mL FM 4-64.
8. To prepare LB medium, weight 5 g of yeast extract, 10 g of tryptone, and 10 g of sodium chloride (NaCl). Dissolve the components in 900 mL of deionized water to a volume of 900 mL. Adjust the pH to 7.0 with 5 N NaOH and make up the volume to 1 L with deionized water. Add 15 g of agar to a solid medium. Sterilize in an autoclave at 121 °C for 30 min on the liquid cycle.
9. Sterilize stock solutions of antibiotics in water by filtering through a 0.22 μm filter. Antibiotic solutions should be aliquoted into 1.5 mL microtubes and stored at −20 °C. Selection dose of the primary antibiotics for *Agrobacterium*: Ampicillin (50 mg/L); kanamycin (100 mg/L); chloramphenicol (50 mg/L); spectinomycin (100 mg/L); streptomycin (300 mg/L); gentamicin (50 m/L); rifampicin (50 mg/L).
10. *A. tumefaciens* GV3101 carries Ti plasmid pMP90 (pTiC58DT-DNA), harboring gentamicin resistance for the transient transformation protocol. Furthermore, to enhance protein expression, a recombinant *Agrobacterium* strain that encodes a viral suppressor of RNA silencing, such as the potyviral helper component-proteinase (HC-Pro) from tobacco etch virus, the P19 protein from tomato bushy stunt virus or the P21 protein of beet yellows virus, may be co-infiltrated.
11. GYT medium is 10% (v/v) glycerol, 0.125% (w/v) yeast extract, 0.25% (w/v) tryptone. Dissolve 0.0125 g of yeast extract and 0.025 g of tryptone in 5 mL of deionized water. Add 1 mL of glycerol. Make up the volume of the solution to

10 mL with deionized water. Sterilize the medium using a 0.22 μm filter. Store in small batches at 4 °C.

12. Prepare acetosyringone stocks in small batches. Weigh 0.392 g acetosyringone and add 99.5% dimethyl sulfoxide (DMSO) to a volume of 5 mL. Make up to 10 mL with DMSO. Store at − 20 °C, and discard after 1 month.
13. The infiltration buffer must be prepared on the day of use. To prepare 100 mL of buffer, add 1 mL of magnesium chloride 100×, 1 mL of MES 100× and 100 μL of acetosyringone 1000× in 98 mL of deionized water.
14. Because PMSF has limited water solubility it must be dissolved in a small amount of solvent, such as ethanol, methanol, or isopropyl alcohol, before addition to a buffer. Store in aliquots at −20 °C.
15. PMSF, benzamidine, and other protease inhibitors should only be added moments before use. PMSF is an irreversible inhibitor of serine and cysteine proteases. It is inactivated in aqueous solutions and has a half-life of approximately 35 min.
16. Antibodies against fluorescent tags can be purchased commercially conjugated to labels such as the HRP enzyme. In this case the use of secondary antibodies is not necessary.
17. For GFP (excitation peak at 489 nm), YFP (excitation peak at 513 nm) and mCherry (excitation peak at 587 nm) excitation, the equipment must contain an Argon (wavelength at 488 and 514 nm) and Helium-Neon (wavelength at 543 nm) laser and barrier filters suitable for the emission lengths of the fluorophores: 500–530 nm band pass filter for GFP (emission peak at 511 nm), 560–615 nm filter for YFP (emission peak at 530 nm) and 608–680 nm for mCherry (emission peak at 610 nm).
18. Use an automatic pipette to remove any remaining drops of water before resuspending the pellet in the GYT medium.
19. Resuspend the cell pellet carefully; vortexing is not recommended.
20. The DNA to be used in electroporation should ideally be resuspended or eluted in ultrapure water or TE buffer (Tris–HCl pH 8.0, 10 mM EDTA pH 8.0) at a concentration of 1–10 ng/μL. Samples with high ion concentrations in the electroporation cuvette increase the conductivity, causing the electrical current to arc or skip through the suspension of cells and DNA. In these cases, the DNA preparation to be electroporated should be diluted or purified by spin-column chromatography.
21. Before placing the cuvette in the electroporator, dry the cuvette with soft paper.

22. Always use fresh *Agrobacterium* cultures for all infiltrations.
23. Resuspend in a smaller volume if the final pellet obtained is small. The most appropriate volume is determined empirically.
24. When the protein expression level is a problem, the OD_{600} value can be increased up to 1.0. Alternatively, co-infiltrate with *A. tumefaciens* that encodes a viral suppressor of RNA silencing (e.g., HC-Pro and P19).
25. Do not pick too old or very young leaves to agroinfiltrate.
26. It is interesting to use a permanent marker pen to delimit the area of the leaf where the agroinfiltration was carried out. This will facilitate the identification of the region when the agroinfiltrated leaves need to be cut for analysis by confocal microscopy or collected to extract proteins or RNA.
27. Perform a mock infiltration with infiltration buffer to assess background fluorescence or protein level.
28. For protein or RNA extraction, it is essential to collect leaf samples, freeze them immediately in liquid nitrogen, and store them at −80 °C.
29. We typically use 72 h. If an RNA silencing suppressor is co-infiltrated with target constructs, it is possible to increase protein expression levels by extending the incubation period.
30. HRP-linked antibodies need substrates that can provide high signal-to-noise ratios for the chosen detection method, whether chemiluminescent, colorimetric, or fluorescent. AP-conjugated antibodies utilize alkaline phosphatase substrates primarily for chemiluminescent or colorimetric detection.
31. When grinding the samples, do not let the material thaw before adding TRIzol.
32. Another essential element for effective RNA isolation is an RNase-free working environment. Wear gloves when handling RNA and RNase-free reagents and consumables (microtubes and tips).
33. Avoid cutting close to the leaf veins; focusing on the images will be more challenging. Also, do not crush the leaf too much when positioning the coverslip, as this will cause cell rupture and distortion in the images.
34. Make sure that the thickness of the coverslip is adequate to the specifications of the objective to be used. We usually use 0.13–0.16 mm coverslips, as objective lenses for transmitted light that are commonly available are made to accommodate a 0.17 mm coverslip between the sample and the lens.
35. The following list shows the most common fluorophores, as well as the laser wavelengths to be used for excitation (value

before the slash) and their respective emission wavelengths (value after the slash). DAPI and CFP: 405/461; GFP: 488/510; YFP: 514/535; mRFP and mCherry: 543/584; Alexa fluor 594 and Texas red: 594/615; Alexa fluor 633: 633/639 [18].

36. To prevent photobleaching or fluorescence saturation, the laser intensity should be as low as feasible while producing the required emission. Scan slides using low intensity for localization and slightly higher for capture. The laser intensity is determined by the output (%) and laser power. For GFP or YFP fluorophore scans, we recommend using 10–20% power (Argon-ion laser). For mCherry fluorophore scans, use 50–100% power (Helium/Neon laser).

37. More recent confocal microscope models, such as the Nikon Eclipse Ti2-E series, have pre-adjusted filter settings for the most common fluorophores. The user simply selects the fluorophore from the list available in the instrument's software, and the filters and dichroic mirrors optical configuration is automatically adjusted based on the selected fluorophores.

38. Confocal microscopes contain a pinhole that prevents light from being detected outside the focal plane. Pinhole adjustment allows optical sections to be made inside thick samples. The ideal size depends on the objective being used and the fluorescence wavelength. A pinhole set to 1 Airy unit will provide optimal resolution, resulting in the best depth/efficiency ratio. To perform this adjustment, open the pinhole during scanning and close it gradually until fluorescence and resolution are adequate. Very important: in colocalization experiments, the size of the pinhole must be adjusted so that the optical slices of the channels for both fluorophores are equal.

39. Images can be optimized by selecting the "Color Palette" option in the Capture window and then the "Range Indicator." In this option, you will once again have access to Detector Gain and Amplifier Offset. Adjusting in Pallete mode makes it possible to remove saturation from the samples. Reduce the Detector Gain until just a tiny portion of the stained regions show red pixels. The Amplifier Offset should be adjusted until the background is a mixture of blue and black pixels.

40. When necessary, the brightness and contrast of the images can be adjusted in the microscope's own image analysis program to obtain images with better resolution. However, such manipulations must be applied to the image as a whole and not just to specific areas of the micrograph. Repositioning, selective augmentation, copying, pasting, removal, and similar actions should never be done.

Acknowledgments

This work was supported by a Technical and Financial Cooperation Agreement for the joint execution of the structuring research project n° 145/2021, signed between the Universidade do Estado de Minas Gerais and the Fundação Arthur Bernardes, the Council for Advanced Professional Training (CAPES), National Council for Scientific and Technological Development (CNPq), and the Minas Gerais Research Funding Foundation (FAPEMIG RED-00205-22). The authors also thank the Research Productivity Scholarship Program—PQ/UEMG and the microscopy facility at Universidade Federal de Viçosa.

References

1. Cooper GM (2019) The cell, a molecular approach, 8th edn. Oxford University Press, New York
2. Jain A, Zoncu R (2022) Organelle transporters and inter-organelle communication as drivers of metabolic regulation and cellular homeostasis. Mol Metab 60:101481
3. Liu Y, Li P, Fan L, Wu M (2018) The nuclear transportation routes of membrane-bound transcription factors. Cell Commun Signal 16:12
4. Yang ZT, Lu SJ, Wang MJ, Bi DL, Sun L, Zhou SF, Song ZT, Liu JX (2014) A plasma membrane-tethered transcription factor, NAC062/ANAC062/NTL6, mediates the unfolded protein response in Arabidopsis. Plant J 79:1033–1043
5. Walter P, Ron D (2011) The unfolded protein response: from stress pathway to homeostatic regulation. Science 334:1081–1086
6. Srivastava R, Deng Y, Shah S, Rao AG, Howell SH (2013) BINDING PROTEIN is a master regulator of the endoplasmic reticulum stress sensor/transducer bZIP28 in Arabidopsis. Plant Cell 25:1416–1429
7. Silva PA, Silva JC, Caetano HD, Machado JPB, Mendes GC, Reis PAB, Brustolini OJB, Dal-Bianco M, Fontes EPB (2015) Comprehensive analysis of the endoplasmic reticulum stress response in the soybean genome: conserved and plant-specific features. BMC Genomics 16:783
8. Hanley-Bowdoin L, Bejarano ER, Robertson D, Mansoor S (2013) Geminiviruses: masters at redirecting and reprogramming plant processes. Nat Rev Microbiol 11:777–788
9. Kumar RV (2019) Plant antiviral immunity against geminiviruses and viral counter-defense for survival. Front Microbiol 10:1460
10. Martins LGC, Raimundo GAS, Ribeiro NGA, Silva JCF, Euclydes NC, Loriato VAP, Duarte CEM, Fontes EPB (2020) A begomovirus nuclear shuttle protein-interacting immune hub: hijacking host transport activities and suppressing incompatible functions. Front Plant Sci 11:398
11. Devendran R, Namgial T, Reddy KK, Kumar M, Zareen F, Chakraborty S (2022) Insights into the multifunctional roles of geminivirus-encoded proteins in pathogenesis. Arch Virol 167:307–326
12. Wang L, Tan H, Medina-Puche L, Wu M, Gomez BG, Gao M, Shi C, Jimenez-Gongora T, Fan P, Ding X, Zhang D, Ding Y, Rosas-Díaz T, Liu Y, Aguilar E, Fu X, Lozano-Durán R (2022) Combinatorial interactions between viral proteins expand the functional landscape of the tomato yellow leaf curl virus proteome. PLoS Pathog 18:e1010909
13. Breves SS, Silva FA, Euclydes NC, Saia TFF, Jean-Baptiste J, Andrade-Neto ER, Fontes EPB (2023) Begomovirus-host interactions: viral proteins orchestrating intra and intercellular transport of viral DNA while suppressing host defense mechanisms. Viruses 15:1593
14. Carvalho CM, Machado JPB, Zerbini FM, Fontes EPB (2008) NSP-interacting GTPase: a cytosolic protein as cofactor for nuclear shuttle proteins. Plant Signal Behav 3:752–754
15. Gouveia-Mageste BC, Martins LGC, Dal-Bianco M, Machado JPB, Silva JCF, Kim AY, Yazaki J, Santos AA, Ecker JR, Fontes EPB (2021) A plant-specific syntaxin-6 protein contributes to the intracytoplasmic route for the

begomovirus CabLCV. Plant Physiol 187: 158–173

16. Zhao W, Wu S, Barton E, Fan Y, Ji Y, Wang X, Zhou Y (2020) Tomato yellow leaf curl virus V2 protein plays a critical role in the nuclear export of V1 protein and viral systemic infection. Front Microbiol 11:1243
17. Zhao S, Gong P, Liu J, Liu H, Lozano-Durán R, Zhou X, Li F (2023) Geminivirus C5 proteins mediate the formation of virus complexes at plasmodesmata for viral intercellular movement. Plant Physiol 193:322–338
18. Goodin MM (2018) Protein localization and interaction studies in plants: toward defining complete proteomes by visualization. Adv Virus Res 100:117–144
19. Calil IP, Quadros IPS, Araújo TC, Duarte CEM, Gouveia-Mageste BC, Silva JCF, Brustolini OJB, Teixeira RM, Oliveira CN, Milagres RWMM, Martins GS, Chory J, Reis PAB, Machado JPB, Fontes EPB (2018) A WW domain-containing protein forms immune nuclear bodies against begomoviruses. Mol Plant 11:1449–1465
20. Schütze K, Harter K, Chaban C (2009) Bimolecular fluorescence complementation (BiFC) to study protein-protein interactions in living plant cells. In: Pfannschmidt T (ed) Plant signal transduction, Methods in molecular biology, vol 479. Humana Press, Totowa
21. Livak KJ, Schmittgen TD (2001) Analysis of relative gene expression data using real-time quantitative PCR and the $2^{-\Delta\Delta Ct}$ method. Methods 25:402–408

Chapter 19

Identification of Interaction Between Geminivirus and Plant Proteins by Bimolecular Fluorescence Complementation (BiFC)

Min Du, Xueping Zhou, and Xiuling Yang

Abstract

Geminiviruses rely heavily on complicated protein-protein interactions between viral proteins and between virus and host plant proteins to establish successful infection. The bimolecular fluorescence complementation (BiFC) assay is based on the in vivo complementation of nonfluorescent component parts of a fluorescent protein through the interaction of proximity target proteins, each fused to a different part of the fluorescent protein. Here, we describe a protocol for the BiFC-based method for the identification of the interaction between geminivirus and plant proteins, which allows for the visualization of protein-protein interactions and the subcellular localization of protein interaction complexes in living systems.

Key words Bimolecular fluorescence complementation, Protein-protein interaction, Geminivirus, Subcellular localization, Confocal microscopy

1 Introduction

Geminiviruses are a group of single-stranded DNA viruses that are attributed to many devastating crop diseases worldwide. As obligate intracellular parasites, geminiviruses generally encode four to six viral proteins and rely heavily on the host plant machinery to fulfill their infection cycles. An increasing body of evidence suggests that geminiviruses employ a complex interaction network with plant proteins to recruit, hijack, and co-opt host proteins or to escape plant antiviral responses [1–3]. Identification and investigation of the interaction between geminivirus proteins and plant proteins can provide crucial information for understanding the pathogenesis of geminiviruses and plant antiviral defense responses and development of antiviral strategies.

Numerous methods have been developed to study protein-protein interaction (PPI), including in vitro pull-down assay, in vivo yeast two hybrid assay, coimmunoprecipitation assay,

Francisco Murilo Zerbini et al. (eds.), *Geminiviruses: Methods and Protocols*, Methods in Molecular Biology, vol. 2912, https://doi.org/10.1007/978-1-0716-4454-6_19,

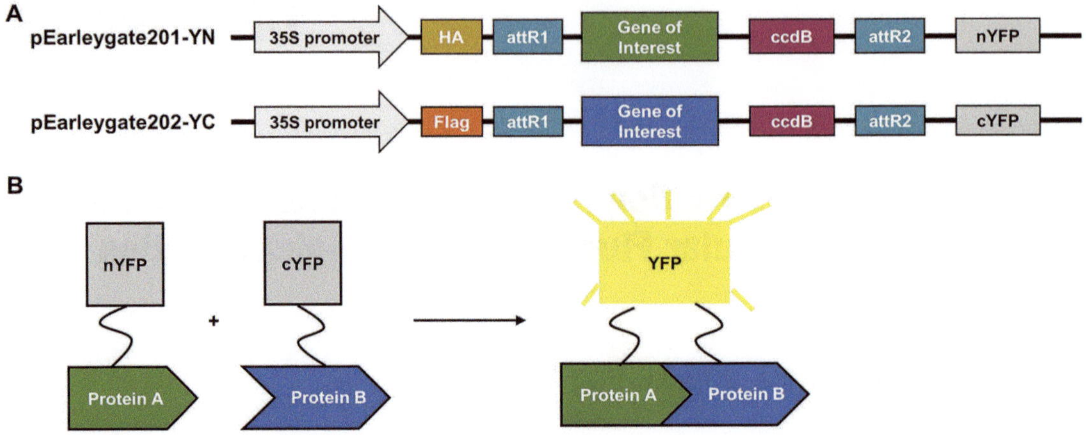

Fig. 1 Schematic representation of the Gateway destination vectors and the principles of the bimolecular fluorescence complementation assay

fluorescence resonance energy transfer (FRET), split luciferase complementation assay, and bimolecular fluorescence complementation (BiFC) assay [4–9]. BiFC is a widely used method to study pairwise protein interactions in living animal and plant cells due to its simplicity, sensitivity, and the merit of revealing subcellular localizations of protein interactions. In the BiFC assay, a fluorescent protein is split into two nonfluorescent fragments and fused to each partner of two proteins under investigation. Upon co-expression of the two fusion proteins in the cell, interaction of the two investigated proteins brings the two nonfluorescent fragments into close spatial proximity and results in reconstitution of an intact fluorescent protein that emits fluorescence under specific wavelengths of light (Fig. 1) [10, 11]. Besides the direct visualization of protein-protein interaction in living plant cells, this method also allows for monitoring the subcellular localization at which protein association occurs. Currently, yellow fluorescent protein (YFP) is the most frequently used fluorescent proteins for BiFC assays. Different sets of plant-compatible BiFC vectors have been generated containing classic multiple cloning sites or Gateway-compatible sequences [12–14].

In this chapter, we described a step-by-step protocol for using the Gateway compatible BiFC vectors to identify the interaction between geminivirus protein and plant host proteins in *Nicotiana benthamiana* cells, which allows for the visualization of protein-protein interactions and the subcellular localization of protein interaction complexes in living systems.

2 Materials

2.1 Plants, Vectors, and Bacterial Strains

1. Wild type *N. benthamiana* seeds.
2. Transgenic RFP-H2B *N. benthamiana* seeds.
3. Pots, pot trays, clear covers, and soil.
4. Insect-free growth chamber at 25 °C under a 16-h light:8-h dark photoperiod.
5. Vectors for plant BiFC assay: pENTR/D-TOPO, pEarleygate201-YN, and pEarleygate202-YC.
6. *Escherichia coli* strain DB3.1, Top 10, and DH5α competent cells.
7. *Agrobacterium tumefaciens* strain EHA105.

2.2 Reagents

1. Lysogeny broth (LB) medium (liquid, solid): 5 g/L yeast extract, 10 g/L tryptone, 10 g/L sodium chloride (NaCl), 16 g/L agar for LB solid medium. Sterilize at 121 °C for 20 min.
2. Antibiotics: kanamycin (Kan) and rifampicin (Rif) (*see* **Note 1**).
3. Agarose gel electrophoresis: TAE buffer and agarose.
4. Enzymes and kits: high fidelity DNA polymerase, restriction endonuclease *Mlu*I, pENTR™/D-TOPO™ Cloning kit (Invitrogen, Catalog no. K2400-20), and LR Clonase™ II Enzyme mix (Invitrogen, Catalog no. 11791-020).
5. Plasmid extraction kit, PCR purification kit, and Gel extraction kit.
6. Infiltration buffer: 10 mM $MgCl_2$, 10 mM β-(N-morpholino) ethane sulfonic acid (MES, pH 5.6), and 100 μM acetosyringone (*see* **Note 2**).
7. Plastic needleless syringe (1 mL).
8. Subcellular localization markers: RFP-H2B is generally used as a nuclear marker, other commercially available dyes or subcellular localization markers listed in [15, 16].

2.3 Equipment

1. Thermocycler.
2. Microwave oven.
3. Agarose and electrophoresis device.
4. Centrifuge.
5. Heated incubator.
6. High temperature autoclave.
7. Spectrophotometer.
8. Electroporation system.

9. Shaking incubator.
10. Stationary incubator.
11. pH meter.
12. Confocal microscopy.

3 Methods

3.1 Preparation of Plant Materials

The seeds of wild type and transgenic RFP-H2B *N. benthamiana* are spread into pots containing wet soil, covered with a clean clear cover, and placed in an insect-free growth chamber at 25 °C under a 16-h light/8-h dark photoperiod. Twelve days later, seedlings are transplanted for growth and the four-week-old plants can be used in the experiment.

3.2 Construction of the BiFC Vectors

1. Design PCR primers and amplify the sequences of geminivirus protein and host plant protein of interest using a proofreading DNA polymerase to produce blunt-end PCR products (*see* **Notes 3** and **4**).
2. Use agarose gel electrophoresis to check the integrity of your PCR products and purify the PCR products by PCR purification kit.
3. Perform the TOPO cloning reaction with your PCR products and the TOPO vector following the manufacturer's instructions, and transform competent cell of *E. coli* Top10 (*see* **Note 5**).
4. Perform colony PCR to screen positive colonies and verify the recombinant by sequencing with the M13F and the M13R primers (Table 1).
5. Linearize entry plasmids with *Mlu*I at 37 °C for 30 min, run the digested products on agarose gel, cut the accurate band, and purify it with gel extraction kit (*see* **Note 6**).
6. Perform an LR recombination reaction to transfer target fragments from the linearized entry vector into the Gateway destination vectors, pEarleygate201-YN, and pEarleygate202-YC, respectively (*see* **Note 7**).

Table 1
Primers used for colony selection and DNA sequencing

Primer name	Primer sequences (5′-3′)
M13F	GTAAAACGACGGCCAGT
M13R	CAGGAAACAGCTATGAC
35S-F	CCTTCGCAAGACCCTTCCTC

7. Transform the LR reaction products into *E. coli* DH5α.
8. Select positive colonies by colony PCR with the 35S-F (Table 1) and the gene-specific reverse primers (*see* **Note 8**).
9. Transform the destination vectors to *A. tumefaciens* (EHA105 strain) by electroporation.
10. Spread the cells on LB agar medium with 50 μg/mL of kanamycin and 50 μg/mL of rifampicin at 28 °C for 2 days.
11. Select positive colonies by colony PCR with the 35S-F and the gene-specific reverse primers.
12. Selected colonies can be cultured overnight at 28 °C and stored as glycerol stocks in a −80 °C freezer.

3.3 Infiltration of N. benthamiana

1. Incubate single colonies of *A. tumefaciens* transformed with recombinant plasmids with a sterile disposable incubating loop into 5 mL of liquid LB medium with 50 μg/mL of kanamycin and 50 μg/mL of rifampicin.
2. Grow the *A. tumefaciens* strains overnight at 28 °C with vigorous shaking (180 rpm).
3. Centrifuge the cell suspensions at 4000 rpm for 10 min. Discard the supernatant, and resuspend the pellets with infiltration buffer to bring the OD_{600} to 1.0.
4. Mix equal volume of two *A. tumefaciens* strains harboring the nYFP and cYFP derivatives in desired combinations.
5. Incubate the suspensions at room temperature for 2–4 h.
6. Infiltrate the agrobacterial suspensions into the abaxial side of young fully expanded leaves of 4-week-old *N. benthamiana* with a 1 mL needle-less syringe (*see* **Note 9**).
7. Place the plants in the growth chamber for 24–72 h before confocal microscopy.

3.4 Confocal Microscopy

1. Take a 1–2 cm^2 segment of leaf tissue from the infiltrated area using a punch or a very sharp blade.
2. Place the excised leaf tissue with the adaxial side facing up on the middle of a microscope slide, drop one drop of water, and cover with a coverslip (*see* **Note 10**).
3. Epidermal cells are visualized with a 63x immersion oil objective in a multitrack mode. The YFP signals are excited with 514 nm laser line and emission are detected at 519–587 nm. The RFP fluorophore is excited with 561 nm laser line and emission is detected at 600–630 nm [17] (*see* **Notes 11** and **12**).

BiFC assay examples are shown in Fig. 2.

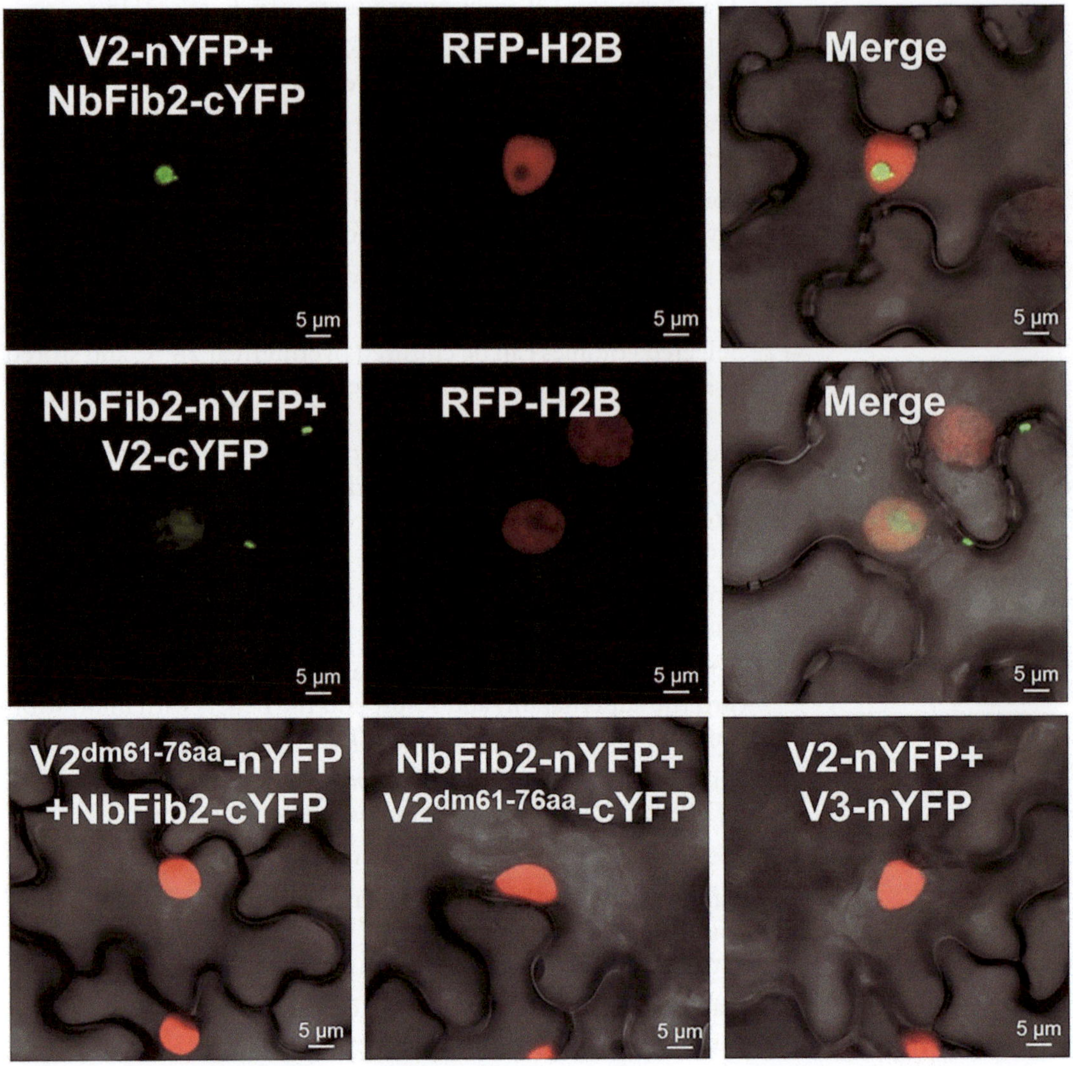

Fig. 2 Reconstruction of fluorescent YFP by its two non-fluorescent fragments mediated by the interaction between the V2 protein of mulberry mosaic dwarf-associated virus (MMDaV) and the Fibrillarin 2 of *Nicotiana benthamiana* (NbFib2) [17]. Constructs containing the nYFP and cYFP fusion proteins were co-expressed in RFP-H2B transgenic *N. benthamiana* via agroinfiltration. YFP fluorescence was observed as a consequence of complementation of YN and YC tagged with MMDaV V2 or NbFib2. Images were captured at 48 h post-infiltration using a Zeiss LSM 980 confocal laser scanning microscope. RFP-H2B served as a nuclear marker. Bars represents 5 μm

4 Notes

1. Concentrations of antibiotics are typically 50 μg/mL of kanamycin, and 50 μg/mL of rifampicin.
2. Prepare all solutions using double deionized water and store infiltration buffer at 4 °C.

3. Include the four base pair sequences (CACC) that is necessary for directional cloning on the 5′ end of the forward primer.
4. For TOPO cloning, using the high-fidelity polymerase that creates a blunt-end PCR product. For C-terminal fusion constructs, the stop codon should be removed in the reverse primers.
5. A BP recombination reaction between the *att*B-PCR products and the pDONR vectors (e.g., pDONR221 or pDONR/Zeo) can also be used to create an entry clone. If you are performing a BP recombination reaction, note that the PCR primers should contain the *att*B sequences. The detailed protocol of Gateway recombination cloning is available at the company website (http://www.invitrogen.com).
6. Select a restriction cutting site that is not contained in the target gene. If the destination vector and the entry vector contain different antibiotic resistances, the linearized step is not required.
7. It is recommended to use YFP fragments truncated at residue 155 (N-terminal amino acid residues 1–154 for YN and C-terminal residues 155–238 for YC) in most cases, since they produce relatively bright fluorescent signals in complexes formed by many interacting partners, but lower fluorescence when fused to noninteracting proteins under the appropriate conditions [10]. Furthermore, Venus is a variant of EYFP, generated from multiple amino acid residue mutations of EYFP. When using Venus in BiFC assays, it is usually more sensitive but prone to self-assembly of the two split fluorescent fragments [18, 19].
8. In general, colony PCR screening of the correct clone represents a successful clone, and it is recommended that final verification can be done by DNA sequencing.
9. Label the infiltration leaf area with a marker pen and gently wipe the excess buffer of the leaf with tissue paper.
10. Make sure there are no air bubbles between the leaf and the coverslip.
11. The image must be optimized by adjusting the pinhole, detector gain, and laser power. It is necessary to include negative control combinations such as beta-glucuronidase (GUS) to avoid false-positive.
12. After the confocal observation, immunoblotting should be performed to ascertain the expression level and integrity of the fusion proteins. Weak interaction signaling due to low levels of protein expression can be enhanced by co-expression with viral RNA silencing suppressors, such as the P19 protein of tomato bushy stunt virus.

Acknowledgments

This work was supported by the National Natural Science Foundation (32272518 and 31972245) to Xiuling Yang.

References

1. Yang XL et al (2019) Geminivirus-associated betasatellites: exploiting chinks in the antiviral arsenal of plants. Trend Plant Sci 24:519–529
2. Aguilar E, Gomez BG, Lozano-Duran R (2020) Recent advances on the plant manipulation by geminiviruses. Curr Opin Plant Biol 56:56–64
3. Li FF et al (2018) The βC1 protein of geminivirus-betasatellite complexes: a target and repressor of host defenses. Mol Plant 11: 1424–1426
4. Hu CD, Chinenov Y, Kerppola TK (2002) Visualization of interactions among bZip and Rel family proteins in living cells using bimolecular fluorescence complementation. Mol Cell 9:789–798
5. Fujikawa Y, Kato N (2007) Split luciferase complementation assay to study protein-protein interactions in *Arabidopsis* protoplasts. Plant J 52:185–195
6. Chen Y, Mills JD, Periasamy A (2003) Protein localization in living cells and tissues using FRET and FLIM. Differentiation 71:528–541
7. Fields S, Song O (1989) A novel genetic system to detect protein-protein interactions. Nature 340:245–246
8. Lee C (2007) Coimmunoprecipitation assay. In: Rosato E (ed) Circadian rhythms, Methods in molecular biology, vol 362. Humana Press, New York
9. Sun Y, Rombola C, Jyothikumar V, Periasamy A (2013) Förster resonance energy transfer microscopy and spectroscopy for localizing protein-protein interactions in living cells. Cytometry A 83:780–793
10. Kerppola TK (2008) Biomolecular fluorescence complementation (BiFC) analysis as a probe of protein interactions in living cells. Annu Rev Biophys 37:465–487
11. Miller KE et al (2015) Bimolecular fluorescence complementation (BiFC) analysis: advances and recent applications for genome-wide interaction studies. J Mol Biol 427:2039–2055
12. Walter M et al (2004) Visualization of protein interactions in living plant cells using bimolecular fluorescence complementation. Plant J 40: 428–438
13. Yang XL et al (2007) Functional modulation of the geminivirus AL2 transcription factor and silencing suppressor by self-interaction. J Virol 81:11972–11981
14. Sun S, Li S, Zhou X, Yang X (2023) WRKY1 represses the WHIRLY1 transcription factor to positively regulate plant defense against geminivirus infection. PLoS Pathog 19:e1011319
15. Tang Z, Bernards MA, Wang A (2022) Simultaneous determination and subcellular localization of protein-protein interactions in plant cells using bimolecular fluorescence complementation assay. In: Wang A, Li Y (eds) Plant virology, Methods in molecular biology, vol 2400. Humana Press, New York
16. Nelson BK, Cai X, Nebenführ A (2007) A multicolored set of *in vivo* organelle markers for co-localization studies in *Arabidopsis* and other plants. Plant J 51:1126–1136
17. Wang D, Sun S, Ren Y, Li S, Yang X, Zhou X (2020) RepA promotes the nucleolar exclusion of the V2 protein of mulberry mosaic dwarf-associated virus. Front Microbiol 11:1828
18. Kodama Y, Hu CD (2010) An improved bimolecular fluorescence complementation assay with a high signal-to-noise ratio. BioTechniques 49:793–805
19. Lee LY, Gelvin SB (2014) Bimolecular fluorescence complementation for imaging protein interactions in plant hosts of microbial pathogens. In: Vergunst A, O'Callaghan D (eds) Host-bacteria interactions, Methods in molecular biology, vol 1197. Humana Press, New York

Chapter 20

Exploring the Effect of Tomato Yellow Leaf Curl Virus Infection on Whitefly Probing and Feeding Behavior by Electrical Penetration Graph (EPG) Technique

Elisa Garzo and Aránzazu Moreno

Abstract

The majority of plant viruses rely on Hemipteran vectors for their survival and transmission. Moreover, many viruses can manipulate their insect vectors. In this context, the Electrical Penetration Graph (EPG) technique is a valuable tool for understanding how plant viruses, such as the begomovirus tomato yellow leaf curl virus (TYLCV), modify the probing and feeding behavior of piercing-sucking insect vectors like the whitefly *Bemisia tabaci* Gennadius (Hemiptera: Aleyrodidae).

Key words Insect-plant-virus interaction, *Bemisia tabaci*, *Begomovirus*, Monitoring feeding activities, Vector manipulation

1 Introduction

Most plant viruses need their insect vectors for transmission to other plants [1]. Different strategies for the transmission of plant viruses by insect vectors have been described based on the length of time that vectors retain the ability to transmit them and the location of the virus retention site within the vector: (1) Non-circulative transmission, which includes non-persistent and semi-persistent transmission modes, is characterized by the short retention of the virus within the vector. Viruses transmitted by the non-circulative mode are also known as "cuticula-borne viruses" because they are carried on the cuticle lining of the vector's feeding apparatus [2]; (2) Circulative or persistent transmission involves the vector remaining viruliferous for a long time or throughout its entire life cycle. Viruses transmitted circulatively circulate within the arthropod body and are not lost after molting, invading the hemolymph and salivary glands of their vectors [3].

Francisco Murilo Zerbini et al. (eds.), *Geminiviruses: Methods and Protocols*, Methods in Molecular Biology, vol. 2912, https://doi.org/10.1007/978-1-0716-4454-6_20,

Viruses that depend on vectors for transmission can induce chemical and physical changes in their vector and/or their shared host plant, affecting vector-host interactions to enhance virus transmission and spread [4–7]. These changes may occur in different ways: through manipulation of the vector—directly mediated by the presence of the virus in the vector's body—or through manipulation of the host plant—indirectly mediated by changes occurring in the plant as a consequence of pathogen infection [8].

In this context, the Electrical Penetration Graph (EPG) technique, developed by McLean and Kinsey [9] and later modified by Tjallingii [10], is a useful tool for understanding how plant viruses can modify the probing and feeding behavior of piercing-sucking insect vectors. In the EPG technique, an insect with piercing mouthparts and a plant are made part of an electrical circuit by connecting each to an electrode, one to the insect and one to the plant. The electrical signal is amplified and digitized by a converter card. Furthermore, voltage fluctuations and electrical resistance are recorded and can be matched to specific feeding events.

The EPG technique has been extensively applied in characterizing host plant resistance [11–14], in physiological and molecular analyses of phloem sap [15–17], and in combination with other techniques such as stylectomy and histology [12, 18, 19]. The EPG technique has also been used to study the transmission mechanisms of plant pathogens by their insect vectors [20–22].

In this chapter, we focus our attention on tomato yellow leaf curl virus (TYLCV), a member of the genus *Begomovirus*, family *Geminiviridae*, that affects several cultivated plants, with domesticated tomato (*Solanum lycopersicum*) as its primary host [23]. TYLCV is transmitted by *Bemisia tabaci* Gennadius (Hemiptera: Aleyrodidae) in a circulative manner. The EPG technique has been used by several researchers to study the direct and indirect effects of TYLCV on the probing and feeding behavior of the whitefly *B. tabaci*. Moreno-Delafuente et al. [24] demonstrated that TYLCV-viruliferous *B. tabaci* fed more frequently from phloem sieve elements and made a larger number of phloem contacts in eggplants than non-viruliferous whiteflies. This probing behavior enhances the inoculation efficiency of TYLCV by its vector. On the other hand, Liu et al. [25] showed that whiteflies of biotypes B and Q appeared to find TYLCV-infected plants more attractive, probing them more quickly and having a greater number of feeding events.

Here, we describe the steps that users should follow to study the probing and feeding behavior of *B. tabaci* on tomato plants infected and non-infected by the begomovirus TYLCV.

2 Materials

Prepare all materials before conducting the EPG recordings.

2.1 Plants, Whitefly Population, and Virus Isolate

1. Healthy and virus-infected tomato plants (*Solanum lycopersicum*). These plants are used as virus sources and experimental plants for the different treatments.
2. Eggplants (*Solanum melongena*). These plants are used for rearing whitefly colonies because they are excellent host plants for *B. tabaci* and are immune to TYLCV.
3. Soil:vermiculite mixture (2:1).
4. Plants fertilizer 20–20–20 NPK.
5. Plastic pots (20 cm of diameter).
6. Plastic Petri dish (10 cm in diameter).
7. Newly-emerged (2–7 days old) *Bemisia tabaci* Mediterranean species individuals.
8. Tomato yellow leaf curl virus isolate.
9. Insect cage covered with insect-proof net with a sleeve opening in the front panel of the cage.
10. Clip-cage: length: 5.5 cm, width: 5.5 cm and height: 2 cm, with a hole (2 cm in diameter) at the top covered with mesh to allow for transpiration (Fig. 1a).
11. Handmade vacuum aspirator: self-made with tip 1000 μL, suction silicon tube and fine mesh to prevent the intake of insects. The user operates the aspirator manually.

2.2 Electrical Penetration Graph (EPG) Technique

1. Ice-bag, Petri dish filled with a layer of minced ice or small insect chill table (BioQuid products, USA).
2. Watch glass (9 cm of diameter).
3. Insect electrodes: brass insect pin, thin cooper extension wire (2 cm length, 0.2 mm in diameter), solder and soldering iron.
4. Gold wire (2 cm length, 12.5 μm in diameter).
5. Water based silver-conducting glue paint: 4 g water, 4 g paper glue, 4 g silver powder (Epg Systems, the Netherlands; https://www.epgsystems.eu/phocadownload/userupload/Add%20ons%20and%20hints.pdf).
6. Eppendorf (1.5 mL) and Falcon (10 mL) tubes.
7. Faraday cage: self-made cage (length: 110 cm, width: 60 cm and height: 100 cm) covered with metal netting. The mesh width between 2 mm and 1 cm.
8. One Giga-8dd DC-EPG system with 1G Ohm (EPG Systems, The Netherlands).

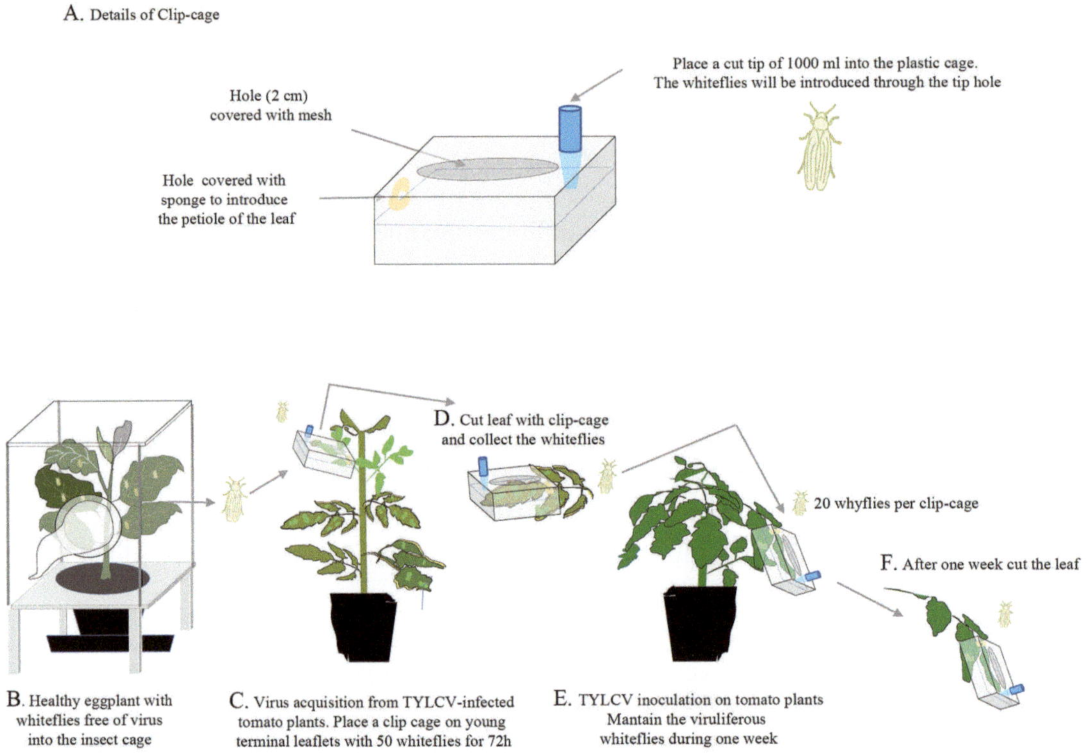

Fig. 1 Generation of TYLCV-infected tomato plants. (**a**) Detail of clip-caged used to confine the whiteflies during acquisition and inoculation access period. (**b**) Whiteflies rearing on potted eggplant into the insect cage. (**c**) TYLCV-acquisition access period by whiteflies. (**d**) Cut the leaf let to collect viruliferous whiteflies. (**e**) TYLCV-inoculation access period by viruliferous whiteflies. (**f**) Cut the leaf where the whiteflies inoculated the virus and remove egg, larvae, and adult of viruliferous whiteflies

9. USB analog-to-digital converter card.
10. Binocular microscope.
11. Computer with Windows OS.

2.3 Software

1. Stylet + software (EPG Systems, The Netherlands) for acquisition (Stylet+d) and analysis (Stylet+a) of EPG waveforms (*see* **Note 1**).
2. NPAC-EPG software for automatic calculation of EPG variables.

3 Methods

3.1 Tomato and Eggplant Growth

1. Germinate tomato seeds in plastic Petri dishes and transplant the plantlets into small pots (8 × 8 cm) after 1 week, using a mixture of soil and vermiculite (2:1). The number of seeds must be calculated according to the experimental design. These plants will be used for EPG recordings.

2. Germinate eggplant seeds every 15 days in a plastic Petri dish. After 1 week, transplant the plantlets into pots of 8 × 8 cm. Three weeks later, transplant the eggplants (4–5 true leaves) into 20 cm pots. After 2 days, these plants will be used to maintain the whitefly colonies.
3. Maintain the plants in a walk-in-environmental growth chamber under controlled conditions of temperature (24:20 °C day: night, photoperiod 16:8 h light:darkness, 80% relative humidity).
4. Water plantlets two–three times a week using 0.25 g/L 20–20–20 (NPK).

3.2 Whitefly Colony

1. Establish a culture of *B. tabaci* colony, which will be reared on potted eggplants (*see* **Note 2**).
2. Place one eggplant (with 4 or 5 true leaves) into the insect cages covered by insect-proof net (Fig. 1b). Introduce 100 adult whiteflies into the cage. Maintain the cage in a greenhouse or growth chamber under controlled conditions (25:21 °C D:N, 80% RH). After 1 month, use the newly emerged adults (2–7 days old) for the experiments.
3. If necessary, confirm the biotype status of the whitefly population by determining the sequence of cytochrome oxidase I mitochondrial gene, following the protocol described by Frolich et al. [26], and performing a BLAST procedure with the reference sequence of interest.

3.3 Generation of TYLCV-Infected Tomato Plants

1. Maintain TYLCV isolate on tomato plant by whitefly-mediated transmission. Generate new TYLCV-infected plants 1 month before conducting the experiment.
2. For viral acquisition from TYLCV-infected plants, place a clip cage (Fig. 1c) on the young terminal leaflets of tomato TYLCV-infected plants exhibiting clear symptoms of infection. Introduce 50 whitefly adults into the clip cage for a 72 h of acquisition access period (AAP). After that, cut the leaflet (Fig. 1d) and open the clip cage and collect the viruliferous whiteflies (*see* **Note 3**).
3. For viral inoculation in healthy plants, place a new clip cage on the second leaflets of young healthy tomato plants (3-leaf stage), and release 20 viruliferous whiteflies for a one-week of inoculation access period (IAP) (Fig. 1e). After that, cut the leaf (Fig. 1f) to remove the whiteflies from tomato plants, and place the plants in an insect-proof cage under greenhouses conditions, as described above (*see* **Note 4**).
4. After a one-month postinoculation period, the infected tomato plants will be evaluated using PCR [27] tissue-print hybridization [28], TAS-ELISA test (according to the manufacturer's protocol) or by observing symptoms.

5. For the generation of non-infected TYLCV tomato plants, used as controls, the same methodology described above will be followed, using whiteflies and plants free of the virus.

3.4 Installation of Stylet + Software

1. Stylet + software (EPG Systems, The Netherlands) is a specialized free EPG data acquisition and waveform analysis program. Download the Setup_2020.exe file from https://epgsystems.eu/downloads-install-files-manuals. Open and run in your PC-computer.

3.5 Making Insect Electrodes

Before insect attachment is necessary to make insect electrodes (EPG Systems, The Netherlands) (Fig. 2).

1. Take thin cooper extension wire (2 cm length, 0.2 mm in diameter) and solder to brass pin.
2. Pieces of gold wire (1.5 cm length and 12.5 μm in diameter) will be prepared using a binocular microscope. Cut the pieces of gold wire with a blade on a black platform.
3. Attach the gold wire to the cooper extension wire using silver glue paint.
4. Self-made silver glue to attach gold wire to the insect. Silver glue is water based. For 10 mL (Falcon tube) of glue, mix 4 g of water (with 1 or 2 droplets of Triton X100 for each 100 mL of water), 4 g of transparent paper glue and silver powder (*see* **Note 5**). The ingredients should be mixed thoroughly. Make small vials for use (1.5 mL Eppendorf tube). Save the stock solution at about 5 °C (*see* **Note 6**).

3.6 Attach the Gold Wire to the Whitefly's Dorsum

1. Collect whitefly adults (2–5 days old) in a 1.5 mL Eppendorf tube using a vacuum aspirator.
2. To facility wiring, whiteflies will be maintained on an ice-bath for a maximum of 10 min. Around 5–6 whiteflies will be placed

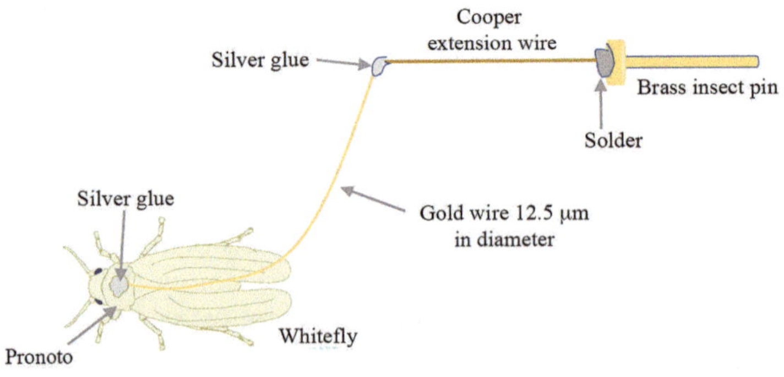

Fig. 2 Insect electrode attached to whitefly pronotum with a small droplet of water-based silver glue

on a glass disc on an insect chill table. Remove the males (*see* **Note 7**) and position the females dorsally using an entomological needle.

3. Attach the insect electrode with a gold wire (1.5 cm length, 12.5 μm in diameter) to whitefly pronotum with a small droplet of water-based silver glue (Fig. 2) (*see* **Note 8**).
4. Insert the electrode into a Styrofoam to store the wired whiteflies to complete the acclimation period (1 h) between the time of wiring and the beginning of EPG recording as described by Johnson and Walker [29].

3.7 Probing and Feeding Behavior on Infected and Non-infected Tomato Plants

1. EPG recordings are made in a Faraday cage (Fig. 3). The position of the plants for each treatment should be randomly assigned in each recording (*see* **Note 9**).
2. Place four TYLCV-infected and four non-infected plants inside the Faraday cage alternately. If the plants are large and come into contact with each other, then use only four plants per cage.
3. Fix the first or second youngest leaf on the abaxial side of each plant with hair clips onto a plastic strip.
4. Insert the soil electrodes into the soil of each potted plant.
5. Connect the wired whiteflies to the input of the Giga-8dd probe and place on the abaxial side of the first or second youngest leaf of infected or noninfected tomato plants. Each

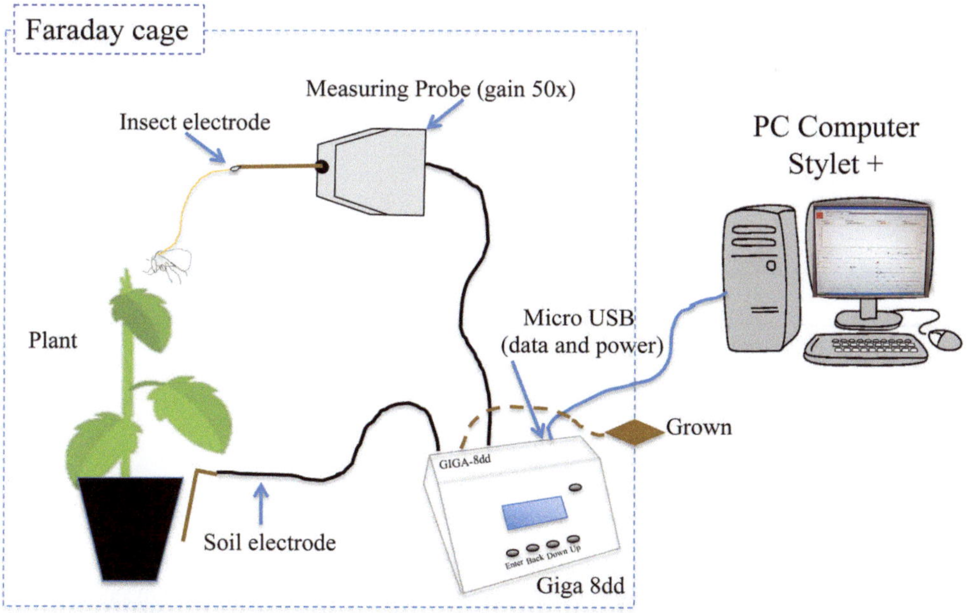

Fig. 3 Experimental EPG configuration. Only one of the eight probes shown

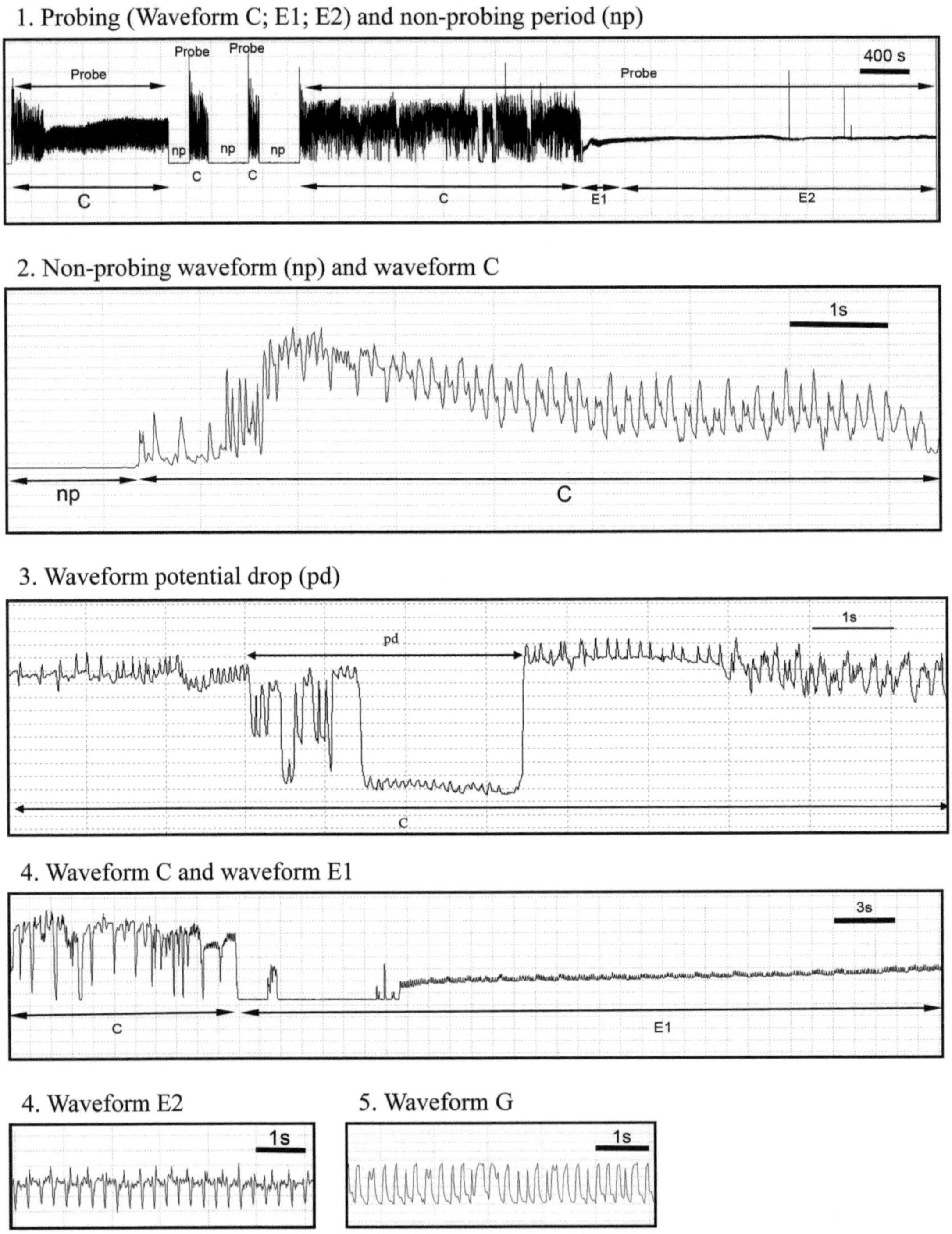

Fig. 4 The image contains the waveforms present in an EPG recording for *Bemisia tabaci*. (*1*) Probing and non-probing period. (*2*) Waveform C, intercellular apoplastic stylet pathway where the insect shows a cyclic activity of mechanical stylet penetration and secretion of saliva. (*3*) Waveform potential drop (pd) represents an intracellular stylet puncture. (*4*) Waveform E1, salivation into the phloem sieve elements at the beginning of the phloem phase. (*5*) Waveform E2, passive phloem sap uptake from sieve elements. (*6*) Waveform G, active intake of xylem sap. Probing period includes the waveforms C, pd., E1, E2, and G

replicate of the experiment should consist of a single whitefly and a single plant that will be used only once per recording (*see* **Note 10**).

6. Eight hours will be an appropriate recording duration (*see* **Note 11**).
7. EPG signals will be digitalized by a USB analog digital converter card and the data will be acquired with the Stylet software (Stylet d+) (*see* **Note 12**). The data will be analyzed with the same software (Stylet a+) after data conversion.
8. Experiments will be carried out at 25 ± 2 °C, 60–70% HR and with additional artificial light during the recording.
9. EPG waveform associated with whitefly probing and feeding behavior are described in Fig. 4, according to [30, 31].
10. Calculate the EPG variables using an MS Excel workbook for automatic parameters calculation of EPG data (NPAC-EPG software) developed by [32] (*see* **Note 13**).
11. Use the output given by the NPAC-EPG software for each whitefly (replicate) to calculate the treatment mean for each variable (*see* **Note 14**). After that, compare all treatment means.
12. Compare the variables means with a parametric test when the variables following normality assumptions before or after transformation and a nonparametric test when variables will not meet normality assumptions.

4 Notes

1. Both software programs are compatible with all Windows platform versions (XP, 7, 8, and 10) and Mac computers running VirtualBox. With a virtual Windows environment running in the MacOS background, only Stylet+a will work; Stylet+d will not.
2. Eggplants are excellent host plants for *B. tabaci* and are immune to TYLCV, preventing virus contamination of the whitefly colonies. However, users can also maintain the whitefly colony directly on tomato plants, provided that TYLCV-infected and noninfected plants are not kept together in the same greenhouse or growth chamber.
3. To facilitate the collection of whiteflies, cut the leaf where the clip-cage is located and place it on ice to immobilize the insects.
4. The optimal inoculation period for TYLCV is approximately 72 h. However, waiting for 1 week before cutting the leaf where the whiteflies are feeding ensures both the inoculation and infection of the plant, while also facilitating the removal of the eggs and larvae present on the leaf.

5. Sometimes the preparation of silver glue has some difficulties because not all samples of glue pens are suitable. First, you need to prepare a small amount of mixture (water, glue and silver powder) on a microscope slide glass and check whether it mixes well with the silver powder. If the smooth suspension is not suitable, then try another glue sample.
6. The silver particles are heavy and will soon sink to the bottom of the Eppendorf. It is important that you thoroughly shake it before use. The silver glue dries very fast, so it is important to close the vial and only use the glue on the inside of the lid of the Eppendorf. Create a support to keep the opened Eppendorf upright. When the silver glue starts to dry, then you can dilute with some drop of stock solution (water with some drops of Triton X100 such as described in Subheading 3.5).
7. Only females are used in this study because they feed better and are more efficient vectors of TYLCV than males [33].
8. Take silver paint with the handled needle and lightly tap the gold wire. Then, take another drop of thicker silver paint and tap the gold wire again until a small ball forms. Immediately place this drop on the pronotum of the whitefly.
9. Randomize of the treatments inside the Faraday cage to reduce any potential effects of external factors such as light, heating, air conditioning, etc.
10. If the whiteflies spend a long time in non-probe activity on tested tomato plants during the recordings, we recommend adapting the whiteflies to the tomato plant host for 2 days before starting the experiment.
11. The appropriate recording duration depends on the research objectives and the feeding behavior of the insect under study. In general, the recordings should be long enough to include all the behaviors relevant to the research objectives [34].
12. The EPG acquisition software (Stylet d+) should be started before placing the insects on the plants. This ensures the recording of the insects' initial behavior on the plant.
13. The NPAC-EPG workbook is able to calculated 127 variables but we recommend to the user a select set of EPG variables (Tables 1 and 2) for study the probing and feeding behavior of whiteflies on TYLCV-infected and noninfected tomato plants. Also these variables can be selected if the users study the probing and feeding behavior of viruliferous and non-viruliferous whiteflies.
14. Replication needs to be appropriate for each experiment, a minimum of 15–20 replicates per treatment is recommended [34].

Table 1
Nonsequential EPG variables used to compare the probing and feeding behavior of whitefly on TYLCV-infected and noninfected tomato plants

Nonsequential EPG-variables	
Waveforms	
Non-probe (np), no stylets contact with the leaf tissue	Number Total duration Mean duration PPW
Probe, stylets contact with the leaf	Number Total duration Mean duration PPW
Intercellular stylet pathway (C)	Number Total duration Mean duration PPW
Potential drop (pd), intracellular stylets puncture included in C waveform	Number Total duration Mean duration PPW
Derailed stylet mechanics (F)	Number Total duration Mean duration PPW
Active intake of xylem sap (G)	Number Total duration Mean duration PPW
Salivation in phloem sieve elements (E1)	Number Total duration Mean duration PPW
Passive phloem sap uptake from the sieve element (E2)	Number Total duration Mean duration PPW
Sustained phloem ingestion (>10 min, sE2)	Number Total duration Mean duration PPW

PPW proportion of individuals that produced the waveform type

Table 2
Sequential EPG variables used to compare the probing and feeding behavior of whitefly on TYLCV-infected and noninfected tomato plants

Sequential EPG-variables
Time to the first probe from start the EPG
Duration of the first probe
Time from the beginning of the first probe to first pd
Time from the beginning of the probe to the
Time to first E from start of first probe
Time to the first E2 from start of first probe
Time to first sE2 from start of first probe
Time from the beginning of that probe to first E
Time from the beginning of that probe to first E2
Time from the beginning of that probe to first sE2
Time in C to 1stE in first probe with E
Time in C to first sE2 in first probe with sE2
Average time in C to 1stE in probes with E
Number of brief probes (<3 min) before first E in the recording
Number of probes before first E in the recording
Number of probes after first E in the recording

References

1. Whitfield AE, Falk BW, Rotenberg D (2015) Insect vector-mediated transmission of plant viruses. Virology 479-480:278–289
2. Fereres A, Moreno A (2009) Behavioural aspects influencing plant virus transmission by homopteran insects. Virus Res 141:158–168
3. Hogenhout SA, Ammar ED, Whitfield AE, Redinbaugh MG (2008) Insect vector interactions with persistently transmitted viruses. Annu Rev Phytopathol 46:327–359
4. Eigenbrode SD, Ding H, Shiel P, Berger PH (2002) Volatiles from potato plants infected with potato leafroll virus attract and arrest the virus vector, *Myzus persicae* (Homoptera: Aphididae). Proc R Soc B 269:455–460
5. Mauck KE, Bosque-Pérez NA, Eigenbrode SD, De Moraes C, Mescher M (2012) Transmission mechanisms shape pathogen effects on host-vector interactions: evidence from plant viruses. Funct Ecol 26:1162–1175
6. Carmo-Sousa M, Moreno A, Garzo E, Fereres A (2014) A non-persistently transmitted-virus induces a pull-push strategy in its aphid vector to optimize transmission and spread. Virus Res 186:38–46
7. Carmo-Sousa M, Moreno A, Plaza M, Garzo E, Fereres A (2016) Cucurbit aphid-borne yellows virus (CABYV) modifies the alighting, settling and probing behaviour of its vector *Aphis gossypii* favoring its own spread. Ann Appl Biol 169:284–297
8. Ingwell LL, Eigenbrode SD, Bosque-Pérez NA (2012) Plant viruses alter insect behaviour to enhance their spread. Sci Rep 2:1–6

9. McLean DL, Kinsey MG (1964) A technique for electronically recording aphid feeding and salivation. Nature 202:1358–1359
10. Tjallingii WF (1978) Mechanoreceptors of the aphid labium. Entomol Exp Appl 24:531–537
11. van Helden M, Tjallingii WF (1993) Tissue localisation of lettuce resistance to the aphid *Nasonovia ribisnigri* using electrical penetration graphs. Entomol Exp Appl 68:269–278
12. Garzo E, Fernández-Pascual M, Morcillo C, Fereres A, Gómez-Guillamón ML, Tjallingii WF (2018) Ultrastructure of compatible and incompatible interactions in phloem sieve elements during the stylet penetration by cotton aphids in melon. Insect Sci 25:631–642
13. Álvarez AE, Tjallingii WF, Garzo E, Vleeshouwers V, Dicke M, Vosman B (2006) Location of resistance factors in the leaves of potato and wild tuber-bearing Solanum species to the aphid *Myzus persicae*. Entomol Exp Appl 121:145–157
14. Escudero-Martinez C, Leybourne D, Bos J (2021) Plant resistance in different cell layers affects aphid probing and feeding behaviour during non-host and poor-host interactions. Bull Entomol Res 111:31–38
15. Will T, Hewer A, van Bel AJE (2008) A novel perfusion system shows that aphid feeding behaviour is altered by decrease of sieve-tube pressure. Entomol Exp Appl 127:237–245
16. Gutiérrez S, Yvon M, Pirolles E, Garzo E, Fereres A, Michalakis Y, Blanc S (2012) Circulating virus load determines the size of bottlenecks in viral populations progressing within a host. PLoS Pathog 8:e1003009
17. Garzo E, Sánchez-López CM, Fereres A, Soler C, Marcilla A, Pérez-Bermúdez P (2023) Isolation of extracellular vesicles from phloem sap by size exclusion chromatography. Curr Protoc 3:e903
18. Tjallingii WF, Esch TH (1993) Fine structure of aphid stylet routes in plant tissues in correlation with EPG signals. Physiol Entomol 18: 317–328
19. Chinchilla-Ramírez M, Garzo E, Fereres A, Gavara-Vidal J, ten Broeke CJM, van Loon JJA, Urbaneja A, Pérez-Hedo M (2021) Plant feeding by *Nesidiocoris tenuis*: quantifying its behavioral and mechanical components. Biol Control 152:104402
20. Martín B, Collar JL, Tjallingii WF, Fereres A (1997) Intracellular ingestion and salivation by aphids may cause the acquisition and inoculation of non-persistently transmitted plant viruses. J Gen Virol 78:2701–2705
21. Jimenez J, Tjallingii WF, Moreno A, Fereres A (2018) Newly distinguished cell punctures associated with transmission of the semipersistent phloem-limited beet yellows virus. J Virol 92:e01076-18
22. Cornara D, Garzo E, Morente M, Moreno A, Alba-Tercedor J, Fereres A (2018) EPG combined with micro-CT and video recording reveals new insights on the feeding behavior of *Philaenus spumarius*. PLoS One 13(7): e0199154
23. Czosnek H, Laterrot H (1997) A worldwide survey of tomato yellow leaf curl viruses. Arch Virol 142(7):1391–1406
24. Moreno-Delafuente A, Garzo E, Moreno A, Fereres A (2013) A plant virus manipulates the behaviour of its whitefly vector to enhance its transmission efficiency and spread. PLoS One 8:e61543
25. Liu B, Preisser EL, Chu D, Pan H, Xie W, Wang S, Wu Q, Zhou X, Zhang Y (2013) Multiple forms of vector manipulation by a plant-infecting virus: *Bemisia tabaci* and tomato yellow leaf curl virus. J Virol 87(9): 4929–4937
26. Frolich DR, Torres-Jerez I, Bedford ID, Markham PG, Brown JK (1999) A phylogeographical analysis of the *Bemisia tabaci* species complex based in mitochondrial DNA markers. Mol Ecol 8:1593–1602
27. Mason G, Caciagli P, Accotto GP, Noris E (2008) Real-time PCR for the quantitation of tomato yellow leaf curl Sardinia virus in tomato plants and in *Bemisia tabaci*. J Virol Methods 147(2):282–289
28. Monci F, Sánchez-Campos S, Navas-Castillo J, Moriones E (2002) A natural recombinant between the geminiviruses tomato yellow leaf curl Sardinia virus and tomato yellow leaf curl virus exhibits a novel pathogenic phenotype and is becoming prevalent in Spanish populations. Virology 303:317–326
29. Johnson DD, Walker GP (1999) Intracellular punctures by the adult whitefly *Bemisia argentifolii* on DC and AC electronic feeding monitors. Entomol Exp Appl 92:257–270
30. Jiang YX, Lei H, Collar JL, Martin B, Muñiz M, Fereres A (1999) Probing and feeding behaviour of two distinct biotypes of *Bemisia tabaci* (Homoptera:Aleyrodidae) on tomato plants. J Econ Entomol 92(2): 357–366
31. Jiang YX, de Blas C, Barrios L, Fereres A (2000) Correlation between whitefly (Homoptera: Aleyrodidae) feeding behavior and

transmission of tomato yellow leaf curl virus. Ann Entomol Soc Am 93(3):573–579

32. Garzo E, Álvarez AJ, MorenoA, Walker GP, Tjallingii WF, Fereres A (2024) Novel program for automatic calculation of EPG variables. Journal of Insect Science 24(3): 28
33. Ning WX, Shi XB, Liu BM, Pan HP, Wei WT, Zeng Y, Sun XP, Xie W, Wang SL, Wu QJ et al (2015) Transmission of *tomato yellow leaf curl virus* by *Bemisia tabaci* as affected by whitefly sex and biotype. Sci Rep 29:10744
34. Walker GP, Fereres A, Tjallingii WF (2024) Guidelines for conducting, analyzing and interpreting electrical penetration graph (EPG). Entomol Exp Appl 172:564

Index

Francisco Murilo Zerbini et al. (eds.), *Geminiviruses: Methods and Protocols*, Methods in Molecular Biology, vol. 2912, https://doi.org/10.1007/978-1-0716-4454-6,